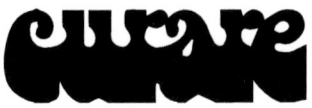

ZEITSCHRIFT FÜR MEDIZINETHNOLOGIE
JOURNAL OF MEDICAL ANTHROPOLOGY

hg. von der Arbeitsgemeinschaft Ethnologie und Medizin (AGEM)
ed. by the Association for Anthropology and Medicine (AGEM)

VOL. 46 (2023) 2

EDITORIAL EDITORIAL	Editorial DIE REDAKTION	3
SCHWERPUNKT THEMATIC FOCUS	Ambivalences of Healing Cooperations in Biomedical Settings EDITED BY CORNELIUS SCHUBERT & EHLER VOSS	5
Einleitung Introduction	Preparing for Patients and Preparing for Physicians. Skills and Values of Healing Cooperations and their Ambivalences CORNELIUS SCHUBERT & EHLER VOSS	7
Artikel Articles	In-Patient Psychiatric Care as a Space of Ambiguity | Therapeutic Encounters from a Sensory and Embodied Perspective ANNA HÄNNI	11
	Patient-Physician-Relationship in Cancer Care | Relevance and Ambivalences as Perceived by Oncologists NICOLE ERNSTMANN, SOPHIE ELISABETH GROSS, UTE KARBACH, LENA ANSMANN, ANDRÉ KARGER, HOLGER PFAFF, MARKUS WIRTZ, WALTER BAUMANN & MELANIE NEUMANN	27
	Digital Healing? Digital Capitalism? | Neoliberalism, Digital Health Technologies, and Citizen Health NICK J. FOX	43
	Feeling out of the Box | Ambivalences of Unexpected Amelioration among Sickened Health Professionals through Displacing Cooperations in Brazil MÁRCIO VILAR	55

UNABHÄNGIGE ARTIKEL / INDEPENDENT ARTICLES

Connected Epistemologies | A Fragmented Review of Post- and Decolonial Perspectives in Medical Anthropology
GIORGIO BROCCO … 77

Healthcare Workers' Experiences during the COVID-19 Pandemic in Argentina | A Syndemic Approach to Hospitals
ANAHI SY … 99

FORUM

Alternative Religiosität und „natürliche" Geburt | Religionswissenschaftliche Bemerkungen zu Robbie Davis-Floyd
JILL MARXER & JOHANNES ENDLER … 115

Radical Applied Clinical Anthropology
JASON WILSON & ROBERTA BAER … 125

BERICHTE / REPORTS

Krisen, Körper, Kompetenzen. Methoden und Potentiale medizinanthropologischen Forschens | Bericht zur 35. Jahrestagung der Arbeitsgemeinschaft Ethnologie und Medizin (AGEM) in Kooperation mit dem 20. Arbeitstreffen der Kommission Medizinanthropologie der Deutschen Gesellschaft für Empirische Kulturwissenschaft (DGEKW), Warburg-Haus Hamburg, 08.–09. September 2023
LEA KOOP-MEYER … 137

REZENSIONEN / BOOK REVIEW

Diana Espírito Santo 2023 | Spirited Histories. Technologies, Media, and Trauma in Paranormal Chile.
HELMAR KURZ … 145

Inga Scharf da Silva 2022 | Trauma als Wissensarchiv. Postkoloniale Erinnerungspraxis in der Sakralen Globalisierung am Beispiel der Zeitgenössischen Umbanda im Deutschsprachigen Europa.
HELMAR KURZ … 147

ZUSAMMENFASSUNGEN / ABSTRACTS / RÉSUMÉS

Zusammenfassungen der Beiträge
Article abstracts
Résumés des articles … 151

Ziele & Bereiche
Aims & Scope … 164

Editorial

Mit dem vorliegenden Schwerpunkt knüpfen die Herausgeber Cornelius Schubert & Ehler Voss an ihr als *Curare* 41 (2018) 1+2 erschienenes Heft zu *Heilungskooperationen* an. Heilung wurde darin als eine Praxis der Kooperation menschlicher und nichtmenschlicher Akteure verstanden, deren Aushandlungen Ambivalenzen entstehen lassen, die sich den zahlreichen Versuchen einer Vereindeutigung immer wieder entziehen und dadurch nicht selten zu Verwerfungen führen. Das vorliegende Heft konzentriert sich in vier Beiträgen auf die jeweils spezifischen Ambivalenzen von Heilungskooperationen in unterschiedlichen gegenwärtigen biomedizinischen Settings, die zeigen, wie diese Ambivalenzen in diesem sich stets wandelnden Feld zwischen Körpern und Technologien individuell verhandelt werden.

In den vom Schwerpunkt unabhängigen Forschungsbeiträgen folgt Giorgio Brocco den Spuren post- und dekolonialer Perspektiven in der Medizinanthropologie und Anahi Sy analysiert mithilfe des Konzepts der Syndemie die Ereignisse in öffentlichen Krankenhäusern Argentiniens während der Covid-19-Pandemie.

In der Rubrik Forum betrachten Jill Marxer & Johannes Endler anhand des Werks von Robbie Davis-Floyd das Verhältnis von alternativer Religiosität und dem Konzept der natürlichen Geburt aus religionswissenschaftlicher Perspektive. Roberta Baer & Jason W. Wilson schlagen in ihrem Beitrag die Implementierung von ethnographischen Methoden im Klinikalltag vor, um der von ihnen diagnostizierten Krise der Gesundheitsversorgung in den USA wirksam zu begegnen. Darüber hinaus berichtet Lea Koop-Meyer von der 35. Jahrestagung der Arbeitsgemeinschaft Ethnologie und Medizin (AGEM), die in Kooperation mit dem 20. Arbeitstreffen der Kommission Medizinanthropologie der Deutschen Gesellschaft für Empirische Kulturwissenschaft (DGEKW) unter dem Titel „Krisen, Körper, Kompetenzen: Methoden und Potentiale medizinanthropologischen Forschens" vom 08.–09. September 2023 im Warburg-Haus in Hamburg stattfand.

Wir freuen uns sehr, dass die *Curare* nun zusätzlich zur gedruckten Version auch als Open-Access-Zeitschrift erscheint und danken der Deutschen Forschungsgemeinschaft (DFG) und dem Fachinformationsdienst Sozial- und Kulturanthropologie (FID SKA) für die finanzielle und organisatorische Unterstützung bei der Umstellung sowie der Universitätsbibliothek Tübingen für das Webhosting der Zeitschrift.

Alle Ausgaben ab 2018 werden veröffentlicht auf www.curarejournal.org. Die Ausgaben von 1978–2017 sind abrufbar unter www.evifa.de/curare-journal.

Die Redaktion

[English version]

With the present thematic focus, the editors Cornelius Schubert & Ehler Voss build on their concept of Healing Cooperations first introduced in *Curare* 41 (2018) 1+2. In that issue, healing was understood as a practice of cooperation of human and nonhuman actors, whose negotiations engender ambivalences that continuously elude the many attempts at unequivocal definition, thus often resulting in ruptures. The present issue devotes four texts to the specific ambivalences of healing cooperations in various contemporary biomedical settings, demonstrating how those ambivalences are individually negotiated within this ever-shifting field between bodies and technologies.

In research articles independent of the thematic focus, Giorgio Brocco traces postcolonial and decolonial perspectives in medical anthropology, while Anahi Sy deploys the concept of syndemics to analyze events in Argentina's public hospitals during the COVID-19 pandemic.

In the Forum section, JILL MARXER & JOHANNES ENDLER draw on Robbie Davis-Floyd's work and religious-studies perspectives in their examination of the relationship between alternative religiosity and the concept of natural childbirth. ROBERTA BAER & JASON W. WILSON suggest bringing ethnographic methods into everyday clinical practice in order to effectively address the healthcare crisis they observe in the United States and LEA KOOP-MEYER reports on the thirty-fifth annual meeting of the Association for Anthropology and Medicine (AGEM), held in cooperation with the twentieth workshop of the Commission Medical Anthropology of the German Society for Cultural Analysis | European Ethnology (DGEKW). Titled "Krisen, Körper, Kompetenzen: Methoden und Potentiale medizinanthropologischen Forschens" ["Crises, Bodies, Competencies: Methods and Potentials of Medical Anthropological Research"], it took place from September 8–9, 2023, at the Warburg-Haus, Hamburg.

We are delighted that the print edition of *Curare* is now complemented by Open Access availability and we would like to thank the German Research Foundation (DFG) and the Specialised Information Service for Social and Cultural Anthropology (FID SKA) for their financial and organizational support during the transformation as well as the University Library of Tübingen for hosting the journal online.

All issues from 2018 are published online at www.curarejournal.org. Issues from 1978 to 2017 are available at www.evifa.de/curare-journal.

THE EDITORIAL BOARD

SCHWERPUNKT
THEMATIC FOCUS

Ambivalences of Healing Cooperations in Biomedical Settings

EDITED BY
CORNELIUS SCHUBERT & EHLER VOSS

Preparing for Patients and Preparing for Physicians

Knowledge, Values, and Skills of Healing Cooperations and their Ambivalences

Cornelius Schubert & Ehler Voss

The complexities of healing cooperations and how they change over time are of central concern in studying healing practices by the social sciences and humanities. Much has already been written, but the ongoing transformations of healthcare warrant a continuous engagement with the topic. In this issue of *Curare*, we focus on a specific aspect of healing cooperations in biomedical settings. The contributions will shed light on the ambivalences that accompany different constellations of patients and physicians, ranging from psychiatry to oncology, general practice, and chronic diseases. Understanding healing as a cooperative practice, the focus lies on multiple agents and how they negotiate different needs and potentials. Each biomedical setting enacts its own sets of knowledge claims, values, and skills (Berg & Mol 1998).

Such negotiations of healing cooperation are usually based on asymmetrical relations between healer and patient. Especially in biomedical contexts, the asymmetry of the patient-physician relationship has long been a main criticism (Pilnick & Dingwall 2011), and empirical studies have time and again reasserted fundamental disparities between those seeking and those providing health services (Begenau, Schubert, & Vogd 2010). At the same time, these asymmetries are constitutive of the healing encounter, because they form a functional difference between healers and clients. Without specific expertise, skills, and knowledge of healing, there would be no need for consultation, and often patients are looking exactly for such an asymmetric relation to put themselves in the hands of an authority they can trust. Nevertheless, this asymmetry has often been criticized, especially in the realm of modern biomedicine and psychology, and especially in the context of chronic and rare diseases. Professional dominance (Freidson 1970) and a paternalistic imbalance in healer-patient relationships have thus led to an increasing claim for shared decision making and informed consent in order to empower the patient vis-à-vis her or his healer. The aim is to develop therapies and forms of interaction that explicitly seek to re-balance the relationship by taking into account the patients' knowledge (e.g. in many psychological therapies), or even trying to turn the asymmetric healer-patient relationship around and calling for full responsibility of patients themselves (e.g. in many esoteric therapies).

How physicians and other healers conduct their encounters with clients is an integral element of their training. Nevertheless, this knowledge is only partly provided by official channels or courses; rather, it is often learned in a subtle and implicit manner during practical apprenticeship. Despite broad investigations of the professional encounters between healers and their clients, few studies have addressed the question how exactly these skills and attitudes are learned. In contrast to biomedical contexts, the encounter of non-biomedical healers with their clients is often conceived as being less hierarchical. Yet, we would assume a similar functional difference between them. We assume that how these asymmetries and differences are managed and performed in daily practice is largely learned in the formative years of apprenticeship.

Since the seminal studies "The Student Physician" (Merton, Reader, & Kendall 1957) and "Boys in White" (Becker, Geer, Hughes, & Strauss 1961), there has been little in-depth research on how students of healing practices acquire such skills and how they are transmitted in learning contexts. These studies have shown how novice physicians learn to cope with the contingencies of daily work and how they learn to balance responsibility and experience. Fine-grained ethnographic fieldwork enabled researchers to show how such skills and attitudes are learned in the processes of becoming a competent member of a healing profession, by observing and imitating role models and by being sensitive to the norms and values displayed by significant others. In line with BECKER, GEER, HUGHES, & STRAUSS, we assume that most of these skills are part of the tacit learning in the "hidden curriculum" (HAFFERTY & FRANKS 1994). The hidden curriculum refers to those aspects of learning contexts that do not figure prominently in official accounts, but are learned as part of becoming a member of a healing profession. Despite (or because of) their informal character, they serve as powerful orientations that slowly become taken for granted, in many cases without explicit recognition by those who teach and learn them.

Irrespective of the given healing cosmology, healing knowledge is ordered in specific systems that are organized in rules, schemes, and procedures that need to be adapted to the individual healing cooperation. Therefore, every healing cooperation is laced with fundamental uncertainties – not only with respect to treatment, but also to interaction (cf. FOX 1980; HENRY 2006). And all healing apprentices learn how to cope with these contingencies. The subtle transmission of a "paternalistic" model of physician-client interaction in biomedical education might account for the longstanding asymmetry that is part of the official program of medical education, despite longstanding calls for "shared decision making" and "informed consent" (STOLLBERG 2008). Consequently, "professional dominance" (FREIDSON 1970) is a skill that needs to be learned before it can be practiced.

But patients also often prepare for contact with healers. The Internet offers new possibilities for getting information and sharing experiences about a perceived inefficacy or even harmfulness of popular and officially accepted therapies, on the one hand, and the efficacy of unknown and unconventional approaches, on the other, which may lead to distrust of professional or institutional authorities. Thus, patients can develop many strategies to carry out their own ideas and plans against a healer's advice, if they disagree about the cause of the illness and the right course of treatment. Such strategies also may include simulating or neglecting specific symptoms to get a desired prescription, to avoid a specific treatment, or to get a temporary or permanent certificate of illness.

But empowerment is ambivalent. Patients are often torn between trust and suspicion, between the wish to be guided by experts and the wish to become an expert on their own, to give up or to keep responsibility for their health. Too much information can turn empowerment into confusion, and empowerment can also turn into manipulation, e.g. when pharmaceutical companies encourage patients to ask their healers for the drugs they sell (cf. DUMIT 2012). Thus, empowerment is hardly straightforward. For instance, in which direction is empowerment oriented? Is it an extension of the patients' biomedical knowledge? Or does it facilitate increasing demands on doctors, who are approached by patients who figure as consumers or customers? Does it include the right to remain a passive patient? Empowerment does not necessarily pit an autonomous patient against a dominant physician. This mélange opens up questions about the modes and means of empowerment. Who, beyond patients, has an interest in empowerment? Are Internet media engines of emancipation or sources of confusion?

The focus on ambivalences offers insights into the contingencies of care and healing and how they are resolved on the micro-level of healing encounters and healing cooperations. The sources of such ambivalences are manifold. First, the general uncertainties connected to medical practice have not decreased through the increase of medical knowledge and technologies (e.g. in surgery, CRISTANCHO, APRAMIAN, VANSTONE, LINGARD, LORELEI, & NOVICK 2013). Second, the emancipation of patients in recent decades has shifted the legitimacy of knowledge claims to include so-called "lay-expertise" (EPSTEIN 2023), while also bringing consumerism into healthcare, at least in the last three decades (LUPTON 1997). Third, current digital devices, such as apps and activity trackers, increase the complexities of healing once again by introducing novel data and metrics that rest in an uneasy space between lifestyle and medicine (WILLIAMS, WILL, WEINER, & HENWOOD 2020). Thus, the ambivalences of healing can be perceived as a threat to medical authority, casting doubt on what is often conceived as biomedical objective truth.

The continuing "social authority" of medicine shows that this is not necessarily the case, however; there might be shifts in the "cultural authority" of medicine (EPSTEIN & TIMMERMANS 2021). The social authority of medicine typically rests on the cooperation of patients and physicians: either patients granting authority based on ascribed expertise and not challenging their physicians' knowledge and skills (Haase, Ajjawi, Bearman, Brodersen, Risor, & Hoeyer 2023) or physicians carefully navigating and negotiating their authority by managing ambivalences in daily interaction (Stivers & Timmermans 2020). Seen on a larger scale, the cultural authority of medicine, i.e., the broader cultural legitimacy of biomedical knowledge, values, and skills, might have lost some of its dominance over the past decades, culminating in a crisis of credibility during the COVID-19 pandemic (Goldenberg 2021; Harambam & Voss 2023).

The contributions to this issue engage with the issues raised above. The first two contributions by Anna Hänni about *In-Patient Psychiatric Care as a Space of Ambiguity* and by Nicole Ernstmann, Sophie Elisabeth Gross, Ute Karbach, Lena Ansmann, André Karger, Holger Pfaff, Markus Wirtz, Walter Baumann, & Melanie Neumann about *Patient-Physician-Relationship in Cancer Care* study the interactions between patients and physicians in psychiatry and oncology and how a stable course of treatment is maintained. They analyze how the social authority of physicians is maintained in heterogenous settings with diverging values and interests. Ambivalence is a constant feature of such complex treatments, where medical authority is not directly under attack, but physicians need to manage the emerging ambivalences in order to remain in control of the trajectory. The following two contributions by Nick Fox about *Neoliberalism, Digital Health Technologies and "Citizen Health"* and by Márcio Vilar about *Unexpected Amelioration among Sick Health Professionals through Displacing Medical Cooperations in Brazil* study how patients engage with biomedical authority and how they try to mobilize knowledge claims that are not part of mainstream biomedical treatment plans. The cultural authority of medicine is at stake, either from outside, through a democratic access to data, or from inside, when physicians themselves become patients and, by off-label use of drugs, start to contest medical assumptions that are taken for granted.

From all four studies, we can see that all major trends that have characterized biomedical healthcare in recent years each create their own ambivalences. The ambivalence of empowerment and emancipation, shifting authority from physicians to patients while at the same time shifting the burden of responsibility. The ambivalence of knowledge and technology, where new insights and instruments may lead to less certainty and credibility. The ambivalences of cooperation, where trust and credibility, skills and values are being disrupted as well as maintained. The ambivalences of care, in the tension between individualized and standardized treatments, in the tensions between personal and profession relations, and in the tensions between participation and domination. How these ambivalences may be resolved is an empirical question in each of the fields under study. What the empirical studies show is that this is hardly an abstract issue, but one that is negotiated in the physical realties of bodies and technologies in biomedical healthcare.

We are grateful for the financial support from the DFG Collaborative Research Center 1187 "Media of Cooperation" at the University of Siegen.

References

Becker, Howard S., Blanche Geer, Everett C. Hughes, & Anselm L. Strauss (eds) 1961. *Boys in White. Student Culture in Medical School.* Chicago: University of Chicago Press.
Begenau, Jutta, Cornelius Schubert, & Werner Vogd (eds) 2010. *Die Arzt-Patienten-Beziehung.* Stuttgart: Kohlhammer.
Berg, Marc, & Annemarie Mol (eds) 1998. *Differences in Medicine. Unraveling Practices, Techniques, and Bodies.* Durham: Duke University Press.
Cristancho, Sayra M., Tavis Apramian, Meredith Vanstone, Lorelei Lingard, Michael Ott, & Richard J. Novick 2013. Understanding Clinical Uncertainty. What Is Going on When Experienced Surgeons Are Not Sure What to Do? *Academic Medicine* 88, 10: 1516–1521.
Dumit, Joseph 2012. *Drugs for Life. How Pharmaceutical Companies Define Our Health.* Durham: Duke University Press.
Epstein, Steven 2023. The Meaning and Significance of Lay Expertise. In Gil Eyal & Thomas Medvetz (eds) *The Oxford Handbook of Expertise and Democratic Politics.* Oxford: Oxford University Press: 76–102.
Epstein, Steven, & Stefan Timmermans 2021. From Medicine to Health. The Proliferation and Diversification of Cultural Authority. *Journal of Health and Social Behavior* 62, 3: 240–254.
Fox, Renée C. 1980. The Evolution of Medical Uncertainty. *The Milbank Memorial Fund Quarterly. Health and Society* 58, 1: 1–49.

FREIDSON, ELIOT 1970. *Professional Dominance. The Social Structure Of Medical Care*. New York: Atherton Press.

GOLDENBERG, MAYA J. 2021. *Vaccine Hesitancy. Public Trust, Expertise, and the War on Science*. Pittsburgh: University of Pittsburgh Press.

HAASE, CHRISTOFFER B., ROLA AJJAWI, MARGARET BEARMAN, JOHN BRANDT BRODERSEN, TORSTEN RISOR, & KLAUS HOEYER 2023. Data As Symptom. Doctors' Responses To Patient-Provided Data In General Practice. *Social Studies of Science* 53, 4: 522–544.

HAFFERTY, FREDERIC W., & RONALD FRANKS 1994. The Hidden Curriculum, Ethics Teaching, and the Structure of Medical Education. *Academic Medicine* 69, 11: 861–871.

HARAMBAM, JARON, & EHLER VOSS (eds) 2023. Corona Truth Wars. Epistemic Disputes and Societal Conflicts around a Pandemic. *Minerva. A Review of Science, Learning and Policy* 61, 3.

HENRY, M. S. 2006. Uncertainty, Responsibility, and the Evolution of the Physician/Patient Relationship. *Journal of Medical Ethics* 32, 6: 321-23.

LUPTON, DEBORAH 1997. Consumerism, Reflexivity and the Medical Encounter. *Social Science & Medicine* 45, 3: 373–381.

MERTON, ROBERT K., GEORGE READER, & PATRICIA L. KENDALL (eds) 1957. *The Student-Physician. Introductory Studies in the Sociology of Medical Education*. Cambridge: Harvard University Press.

PILNICK, ALISON, & ROBERT DINGWALL 2011. On the Remarkable Persistence of Asymmetry in Doctor/Patient Interaction. A Critical Review. *Social Science & Medicine* 72, 8: 1374–82.

STIVERS, TANYA, & STEFAN TIMMERMANS 2020. Medical Authority under Siege. How Clinicians Transform Patient Resistance into Acceptance. *Journal of Health and Social Behavior* 61, 1: 60–78.

STOLLBERG, GUNNAR 2008. Informed Consent und Shared Decision Making. Ein Überblick über medizinische und sozialwissenschaftliche Literatur. *Soziale Welt* 59, 4: 394–408.

WILLIAMS, ROS, CATHERINE WILL, KATE WEINER, & FLIS HENWOOD 2020. Navigating standards, encouraging interconnections. Infrastructuring digital health platforms. *Information, Communication & Society* 23, 8: 1170–1186.

Cornelius Schubert, Prof. Dr., is Professor of Sociology of Science and Technology at the University of Technology Dortmund. His areas of expertise are in the sociology of technology, the sociology of medicine, innovation studies, and qualitative methods. His research focus lies on the relations of bodies and technologies in healthcare. He currently is the chair of the board of the German Society for Science and Technology Studies (GWTF) and member of the board of the interdisciplinary journal NOvation.

TU Dortmund
University Department of Social Sciences
Emil-Figge-Str. 50
44227 Dortmund, Germany
e-mail: cornelius.schubert@tu-dortmund.de

Ehler Voss, PD Dr. phil., is an anthropologist working at the intersections of medical anthropology, media anthropology, political anthropology, and the anthropology of religion. He is Managing Director of the collaborative research platform Worlds of Contradiction (WOC) and Private Lecturer at the Department of Anthropology and Cultural Research at the University of Bremen; Chair of the Association for Anthropology and Medicine (AGEM); Editor-in-Chief of *Curare*; and Co-founder and Co-editor of boasblogs.org.

University of Bremen
Worlds of Contradiction (WOC)
Universitäts-Boulevard 13
28359 Bremen, Germany
e-mail: ehler.voss@uni-bremen.de

In-Patient Psychiatric Care as a Space of Ambiguity
Therapeutic Encounters from a Sensory and Embodied Perspective

ANNA HÄNNI

Abstract In social anthropology, there exists only little research about the sensory and intersubjective aspects of in-patient psychiatric care. Proceeding from vignettes from ethnographic fieldwork in two psychiatric clinics in Switzerland, this article outlines two empirical research interests and puts them into dialogue. On one side, therapeutic interactions and practices within the clinical setting are analyzed through the lenses of sensory ethnography and embodiment. On the other side, a multiplicity of "therapeutic cultures" and spaces co-exist within clinical premises. In some cases, they encompass diverging or even conflicting aims and basic assumptions about psychopathology and healing. As a result, various possibilities of human sociality and interaction open up to psychiatric sufferers, many of them characterized by ambivalence. What is being perceived as "therapeutic" and what, to the contrary, as a threat to human integrity and health can lie close together and can vary individually. I discuss how closely experiences of ambivalence – be it among psychiatric sufferers or staff members – are related to spatiality, embodied perception and to temporality. Referring to sensory ethnography and Hartmut Rosa's writing on resonance, I argue that, in in-patient psychiatric settings, the human social is inextricably intertwined with the nonhuman.

Keywords sensory ethnography – psychiatry – medical anthropology – phenomenology – therapy

Introduction

The following reflections are based on 4 months of ethnographic fieldwork within two Swiss public psychiatric clinics[1] in 2022, followed by several follow-up interviews. In both clinics, I did my research in the position as a research student and participated in the ward's daily life. In both cases, in-depth access was restricted to one specific ward (one acute ward and one therapy ward). Beyond that restriction, many other therapeutic and institutional spaces beyond wards were accessible to me. During my research, I became interested in different professional understandings of care. Namely, in cultures of medical and non-medical care, and the concomitant sensory and affective lifeworlds. I speak of "cultures" of psychiatric care because I encountered sometimes blurry, sometimes profound differences between therapeutic settings within one and the same institution, accompanied by psychiatric sufferer's ambivalence around the question of what "the therapeutic" entailed in specific instances. My interest led me to follow Jenkins' call to investigate more thoroughly how culture – in this case therapeutic cultures ranging from the biomedical to embodied and creative therapies – shape every aspect of mental illness (JENKINS 2015: 249). My research is driven by the joy of bringing experimental and experiential insights into spaces hardly recognized by social anthropologists: the sensory and atmospheric microcosms of in-patient psychiatric care. This research also attends to the crisis and reorientation towards the cultural and social in which academic psychiatry currently finds itself in (KLEINMAN 2012; DI NICOLA & STOYANOV 2021).

During my fieldwork in both clinics, I had access to wards which accommodated varied clientele: I met privately and publicly insured service users (while there exist exclusively "private" clinics, many provide services for both) and accompanied them, as well as staff members, in their daily activities. This included that I accompanied service users to non-medical therapies that, in many cases, took place outside wards in other buildings of the clinic. What I subsume here under the broad term "alternative therapies" includes a wide range of methods such as art, movement and music therapy, animal-supported therapies, and group-sessions in spiritual care. Every clinic had its own unique way of treating psychiatric sufferers and staff, and even every ward presented an entirely different picture of what "in-patient psychiatric care" looks, feels and sounds like. Note that, due to the limited scope of this article, I won't focus on conversational psychotherapy here – one of the most institutionalized non-medical therapies in both clinics.

Two issues emerged during my fieldwork. First, it struck me how partial and individually different the knowledge seemed that the ward's doctors and nurses had about alternative therapies. It all depended on the people in charge in the wards (typically doctors and nurses), whether non-medical therapies were integrated or rather sidelined in treatment. In interviews with doctors and nurses, this inconsistency surfaced as some cherished alternative therapies as "equally important as medication", while other relegated them to the realm of "day-structuring activities" or "unspecific therapies". The latter is borrowed from medical jargon and could be paraphrased as "there's no harm in trying". In this case, a kind of wellness effect was expected but no significant impact on individual pathology. In contrast to that, the importance of psychopharmaceutical treatment and electroconvulsive therapy seemed considerably less questioned within wards. While "alternative" therapies were an important part of institution's marketing, of therapy plans and even received funding from health insurances, their standing seemed more complicated. Obviously, this reflects the ongoing prevalence of biomedical models of mental illness within western psychiatry (ROSE 2019). Tellingly, many non-medical therapists questioned the institution's biomedical bias. In one clinic, a new ward was on the verge of being opened and, according to alternative therapists, "the management" had not granted any budget for their involvement into therapeutic plans. Tellingly, a considerable amount of service users used and mentioned alternative therapies as an important part of their experience of in-patient treatment. Some of them continued to attend to them as outpatients.

The second issue that emerged from my research material: many users on acute wards complained to me that they felt "not being seen" and "not being listened to" in situations when they would have needed it the most. I was puzzled by both, the sufferer's feeling of invisibility and the complex coexistence of different therapeutic ontologies. Those varied possibilities of human sociality and "choreographies" of *doing* mental affliction and therapy (KLAUSNER 2015: 121) complicate simple notions of "care" and point towards the ambivalence tied to giving and receiving care. I ask: How do structural aspects of the clinic relate to the sensory and embodied dimensions of *experiencing* in-patient psychiatric care? How are psychiatric sufferer's and staff's ambivalent entanglements between healing, harm and affliction connected with the sensory, material and immaterial dimensions of the everyday?

Doing phenomenological anthropology in the psychiatric clinic

My research is influenced by Byron Good's call for "the development of critical studies of how illness comes to meaning, of how reality (not simply beliefs about it) is organized and experienced in matters of sickness and care" (GOOD 1993: 63). It is precisely my attempt to understand the multiplicity of realities I encountered within the microcosm of the psychiatric hospital, indebted to a "critical phenomenology" (GOOD 1993: 63). This radical prioritization of experience allows me to trace how concepts of mental illness and normality, even the very definition of "reality" and the normal are fluid, contested (JENKINS 2015: 9) and performatively constituted in social context (ROSE 2019: 9). I encountered a stunning variety of different (sub-)cultures of therapy and of illness within the very same institutions and even within wards, depending on the people and spaces I found myself interacting with. While I perceive the picture that Erving Goffman draws of the psychiatric clinic in his 1960s-work *Asylums* (GOFFMAN 1961) as too structurally static, it certainly captures the huge impact that institutional structures and hierarchies have on the self, social roles and everyday interactions. While *Asylums* falls short on the changed landscape of psychiatric care today, Goffman's insights into the embodied and performative nature of clinical interactions remain inspiring. Used with caution towards his structuralist generalizations, Goffman's concepts deliver a theoretical background tending to the epistemic hierarchies, social performativity and the entanglement of care and constraint within psychiatric clinics (GOFFMAN 1961). Bearing Foucauldian concepts of psychiatric power in mind, institutional ethnography (SMITH 2005) seems more apt to capture the diverse, often ambiguous, experiences present in day-to-day life. My focus on embodiment and the sensory allows me to understand the "extraordinary conditions" of mental illness (JENKINS 2015) as a complex, fluid entanglement between lived experience, materialities and embodied practices.

Foucault's writings on the emergence of psychiatric practice as normalizing power (FOUCAULT 1988a) capture the history of my research sites. Still, this representationalist, textualized view of psychiatric power does not do justice to the phenomenological richness I encountered in the field. I agree with Csordas' critique that Foucauldian approaches view social reality as "inscribed" into individual bodies and subjugate the body to the semantic (CSORDAS 1993: 136). Ambiguity and not-knowing are omnipresent in day-to-day interactions within in-patient psychiatry; mental illness can be incommensurable, unbearable and incomprehensible, both for the afflicted and those who are not (JENKINS 2015: 261). Practicing phenomenological anthropology allows us to appreciate indeterminacy in psychiatric practice as a matter of intersubjectivity:

> Beginning from perceptual reality, however, it then becomes relevant to ask how our bodies may become objectified through processes of reflection. [...] What is revealed by a return to the phenomena – and the consequent necessity to collapse dualities of mind and body, self and other – is instead a fundamental principle of indeterminacy that poses a profound methodological challenge to the scientific ideal. The "turning toward" that constitutes the object of attention cannot be determinate in terms of either subject or object, but only real in terms of intersubjectivity. (CSORDAS 1993: 149).

I argue, that doing phenomenological ethnographies about in-patient psychiatric care is a more than human matter. Integrating the environmental and material into the scope of "experience" allows for insights that go beyond cartesian dualisms between "mind" and "body" and the tendency in the field of psychiatry to treat the human brain as an isolated entity (ROSE 2019: 95, 189). As a phenomenologist, I am inspired by Kavedžija's approach to human wellbeing as a processual, more-than-human matter of conviviality (KAVEDŽIJA 2021) and by Navaro's ethnographic exploration of how feelings (in this case "spatial melancholia") emerge as entanglements between (human) subjects, objects and non-human environments (NAVARO-YASHIN 2009: 16). On a conceptual level, I draw from environmental anthropology (INGOLD 2002; 2011) and postphenomenological thinking that sharpens ethnographer's awareness not only of the "ontological unity of people and things" (IHDE & MALAFOURIS 2019: 204) but also of how people are *changed* by things and technologies (IHDE & MALAFOURIS 2019: 209).

Besides my theoretical interest in human and other-than-human relationalities, intersubjectivity figures also as an important emic category in my field. It is not only at the core of suffering and the provision of care, but often comes with ambiguity, both for psychiatric sufferers and staff members. A decisive factor which determines whether psychiatric sufferers experience clinical interactions as healing or, to the contrary, as harmful, resides in experiences of intersubjectivity. Joan Tronto (TRONTO 2015) argues that good care involves much more than just organizing acts of caregiving. It involves the identification of caring needs (*caring about*), accepting one's own responsibility to do something about that need (*caring for*) and finally an assessment if needs have been met by the caregiving (*care-receiving*). Those are not instrumental interactions, but involve morality and value commitments. Those who deliver "good care" cultivate being attentive, responsible, competent and responsive towards other's needs (TRONTO 2015: 3–9). Seen through Tronto's theoretical lens and Csordas' paradigm of embodiment, in-patient psychiatric care emerges as a deeply intersubjective practice that enfolds as an embodied entanglement between caregivers and psychiatric sufferers. I add to that point that in-patient psychiatric care does not merely entail human interactions but is equally co-created by sensory, material and other nonhuman aspects that are fundamentally shaped by institutional and political surroundings. The multitude of ambivalent experiences I encountered in the field relate partly back to what Goffman (GOFFMAN 1961) and Foucault (FOUCAULT 1977; 1988a; 2003) have already exhaustively discussed: the institution itself is a place of power-infused hierarchies and social performativity that directly mirrors how a society deals with "troubled" individuals. Following Jenkins' reference to feminist thought, I approach mental illness and clinical practices as a condensation of the personal and the political (JENKINS 2015: 3).

Of atmospheric ambiguities: sensory ethnography and therapeutic encounters

In order to do justice to the ambiguity experienced by interlocutors as well as the indeterminacy of scientific reasoning, sensory ethnography offers methodological inspiration (PINK 2009; INGOLD 2011). Pink frames ethnographic research as a mode of "emplaced knowing" (PINK 2009: 40) which is embodied, but includes materiality, the senses, imagination, reverie and remembrance (PINK 2009: 25 ff). The attunement to the imaginary, remembered and sensory dimensions of therapeutic encounters is crucial to prevent reproducing rationalist medical discourses that presuppose a dichotomy between "objective" reality and seemingly irrational beliefs (GOOD 1993: 194). My interest in ambivalence within in-patient therapeutic encounters draws on a "politics of atmospheres":

> Atmosphere does not so much reside in place as emerge from our ongoing encounters with it, opening up potential as we feel our way through the world, a process animated by affect (but not completely defined by it), a "spatially extended quality of feeling" (BÖHME 1993: 117–118) [...] Accordingly, we argue that atmosphere must be thought of as pulling together affect with sensation, materiality, memory and meaning [...] (SUMARTOJO & PINK 2019: 30).

Atmospheres are political because they are not simply there, but continually emerge as contested, fluid entanglements. They are subject to constant appropriation, change and subversion by all actors involved (SUMARTOJO & PINK 2019: 31). This view of atmospheres as potentialities for change and transformation resonates with an emic category that was omnipresent and often contested in the field: the aim at psychological change and transformation, be it among psychiatric sufferers or as a narrative deployed by therapists and clinicians. Inspired by Ansdell and DeNoras' research on music therapy (ANSDELL & DENORA 2012), I suggest an ecological view of clinical practices and their ambivalences. Walking fieldwork (Irving 2005; 2011) is crucial in that endeavour as it allows interlocutors, who often experienced different wards and treatments during their stay, to retrieve associations and memories tied to clinical spaces and their materiality. In return, accessing memories through walking fieldwork proved ethically challenging in the field as spaces like the emergency reception or a closed unit were associated with unresolved, unspoken trauma for several sufferers. Stasis and the inability to move – for example during acute depression – was equally part of my embodied encounter with in-patient sensory lifeworlds. Others I accompanied to therapy sessions beyond the ward and walks in the park. I rushed with senior psychiatrist's from ward to ward during their "rounds" as they replaced others in times of incessant personnel shortages, talked through lunch breaks with the nurses, and sat in staff meetings. Researching atmospheres requires an attunement to the rhythms, sounds, smells and aesthetics of clinical day-to-day lifeworlds.

Situating ambiguity within a theory of resonance

How can we theoretically situate experiences of ambivalence within the sensory and the embodied dimensions of therapeutic spaces? And how are subjective experiences tied to the political and cultural context of the psychiatric clinic? Even though I can only hint at his complex and large body of writing here, I find inspiration in German sociologist Hartmut Rosa's writing on what he calls resonance (ROSA 2016). Rosa opens his book *Resonanz. Eine Soziologie der Weltbeziehung* with the claim that, "If acceleration is the problem, then resonance may well be the solution" (ROSA 2016: 14, translated by AH). In the tradition of critical theory, he formulates a critique of neoliberal societies and the alienation they produce in various aspects of our everyday lives (ROSA 2016: 253 ff; PETERS & MAJID 2022: 8). Rosa defines alienation as "relation of relationlessness" (ROSA 2016: 438) which is driven by "instrumental reason" (ROSA 2016: 74). He understands experiences of resonance as a powerful counterforce that enables experiences of aliveness. Resonant experiences create meaning in a modern existence otherwise characterized by interpersonal distance, coldness and unresponsiveness (ROSA 2016: 418; PETERS & MAJID 2022: 14). The adaption of Rosa's thinking to my research field is inspired by his claim that institutions embody the most powerful social force that shapes whether we experience states of resonance or alienation (ROSA 2016: 948). Rosa's theory also comes with its problematic aspects. As Peters and Majid point out, he entwines descriptive and normative elements of resonance (PETERS & MAJID 2022: 9) which, from an anthropological point of view, remains too far away from the intricacies and ambivalences of lived in-patient experience. By interweaving Rosa's theory with my phenomenological approach to psychiatry, I hope to creatively enrich those normative aspects with the complexity of lived human sociality. I shed light on the entanglement between intimate, embodied experience and the political that so fundamentally characterizes every facet of mental illness (JENKINS 2015: 3).

State of research

There is a rich body of anthropological research in the field of mental illness (see for example GOOD 2012; JENKINS 2018; KHAN 2017; LESTER 2007; LITTLEWOOD 2000) and global mental health (KOHRT & MENDENHALL 2015; WHITE et al. 2017) and I can only name a few of them here. But there has only recently been a surge in phenomenological ethnographies on the embodied experience of psychiatric in-patients within clinical premises (GARCIA 2010; KLAUSNER 2015; HEYKEN et al. 2019; MEWES 2019; VARMA 2020) and research specifically on non-medical therapies in in-patient settings is still scarce (MATTINGLY 1998; LUHRMANN 2000; MEWES 2019; SCHMID 2020; BRUUN & HUTTEN forthcoming). Albeit not primarily anchored in social anthropology or ethnography, there are important basic works – ranging from ROSE, GOFFMAN and FOUCAULT to SMITH – that focus on the genealogy of psychiatric practices and institutional ruling relations (GOFFMAN 1963; ROSE 1979, 2019; FOUCAULT 1988a, 2003; SMITH 2005). Recent publications in sensory and environmental anthropology intersect partly with my research interest as they focus on in-patient lifeworlds (DUQUE et al. 2021). In an inspiring article, Pink and Hogan trace the intersections between art therapy and anthropology (HOGAN & PINK 2010; PINK et al. 2011; PINK & LEDER MACKLEY 2014), while not emplacing their findings specifically within in-patient experiences and institutions. Conceptually, I am inspired by Luhrmann's outstanding ethnography, *Of Two Minds*, where she traces different professional practices and ontologies of mental illness within clinical practice in the US (LUHRMANN 2000). DeNora and Ansdell's sociologically oriented work explores music therapy in community psychiatry. They ethnographically argue for the importance of research on music therapy beyond biomedical models of treatment and evidence-based assessment (ANSDELL & DENORA 2012) and propose, similar to others, an ecological perspective on in-patient psychiatric care and its socio-material entanglements (KLAUSNER 2015; BISTER et al. 2016; MEWES 2019). Winz and Söderström discuss the sensory experience of psychosis in urban spaces through "biosensory ethnography", which defines the sensory in a more biological manner than I do here (WINZ & SÖDERSTRÖM 2021). In nursing research, there has recently been published an article that adapted Rosa's theory of resonance to nursing as "a new and inspiring phenomenological and critical lens" (LÓPEZ-DEFLORY et al. 2023). I hope to contribute to a growing body of ethnographic, phenomenological research about non-medical therapies within psychiatric clinics.

"We are not a wellness temple here": the institution as a site of trouble

"We are not a wellness temple here" – this quote from a clinic director re-surfaced in several conversations with staff and service users. This emic narrative positioned "the" public clinic as a counter-space to "better" (private) psychiatric care because, to come back to the director's narrative, "here, we have to treat the most severely ill patients because we have to fulfil the performance mandate towards the general population". Nevertheless, there existed a number of private wards within public clinics, which figured as substantially "better" in both user's and staff member's accounts. But even among the privately insured users, the overall impressions they related to me about their treatment could not have been more contradictory. The psychiatric clinic figured for many partly – for some fully – as site of healing, introspection and "hard work on the self".[2] Others, especially those stationed within public acute wards, experienced the clinic as a site of violence and violation of personal boundaries. During the long hours I spent with psychiatric sufferers, a common preoccupation among them became salient: they missed "being seen" and "being listened to". Most nurses and doctors mentioned the density of acutely ill people in overcrowded wards, combined with the lack of professionals and the growing scarcity of financial resources as underlying causes for institutional trouble. An increasingly austere and neoliberal atmosphere in healthcare characterized day-to-day life within wards. This reflects what Disney and Schliehe recently theorized: Institutions dealing with human trouble have become increasingly troubled spaces themselves (DISNEY & SCHLIEHE 2019). One male nurse, who had been working in acute psychiatric care for nearly 30 years at that time, compared the clinic with a car factory: "nowadays, you have to treat as much patients in as little time as possible here". While those narratives of austerity seem plausible from a structural perspective, speculations about the causes for the "troubled institution" can look entirely different in service user's accounts. In a conversation with a user affected by psychosis and hospitalized against his will, he mentioned the "malignancy", "cold-heartedness" and "sadistic" nature of certain nurses as causes of his suffering. Still, this problematic background did not prevent a considerable number of service users from perceiving the clinic also as space of healing.

Biomedical cultures of care: psychotropic medication

Clearly, the advances in psychotropic medication have saved many lives and are, for some people, an indispensable part of recovery. While I don't engage primarily with the anthropology of psychopharmacology in this article, I shall discuss medication critically as a part of the sensory, ontologically diverse therapeutic landscape of the clinic.

Biomedical models of mental illness seemed both hierarchically and institutionally dominant in the clinics I was present. For example, in one ward, which was an institutional flagship for the "best" psychiatric care in the whole clinic, the term "therapy" referred first and foremost to the evaluation and adjustment of psychotropic medication. Psychotherapy was – contrary to official mission statements – not provided for everyone who received medical treatment. This bias towards medication seems to characterize the whole landscape of public psychiatric care in Switzerland.[3] In the majority of cases, this shortcoming was not questioned by staff and commonly explained to me with the argument that clients were "too acutely ill" to undergo psychotherapy and that they had to "stabilize" first. As I oscillated between the ward and alternative therapeutic services, the specificity of discursive, affective and sensory registers between biomedical and other interactions of psychiatric care became salient. Psychiatric sufferers' encounters with head psychiatrists were often biased towards verbal exchange and abstraction. In some clinics, doctors wore white coats, which instantly created a more distanced, distinctly "medical" atmosphere resounding with Goffman's analysis of the psychiatric hospital as a space of highly stratified social performativity (GOFFMAN 1961). The digital documentation platform that operated at the core of the clinical everyday was important during the head psychiatrist's visit. Nurses and lower ranking doctors used it in order to inform head psychiatrists about medical compounds and treatment plans or make adjustments to them. Receiving "the best" care equalized the head psychiatrist's visit and the presence of a relatively stable team of nurses. The head psychiatrist's visit lasted around 10 minutes per client and took place once or twice each week. The head psychiatrist was usually accompanied by an entourage of as many as 12 persons, comprising other psychiatrists, students, nurses, interns, people from other divisions of the clinic, and figures like me, an anthropologist.

This typical conversation, that took place during the head psychiatrist's regular visit, might seem trite when considered by itself, but continued to re-emerge in various nuances during his rounds:

Head psychiatrist: "How are you today? You look a bit low-spirited compared to last week."

Psychiatric sufferer: "I feel sometimes foggy in the morning and don't know how to start my day. Shouldn't I be better by now? It's been three weeks!"

Head psychiatrist: "I see that you are suffering. This is part of your illness; It's an emotional blockage. We will adjust your medication and try out another compound. This will give you more motivation in the mornings."[4]

Despite the leading doctor's known expertise in psychotropic medication, psychiatric sufferers and some staff members questioned the format of his visits in conversation with me. The visit presented a moment of social stress for psychiatric sufferers as it offered too little privacy and time for them to communicate about their psychological state.

The magic pill as realm of the uncertain

Another paradox that became salient was tied to psychotropic medication: On one hand, psychotropic drugs were handled as omnipotent actors at the core of therapeutic treatment in medical discourses. On the other hand, psychiatrists stressed during their day-to-day work, that if and how an individual would react to a compound was in many ways unforeseeable.

The ambivalence and uncertainty tied to biomedical treatment reflects in Renata's tale, who suffered from frequent relapses into illness, accompanied by hospitalization. Medication figured as a reference point in her account of "regaining stability" and losing it. When she told me about one relapse after being discharged from the former clinic, she mentioned similar reasons as many other interlocutors: the lack of ambulant therapeutic treatment and that her medication had not been "well adjusted" at that time. As she depended on a psychiatrist when it came to adjusting or changing psychotropic medication, it becomes salient how biomedical models of treatment are inextricably entwined with medical hierarchies: It's the doctors who are granted the authority to explain and manage the effects and side-effects of psychotropic medication. As she relied on psychotropic medication, Renata perceived an intensive medical surveillance and biochemical treatment of her illness as an indispensable part of her healing journey. At the same time, she uttered a deep ambivalence about medication due to massive side effects. One compound had come with several hair loss. She also suffered from lethargy and pervasive tiredness. Renata granted psychotropic drugs the power to change her life for the worse and for the better – in a way she could hardly control herself. She relied, as many users who take psychotropic drugs, to doctors to orchestrate the array of biochemical actors whose impact on her body and her psyche was not foreseeable for her (see also KLAUSNER 2015: 181–246). Other psychiatric sufferers told me that certain psychotropic drugs robbed them entirely of their sexual life and sense of bodily self – with destructive effect for their romantic relationships.

I met Beat when he had an argument with his ward's head psychiatrist. He was furious about both his medication and his involuntary return to the clinic after a weekend of stress endurance vacation (*Belastungsurlaub*) at home. Angrily, he shouted: "The medication does not help at all! Nothing! You [to the doctor] can eat them by yourself!" The doctor replied calmly: "Yes, I would take the medication if I needed it." Curious about his personal view, I met Beat shortly before his dismissal from the ward. I asked him what he perceived as most healing during his stay at the clinic. I was surprised by his immediate answer: the paintings and flower arrangements in the ward corridor had been, for him, facilitators of healing:

> I have suffered from insomnia for years and I have become suspicious of medication. When the doctor discusses with his assistants for the nth time what medication they could try out on me, I just can't take it anymore. At first, when I arrived here, I suffered from a terrible inquietude – I could not stand still. Then, I made a sport out of contemplating the paintings on the walls of the ward – they are beautiful. I started to meditate, to really contemplate those paintings. With the help of the artworks I regained focus. Later, I did the same with the flowers in the ward. Sadly, people did not understand. The nurses laughed at me in a friendly but belittling way – "so you are again meditating, yeah, yeah …"

The bio-medicalization of the psyche as hardening process: a short reflection

Meandering from the realm of medication into the sensory and the embodied, I end this brief insight into sensory, embodied and discursive experiences tied to psychotropic medication. I illustrated how psychotropic medication figures as both, omnipotent but potentially unpredictable actor in struggles for healing. The omnipresent, ambiguous agency of psychotropic drugs resonates with an era in which "neuroscience seeks to understand mental illness as a brain disorder instead of as behavioral disorder" (JENKINS 2015: 4–5). Medical narratives entail both the explanation and recollection of deranged, sometimes uncanny experiences of mental illness into psychiatric categories and the biomedical. Bearing in mind the messiness and ambiguity of the experience of mental illness itself (JENKINS 2011; 2015), psychotropic medication figures as an institutionalized gateway towards both, controlling the messiness of deranged experience and abstract discourses around "biochemical imbalance" (JENKINS 2015: 57). The concomitant interactions with doctors take place in temporally highly limited phases, often biased towards verbal exchange and visual perception. Medical narratives unite a paradox between biochemical incertitude and what Jenkins called "a religious metaphor of miraculous healing" (JENKINS 2015: 26). In some, but not every, aspect the atmospheric and sensory dimensions of concomitant medicalized interactions are reminiscent of what Arthur Kleinman described as "instrumental rationality in medicine" (KLEINMAN & KLEINMAN 1991).

Service user's accounts resonate, in many ways, with insights from Jenkins' in-depth ethnography of psychotropic medication in the US. Psychotropic medication comes with various critical aspects, one of them being long term sufferer's experience of "recovery without cure". While symptoms might improve significantly due to psychotropic medication, many sufferers perceive themselves as being far from healthy, and experience massive side-effects and social stigma (JENKINS 2011: 9). While I don't go further into that topic here, I want to stress the massive sensory and embodied impact that psychotropic drugs can have on user's self-perception and embodied, affective states of being.

Violence as multisensory entanglement

For service user Claire, "the ward" – which figures as the institutional epicentre of the "neurochemical self" (ROSE 2009) – emerged as a conglomerate of intersubjective, subjective and sensory matters. According to law and institutional discourses, forced measures always had to be ordered by doctors and implemented through strict institutional regulations. In contrast to this legal framework, Claire perceived the fine lines between care-receiving, violence and coercion as a much more ambivalent matter. For her, this was also a matter of the senses – and a complex array of interpersonal relationships with staff members and service users. During a walking interview across the clinical premises, we crossed the building where the emergency reception and acute wards were located. The sight of the building led her to reflect on her initial hospitalization:

> I was first hospitalized in the psychiatric unit of a general hospital. I was in a very bad condition – starving and in the middle of psychosis. I was not sure if I was going to survive. When I first arrived there, they put me in a completely isolated room where there was nothing. Literally nothing. They told me that I needed to sleep and calm down – in a completely isolated room! It was in this room where I almost lost my mind. There, my condition worsened. Only after hours of waiting, I was transferred here, where I was locked in the acute ward for ten days [points towards the building's second floor]. I was not even allowed to go out for a smoke. The toilets were a mess in the women's ward and the door locks not working. I was put in a room with other people. One of them was a kleptomaniac, you always had to watch your stuff. Even after she had been transferred to another room, she sneaked into my room at night. I was afraid and could not sleep, until I begged the nurses to be transferred into the isolation room. I just wanted to be alone, to feel safe. They did not allow me.
> At one point I told them "If you aren't going to listen to me, I'm going to die here". They misunderstood me and thought that I must be suicidal. So they put even more restrictions on me. But that

was not my point at all, I always wanted to live! I just wanted to feel seen!

I have never been to the isolation room in this ward, but I often heard the screams of those who were in there. They tell me that it feels like prison. In wards, there are many rules, which often creates conflicts between patients and nurses. As a patient, you have to learn how to navigate these rules. If you don't obey, they will put you into an isolation cell. It all depends on how you click with the nurses, if you get along with them.

In contrast to Claire's account, nurses almost univocally stressed that their duty to exert forced measures went back to doctor's orders and was one of the most difficult parts of their job. Not only in the account above, but also in a senior nurse's account from the same ward, the isolation room figured as an ambivalent place. The nurse described it as a problematic, but sometimes inevitable "low-stimulus room" for those who needed to "calm down". Nevertheless, she was convinced that, If the ward would be able to provide one on one care, isolation cells would be unnecessary.

Instrumental reason and the sensory: a reflection

During her stay in the closed ward, Claire felt an atmosphere of "instrumental reason" (ROSA 2016: 74) extend into her material and human surroundings. While she had been treated correctly according to institutional procedures, some sensory and interpersonal aspects of her experience catapulted her into invisibility, anger and mistrust. Her experience is inseparable from the carceral materiality she associates with certain clinical spaces. Her experiences of being forced to spend time in different places that felt unsafe for her condensate into a feeling of not being seen. Her awareness of the paradox, that a caring site could potentially turn into a place of violence, coined her interaction with staff members. What she experienced could be described as "looping" in Goffman's terms, a "disruption of the usual relationship between the individual actor and his acts" (GOFFMAN 1961: 35–38). The ambiguity underlying low-stimulus rooms and other clinical spaces results from an entanglement of both the social and the sensory. In Griffero's terms, the experience of social *and* materially enacted violence in this specific room is an instance of atmospheric "feelings poured out into space" (GRIFFERO 2014: 108). This becomes even more salient if we analyze Claire's account through this lens of the atmospheric, "pulling together affect with sensation, materiality, memory and meaning" (SUMARTOJO & PINK 2019: 30). Low-stimulus rooms for forced treatment are institutionally legitimated healing spaces, but can come, paradoxically, with a feeling of dehumanization and isolation for psychiatric sufferers precisely *because* they deprive them from the very foundations in which atmospheric presence is anchored: sensory, material and significatory diversity. Human beings – and to an even greater extent psychiatric sufferers (WINZ & SÖDERSTRÖM 2021) – both live and feel enmeshed with sensory and material environments. Jenkins refers to mental illness as "complex processes of struggle" whose multidimensionality is more aptly described with the term "extraordinary conditions" than in the categories of psychiatric pathology (JENKINS 2015: 2).

With this theoretical background, I argue that the mute or even harmful interactions of in-patient care are entangled with the politics of atmosphere. The extraordinary experience of forced seclusion creates a "counter-atmosphere" that can destabilize the very experience of feeling alive and of dignity. This focus on the atmospheric and the sensory critically introduces a largely absent dimension within biomedical psychiatric discourses and ontologies of care. I argue that there is a need to complement biomedical spaces, practices and ontologies of psychiatric care with the ephemeral and the sensory. This acknowledges, to use Ingold's words, that "we do not then look beyond the material constitution of objects in order to discover what makes them tick; rather the power of agency lies with their materiality itself" (INGOLD 2011: 28).

Resonance as analytical lens on inconsistent encounters

How can we relate the atmospheric dimensions of the clinical back to the emic notions of "being seen" and "being listened to"? Here, I relate these atmospheric micropolitics to Rosa's theory of resonance that situates "mute" and "resonant" interactions within a larger sociopolitical context

(ROSA 2016). Rosa outlines, through the course of his extensive writing, four criteria of resonant experience, the first two of them being deeply intersubjective: *affection* and *emotion* (PETERS & MAJID 2022: 18). Individuals are moved emotionally while being affected by something "other" outside the self. The emotional aspect of resonance opens us, according to Rosa, to putting some of our emotional energy into the experienced "other" in return, to give something of us back into the outer world of experience (ROSA 2020: 398). As a third criterion, which results directly from affection and emotion, Rosa names *transformation*: the self changes during resonant experiences in a fundamental way. The fourth aspect of resonance is especially important in my discussion of ambivalent experiences of care within psychiatric wards: *elusiveness*. Resonant experiences can't be planned or forced because they entail "uncontrollable relational experiences of Otherness" (PETERS & MAJID 2022: 18ff, 142).

The resonant experience of mutual attention can be destabilized or even thwarted by institutional structures and practices of care. This became salient by the example of the intricacies underlying practices of abstraction and management within the biomedicalized institution. Even more, the structural intricacies of the "troubled institution" that operates with a nexus between care and control fundamentally limit instances in which resonant experiences are facilitated. *Elusiveness* and *uncontrollability* (ROSA 2016: 1063) stand in direct contradiction to many demands that biomedicalized, increasingly neoliberal psychiatric care in Switzerland puts onto psychiatric sufferers. Time plays a crucial role in enabling resonant experiences in the realm of the uncontrollable and unforeseeable. Time is a dimension that has, according to Rosa, become increasingly scarce in the wider scope of neoliberal societies due to different sociocultural acceleration processes. It is a paradox that characterizes the experience of time in late modernity: while suffering social acceleration, a "frenetic standstill [...] in the development of ideas and deep social structures" takes place (ROSA & TREJO-MATHYS 2013: 15). This paradoxical co-presence of stasis and increasing temporal acceleration manifests in the very intimate experience of psychiatric sufferer's interactions with staff and the materialities of the clinic itself. The lack of resonant experience in clinical interactions resonates with Rochelle Burgess' critique of biomedically biased psychiatry: Attending to the diversity and social embeddedness of mental illness requires the capacity to "hold complexity"[5]. It means refusing the violent act of simplifying lived experience into neat clinical categories and to strip sufferer's accounts off their lived socio-political context.

Ontologies of care beyond the biomedical: alternative therapies

In contrast to the entwinement of (bio-)medical expertise and psychotropic medication, non-medical therapies operated on different atmospheric levels. They took place in sensory, material and social settings that phenomenologically differed from wards – mostly in especially assigned rooms within clinical premises. Some psychiatric sufferers regularly attended alternative therapies, while others only went once or not at all because it seemed "too esoteric" for them. Those who participated, experienced a spatial and atmospheric change as they mingled with persons from other wards in fitness studios and in craft studios, while walking towards the dance and movement therapy rooms through the garden, gathered in music studios or walked through the nearby forest. Alternative therapies involved paint and canvas, plants, animals, body-centred practices, instruments, artworks, music, and many other sensory aspects.

One of the most salient observations was how the therapy rooms and other nonhuman aspects were actively created and used as therapeutic tools by therapists. One art therapist referred to his studio specifically as a "safe space" which he created by arranging shelves, plants and easels in a way "that gives patients a feeling of security but still harnesses the lightness and openness of the room". A movement therapist referred to the therapy room as "offering something different than the atmosphere in the ward" to psychiatric sufferers. Furniture, light, sounds, smells and objects were actively harnessed as atmospheric actors by therapists. Some therapists used parks and nearby forests as sites for group therapy. What stood out in many group sessions in alternative therapies was both, an atmosphere of the experimental, open-endedness and a fundamental attitude of "not having to perform". This stood in stark contrast to everyday interactions within the wards, which were usually permeated by the nexus between care and control (GOFFMAN 1961; FOUCAULT 1977, 1988a). During group settings, psychiatric sufferers often adopted a meta-perspective on their stay in the clinic and voiced how they "really felt at the moment".

Besides casual conversation, therapists actively encouraged psychiatric sufferers to express ambivalent feelings about the therapeutic interaction and the group setting immediately. As a result, shame, insecurity and non-compliance were voiced often more openly in alternative therapy spaces than within wards. At the same time, users did not have to expect direct consequences therefore because these encounters were explicitly taking place at the margins of the nexus between care and control that characterized wards. Several psychiatric sufferers referred to music, movement and dance therapy sessions as "challenging" because, often, shame and insecurity surfaced for them during group activities. Even if physical touch was never part of the sessions, the therapists centred sessions around both self-perception and the exploration of interpersonal boundaries. Frequently, participants left the room during the sessions, voicing that they needed a break or "had a crisis". Sometimes they came back, sometimes they didn't. This illustrates, that ambivalence surfaced no less than within wards in alternative therapies, but in fundamentally different ways.

Encounters in art- and movement therapy and spiritual care

Peter, a client diagnosed with autism, became one of my main interlocutors. Reflecting on our previous interview, he wrote to me via e-mail:

> One sees a doctor in this clinic for five minutes per week, at the very most. During this meeting, one or two questions are being asked. The movement therapist, on the other hand, observes a person for over 90 minutes and can try to give inputs to patients. But this requires an effort; this is real work. Sadly, for doctors and the pharma industry it is definitely more convenient to prescribe pills, to make profit…

This account resonates with a key issue that emerged within the contradictions between medical and non-medical care: temporality. Time to "observe" and "give inputs" was precisely what most doctors and nurses on the wards were short of and, paradoxically, what many psychiatric sufferers would have needed. In one-on-one settings, they had 50 minutes of face-to-face time with therapists. As group sessions centred around more casual topics, art and movement therapists told me that a considerable number of psychiatric sufferers used one-on-one sessions entirely for conversation. A movement therapist described her therapeutic approach towards clients as threefold: on an emotional, embodied and intellectual level. Thereby, an alternative experience to the feeling of "not being listened to" and "not feeling seen" was encouraged.

A physiotherapist told me:

> Patients are expected to relate their deepest issues to 'the god in white' [head psychiatrist] and his entourage of 10 persons in only 10 minutes. Once, a patient cried out his soul in my one-on-one session. Later that day, I followed the head physician's visit and saw the patient sitting on the bed, mumbling, 'I'm okay'. I totally understand him: how could one open up his heart in such an intimidating interaction?

She actively framed physiotherapy as a counter-space, an instance of mutual listening:

> When patients come to physiotherapy, they'll tell you every secret they haven't told anybody before. Sometimes heavy stuff – a woman voiced for the first time that she had been sexually assaulted. When the body moves, emotions and words start flowing.

When I asked the physiotherapist what she "does" with those narratives, she told me that she sometimes refrains from documenting everything in the hospital software, which contradicted the institutional protocol. She felt ambivalent about it because she was both committed to professional secrecy but also had a reporting obligation towards the clinic.

Pastoral workers were among the most critical interlocutors within many clinics as they inhabited an in-between position: they took part in day-to-day life of the clinic but organizationally, inhabited an outsider position because they were still part of the parish. This hybrid position had the effect that some pastoral workers were – although there was a change planned in the near future – the only staff group who did not have access to the clinic's digital documentation system. One pastoral worker pointed towards the importance of that position, as it allowed her to clearly work "in the interest of the patient and not of the institution". She questioned notions of illness and psychiatric treatment models during an interview:

> Depression is a healthy response to unhealthy living conditions and behavioural patterns. It urges people to pause, to introspect. But see what happens in the clinic: Patients come here, get pathologized as 'ill', and the only goal of therapy is to make symptoms disappear.

She highlighted that pastoral workers were "probably the only staff group which patients – especially in the forensic wards – are allowed to send away. I like to offer patients that option. It can create a basis of trust if patients are allowed to send me away anytime". The pastoral worker organized group discussions on the ward that explored philosophical, open-ended questions involving the reception of artworks and literature. One example was, when she explored with a group of sufferers the feeling of disappointment via discussing an artwork by the Swiss painter Ferdinand Hodler. Many of the persons present referred to the pastoral worker, in general, as "someone who really listens".

When I asked Beat, what had helped him most while recovering from depression in the clinic, he mentioned art therapy and ergotherapy. Aesthetic perception and creative practice had supported him during a long phase of recovery from the "complete isolation" of depression. As mentioned in the vignette above, he had found relief by "meditating on drawings", but also by attending the arts and crafts studio. When he started to talk about the studio, his eyes lightened up:

> One of my favourite places is the crafts studio. You can weave, you can make your own leather belt, you can sew, you can carve – whatever you want. You meet real artists there. You don't have to talk to anyone If you don't want to, but still you are together with other people. After my worst phase of depression, I had lost contact with my family, with my loved ones. This was the hardest part of it all.

> In the studio, I carved stone figures, which I then gave to my grandchildren.

For Beat, overcoming depression was inseparably connected to materiality and the senses – dimensions of experience that he directly connected to his experience of illness and recovery, isolation and reconnection. The arts and crafts studio was bright, colourful and cozy. In a corner, there was a table for service users to sit and drink tea together. Some worked silently, while others talked while painting or doing manual labour, often commenting other's work. One especially quiet person from another ward discovered her talent for handcraft there, which came with conversations and social contacts. This way of "being seen" differed from what it was commonly associated with in the clinic. In this setting, psychiatric sufferers could, for a short time, leave their categorization within clinical pathology by, as Hogan and Pink call it, creatively harnessing "interior states as ways of *knowing* and *experiencing*" (HOGAN & PINK 2010:158, emphasis in original).

Embodied therapies at the margins of the biomedical hegemony: conclusions

I return to the enmeshment between atmospheric traits of in-patient experience and the – sometimes alarmingly – fine line between mute and resonant interaction. First, it becomes salient that therapies beyond the biomedical treatment model can offer in-patients an enmeshment into distinct "currents of materials" (INGOLD 2011: 31). I argue that psychiatric sufferer's ambivalence towards their in-patient treatment is not simply a matter of affect, but much more a materially and sensorially entangled existential experience. It is precisely during a walking session in the forest or by engaging in creative practices when spaces are created that grant the body, as Csordas puts it, the status as subject and existential ground of culture (CSORDAS 1990: 5). In these instances, politics of atmospheres beyond medical hierarchies are co-created among psychiatric sufferers, therapists and environments. Light, sound and feeling do not merely enfold within human bodies but "take possession of it, sweeping the body up into their own currents" (INGOLD 2002: 134f). If we re-conceptualize the sensory as a pivot point of in-patient experience, service user's experience of the institution as a caring site seems coined by ambivalence. Medical and other ontologies of care coexist therein in sometimes separate sensory and social microcosms. The professionalization of human problems as psychiatric disorders can create a fundamental contradiction between lay, psychodynamic and biomedical views of "what life means and what is at stake in living" (KLEINMAN & KLEINMAN 1991: 293). The concomitant spatial and sensory embeddings of biomedical models of psychiatry reflect a Cartesian bias toward the privileging of mind and discourse which figures in an abstract, disembodied sphere. In a biomedical ontology of facticity and nosological order, indeterminacy is managed and controlled in favour of "hard science" which is, as Csordas puts it, always a result of a "hardening process, a process of objectification" (CSORDAS 1990: 38). I argue that non-medical therapies facilitate, precisely *because* they figure at the margins of clinical prestige, resonant experience by allowing uncertainty to enfold in its multi-layered multisensorial facets.

This leads me to my second conclusion, which centres around the experience and management of care and suffering, by both psychiatric sufferers and therapists. I complicate a uniform picture of "the" institution by suggesting, in its stead, that a variety of therapeutic cultures is actively co-created by the different actors in clinical space, resulting in a multiplicity of "politics of atmospheres". Of course, alternative therapies do not operate beyond the nexus between care and control that is written into the very fundament of the clinic (FOUCAULT 1977, 2003). Nevertheless, they can be subsumed as spaces of resonance that foster human sociality, take psychiatric sufferer's embodied, sensory experience seriously and allow open-ended experiences beyond the social performativity of the wards. The crucial factor that determined whether users perceived a therapeutic setting as boundary-transgressing or as resonant was not the absence of ambivalence, but the sensory and intersubjective resonance offered to it. The embodied, explorative and open-ended attitude behind non-medical therapies attend to the existential ambiguity of being alive, and thereby, they address an existing caveat within medicalized ontologies of psychiatric treatment (DI NICOLA & STOYANOV 2021). I argue that interactions that allow an unfolding of a mutual being-human within in-patient psychiatric care accept that humans are "constantly struggling to sustain and augment [our] being in relation to the being of others, as well as the nonbeing of the physical and material world, and the ultimate extinction of being that is death" (JACKSON 2013: xiv).

This multisensory facilitation of resonance happens, paradoxically, often at the margins of institutionally privileged caring interactions. The complementation of the biomedical epicentre of the psychiatric clinic with embodied, multisensory therapies speaks to the embodied, indeterminant nature of being alive (INGOLD 2002: 92–95) and of wellbeing as such. I have discussed ambiguity within psychiatric care from a sensory, environmental perspective because I argue, as others in similar research areas (ANSDELL & DENORA 2012; DENORA 2013; KLAUSNER 2015; BISTER *et al.* 2016) that, for mentally afflicted people, illness and wellbeing are entangled with "things outside individuals" (DENORA 2013: 9) – embedded in human, nonhuman and cultural ecologies of being.

With these conclusions, I do not argue against biomedical psychiatry as such, but suggest a re-focusing of ethnographic research and practice within in-patient psychiatric care towards affective, sensory and intersubjective aspects of healing. The sidelining of the sensory, embodied and atmospheric dimensions in public psychiatric services is not merely a matter of aesthetics. It is one of the multifaceted factors that can make a huge difference for psychiatric sufferers during times of affliction. Atmospheric entanglements might be decisive points which determine, whether a psychiatric sufferer feels genuinely cared for or caught in violent, mute social interaction. Extending Csordas' claim that the body is the ground of human culture, I argue that we must situate experience within the politics of atmospheres in order to more fully understand the intricacies of in-patient psychiatric care.

Acknowledgments

This work is part of the SNSF funded project Coercive Space-Time-Regimes: Comparing Configurations of Care and Constraint in Different Institutions (project number 192697). Warm thanks to the project members for their support, to the interlocutors in the field and all members of the "group-analytic supervision group for ethnographic fieldwork", led by J. Bonz.

Notes

1 In Switzerland, there is a basic healthcare insurance model, which is mandatory for everybody and entitles for access to "public" healthcare services. Only those who pay a higher monthly insurance fee, have access to the benefits that come with "private" health services within clinics.
2 Emic notions of "work on the self" and narratives of stasis and "being stuck" invite for further reflection within Foucault's framework of "technologies of the self" (Foucault 1988b).
3 Conversation about a recent survey with the head of the Swiss association of Relatives of people with psychological disorders (www.vask.ch) in March 2023.
4 This and the following vignettes date back to ethnographic fieldwork conducted in 2022, including various follow-up interviews. They are paraphrased and translated from German into English by the author. All names have been changed.
5 Rochelle Burgess. The gifts that context give: Reflections on ethnographic encounters in Global Mental Health. Plenary Lecture, ASA-Conference 2023, SOAS London. April 12, 2023.

References

Ansdell, Gary & DeNora, Tia 2012. Musical Flourishing: Community Music Therapy, Controversy, and the Cultivation of Wellbeing. In MacDonald, Raymond; Kreutz, Gunter & Mitchell, Laura (eds) *Music, Health, and Wellbeing*. Oxford: Oxford University Press: 98–112.
Bister, Milena; Klausner, Martina & Niewöhner, Jörg 2016. The Cosmopolitics of 'Niching': Rendering the City Habitable along Infrastructures of Mental Health Care. In Anders Blok & Ignacio Farías (eds) *Urban Cosmopolitics: Agencements, Assemblies, Atmospheres*. London; New York: Routledge, Taylor & Francis Group: 187–206.
Bruun, Mikkel Kenni & Hutten, Rebecca (eds) forthcoming. *Towards an Anthropology of Psychology. Ethnographies of Mental Health and Psychotherapy*. Oxford: Berghahn Books.
Csordas, Thomas J 1990. Embodiment as a Paradigm for Anthropology. *Ethos* 6, 2: 5–47.
---- 1993. Somatic Modes of Attention. *Cultural Anthropology* 8, 2: 135–156.
DeNora, Tia 2013. *Music Asylums: Wellbeing through Music in Everyday Life*. Burlington, VT: Ashgate.
Di Nicola, Vincenzo & Stoyanov, Drozdstoj 2021. *Psychiatry in Crisis: At the Crossroads of Social Sciences, the Humanities, and Neuroscience*. Cham, Switzerland: Springer.
Disney, Tom & Anna Schliehe 2019. Troubling Institutions. *Area* 51, 2: 194–199.
Duque, Melisa; Annemans, Margo; Pink, Sarah & Spong, Lisa 2021. Everyday Comforting Practices in Psychiatric Hospital Environments: A Design Anthropology Approach. *Journal of Psychiatric and Mental Health Nursing* 28, 4: 644–655.
Foucault, Michel 1977. *Discipline and Punish*. 2nd ed. New York: Pantheon Books.
---- 1988a. *Madness and Civilization. A History of Insanity in the Age of Reason*. Translated by Richard Howard. New York: Vintage Books.
---- 1988b. *Technologies of the Self. A Seminar with Michel Foucault*. Edited by Martin, Luther H.; Gutman, Huck & H. Hutton, Patrick. London: Tavistock Publications.
---- 2003. *The Birth of the Clinic an Archaeology of Medical Perception*. Translated by Alan Sheridan. London; New York: Routledge.
Garcia, Angela 2010. *The Pastoral Clinic: Addiction and Dispossession along the Rio Grande*. Berkeley: University of California Press.
Goffman, Erving 1961. *Asylums: Essays on the Social Situation of Mental Patients and Other Inmates*. Garden City, N.Y.: Anchor Books.
---- 1963. *Stigma: Notes on the Management of Spoiled Identity*. Englewood Cliffs: Prentice-Hall.
Good, Byron 1993. *Medicine, Rationality and Experience. An Anthropological Perspective*. Cambridge: Cambridge University Press.
---- 2012. Theorizing the 'Subject' of Medical and Psychiatric Anthropology. *The Journal of the Royal Anthropological Institute* 18, 3: 515–535.
Griffero, Tonino 2014. *Atmospheres: Aesthetics of Emotional Spaces*. Farnham Surrey, England; Burlington, VT: Ashgate Publications.
Heyken, Edda; von Poser, Anita; Hahn, Eric; Nguyen, Thi Mai Huong; Lanca, Jörg-Christian & Ta, Thi Minh Tam 2019. Researching Affects in the Clinic and beyond: Multi-Perspectivity, Ethnography, and Mental Health-Care Intervention. In Kahl, Antje (ed) *Analyzing Affective Societies. Methods and Methodologies*. London: Routledge: 249–264.
Hogan, Susan, & Pink, Sarah 2010. Routes to Interiorities: Art Therapy and Knowing in Anthropology. *Visual Anthropology* 23, 2: 158–174.
Ihde, Don & Malafouris, Lambros 2019. Homo Faber Revisited: Postphenomenology and Material Engagement Theory. *Philosophy & Technology* 32, 2: 195–214.
Ingold, Tim 2002. *The Perception of the Environment: Essays on Livelihood, Dwelling and Skill*. London and New York: Routledge.
---- 2011. *Being Alive: Essays on Movement, Knowledge and Description*. London; New York: Routledge.
Irving, Andrew 2005. Life Made Strange: An Essay on the Re-Inhabitation of Bodies and Landscapes. In James, Wendy & Mills, David (eds) *The Qualities of Time. Anthropological Approaches*. London: Routledge: 317–333.
---- 2011. Strange Distance: Towards an Anthropology of Interior Dialogue. *Medical Anthropology Quarterly* 25, 1: 22–44.

Jackson, Michael 2013. *Lifeworlds: Essays in Existential Anthropology.* Chicago: The University of Chicago Press.

Jenkins, Janis 2011. *Pharmaceutical Self: The Global Shaping of Experience in an Age of Psychopharmacology.* Santa Fe, N.M.: School for Advanced Research Press.

---- 2015. *Extraordinary Conditions. Culture and Experience in Mental Illness.* Oakland, California: University of California Press.

---- 2018. Chapter: Anthropology and Psychiatry. In Bhugra, Dinesh & Bhui, Kamaldeep (eds) *Textbook of Cultural Psychiatry.* Cambridge: Cambridge University Press: 18–34.

Kavedžija, Iza 2021. *The Process of Wellbeing: Conviviality, Care, Creativity.* Cambridge: Cambridge University Press.

Khan, Nichola 2017. *Mental Disorder. Anthropological Insights.* Toronto: University of Toronto Press.

Klausner, Martina 2015. *Choreografien psychiatrischer Praxis: Eine ethnografische Studie zum Alltag in der Psychiatrie.* Bielefeld: Transcript.

Kleinman, Arthur 2012. Rebalancing Academic Psychiatry: Why It Needs to Happen - and Soon. *British Journal of Psychiatry* 201, 6: 421–422.

Kleinman, Arthur & Kleinman, Joan 1991. Suffering and Its Professional Transformation: Toward an Ethnography of Interpersonal Experience. *Culture, Medicine and Psychiatry* 15, 3: 275–301.

Kohrt, Brandon A. & Mendenhall, Emily (eds) 2015. *Global Mental Health: Anthropological Perspectives.* Vol. 27. Walnut Creek, CA: Left Coast Press.

Lester, Rebecca J 2007. Critical Therapeutics: Cultural Politics and Clinical Reality in Two Eating Disorder Treatment Centers. *Medical Anthropology Quarterly* 21, 4: 369–387.

Littlewood, Roland (ed) 2000. *Cultural Psychiatry and Medical Anthropology: An Introduction and Reader.* London: The Athlone Press.

López-Deflory, Camelia; Perron, Amélie & Miró-Bonet, Margalida 2023. Social Acceleration, Alienation, and Resonance: Hartmut Rosa's Writings Applied to Nursing. *Nursing Inquiry* 30, 2: e12528.

Luhrmann, T. M. 2000. *Of Two Minds: The Growing Disorder in American Psychiatry.* New York: A. A. Knopf.

Mattingly, Cheryl 1998. *Healing Dramas and Clinical Plots: The Narrative Structure of Experience.* West Nyack: Cambridge University Press.

Mewes, Julie Sascia 2019. *Alltagswerkstatt: Alltagsbefähigungspraktiken in der psychiatrischen Ergotherapie.* Bielefeld: Transcript.

Navaro-Yashin, Yael 2009. Affective Spaces, Melancholic Objects: Ruination and the Production of Anthropological Knowledge. *Journal of the Royal Anthropological Institute* 15, 1: 1–18.

Peters, Mathijs & Majid, Bareez 2022. *Exploring Hartmut Rosa's Concept of Resonance.* Cham: Springer International Publishing.

Pink, Sarah 2009. *Doing Sensory Ethnography.* London: Sage Publications.

----; Hogan, Susan & Bird, Jamie 2011. Intersections and Inroads: Art Therapy's Contribution to Visual Methods. *International Journal of Art Therapy* 16, 1: 14–19.

---- & Mackley, Kerstin Leder 2014. Re-Enactment Methodologies for Everyday Life Research: Art Therapy Insights for Video Ethnography. *Visual Studies* 29, 2: 146–154.

Rosa, Hartmut 2016. *Resonanz. Eine Soziologie Der Weltbeziehung* (eBook). Berlin: Suhrkamp.

---- 2020. Beethoven, the Sailor, the Boy and the Nazi. A Reply to My Critics. *Journal of Political Power* 13, 3: 397–414.

---- & Trejo-Mathys, Jonathan 2013. *Social Acceleration: A New Theory of Modernity.* New York: Columbia University Press.

Rose, Nikolas 1979. The Psychology Complex: Mental Measurement and Social Administration. *Ideology and Consciousness* 5: 5–68.

---- Rose, Nikolas 2009. *The Politics of Life Itself: Biomedicine, Power, and Subjectivity in the Twenty-First Century.* Princeton: Princeton University Press: 87–223.

---- 2019. *Our Psychiatric Future: The Politics of Mental Health.* Cambridge, UK: Polity Press.

Schmid, Christine 2020. *Ver-rückte Expertisen: Ethnografische Perspektiven auf Genesungsbegleitung.* Bielefeld: Transcript.

Smith, Dorothy E. 2005. *Institutional Ethnography a Sociology for People.* Walnut Creek, CA: AltaMira Press.

Sumartojo, Shanti & Pink, Sarah 2019. *Atmospheres and the Experiential World.* New York: Routledge.

Tronto, Joann 2015. *Who Cares? How to Reshape a Democratic Politics.* Ithaca: Cornell University Press.

Varma, Saiba 2020. *The Occupied Clinic: Militarism and Care in Kashmir.* Durham: Duke University Press.

White, Ross G.; Jain, Summet; Orr, David M.R. & M. Read, Ursula (eds) 2017. *The Palgrave Handbook of Sociocultural Perspectives on Global Mental Health.* London: Palgrave Macmillan.

Winz, Marc & Söderström, Ola 2021. How Environments Get to the Skin: Biosensory Ethnography as a Method for Investigating the Relation between Psychosis and the City. *BioSocieties* 16, 2: 157–17.

This article has been subjected to a double blind peer review process prior to publication.

Anna Hänni, M.A., is a PhD student in social anthropology at the University of Bern. She works at the intersection between medical anthropology, other-than-human ethnography and the senses. Currently, she is a member of the SNSF funded project *Coercive Space-Time-Regimes: Comparing Configurations of Care and Constraint in Different Institutions* (project number 192697), where she explores aesthetics and therapeutic multiplicity in in-patient psychiatric care in Switzerland. Thereby, she focuses on the sensory and embodied dimensions of medical and non-medical caring encounters. She explores feminist and reflexive methods in ethnography and the intersection between the anthropology of religion and medicine.

University of Bern
Institute of Social Anthropology
Lerchenweg 36
3012 Bern, Switzerland
e-mail: annemarie.haenni2@unibe.ch

Patient-Physician-Relationship in Cancer Care
Relevance and Ambivalences as Perceived by Oncologists

NICOLE ERNSTMANN, SOPHIE ELISABETH GROSS, UTE KARBACH, LENA ANSMANN,
ANDRÉ KARGER, HOLGER PFAFF, MARKUS WIRTZ, WALTER BAUMANN & MELANIE NEUMANN

Abstract A major function of patient-physician-communication is building a trustful relationship and a therapeutic alliance between patient and physician. However, building trustful relationships to patients is subject to ambivalences. There are role expectations including affective neutrality, that stand in contrast to this function. Moreover, translation into every day routine is constricted by lack of time or lack of tools, and building a trustful relationship with the patient is a personal challenge. This qualitative study based on semi-structured interviews with oncologists was conducted to explore oncologists' perceptions and experiences of the relevance of trusting relationships to their patients and to examine sources of ambivalences. The results show that a trusting patient-physician-relationship is for oncologists an important prerequisite for successful cancer treatment in terms of open communication, adjustment of treatment to patients' needs, compliance, control of adverse events, activation of patient's resources, patients' treatment confidence, reduction of patients' anxiety, meeting family and caregiver needs and patients' coping efforts. Supporting critically ill patients can be both enriching and stressful. Being rejected by patients in case the therapy does not work was experienced as painful by some oncologists. There is a need for support for oncologists to establish trustful patient-physician-relationships during their patients' cancer journey. The support will have to address contextual factors, communication skills and the attitude needed to face the personal challenge of building trustful patient-physician-relationships. It should provide a protective environment to reflect on one's own fears and challenges in building relationships with patients.

Keywords trust – relationship – therapeutic alliance – oncology – ambivalences

Background

The relationship between patient and physician is at the heart of medicine. A major function of patient-physician-communication is building a trustful relationship and therapeutic alliance between patient and physician (HAES & BENSING 2009: 287–294). Following WEBER (1921), social behavior includes meaningful behavior of actors that is mutually related. A social relationship is built by social behavior of actors with the actor expecting a certain attitude of his counterpart and orientating his action towards this expectation (WEBER 1921). The patient-physician-relationship is a particular form of social relationship. It is characterized by a fundamental asymmetry in terms of expert authority, defining authority, and management authority: The physician knows symptoms, diagnosis, prognosis, and treatment plans – the patient is the layperson. The physician has the power to define, diagnose, classify, differentiate between healthy and ill, or decide about sick-leave. And the physician determines care structures and processes, appointments and diagnostic procedures, and treatment recommendations (SIEGRIST 2005). Moreover, the patient-physician-relationship is characterized by involuntariness in most encounters which is especially true for the physician perspective (BEGENAU, SCHUBERT & VOGT 2010: 7–33).

A conceptual model to reduce this asymmetry and its consequences is patient-centred care. In oncology, where patients experience physical burden, emotional distress, anxiety, depression, or decisional uncertainty during the cancer journey, patient-centred care is of particular importance. Patient-centred care has been defined as "respectful of and responsive to individual patient preferences, needs, and values and ensuring that patient values guide all clinical decisions" (COMMITTEE ON QUALITY OF HEALTH CARE IN AMERICA, INSTITUTE OF MEDICINE 2001). Patient-centred care respects the patient as a unique person, emphasizes communication and information, involves and empowers the patient, promotes a partnership between patient and provider, and gives emotional support (ZILL, SCHOLL, HÄRTER & DIRMAIER 2015). According to the integrative model of patient-centeredness (SCHOLL, ZILL, HÄRTER & DIRMAIER 2014) a central principle of patient-centeredness is a patient-physician-relationship characterized by trust and caring. Such a relationship then allows central activities of patient-centred care, i.e. patient information, patient involvement in care, involvement of family and friends, patient empowerment, and emotional support (SCHOLL, ZILL, HÄRTER & DIRMAIER 2014). Following SCHOLL, ZILL, HÄRTER & DIRMAIER (2014) enabling factors for patient-centred care are communication skills, the integration of medical and non-medical care, access to care, continuity of care, teamwork and teambuilding.

Ambivalences

The physicians' decision and the process of building and maintaining trustful relationships with cancer patients (HILLEN, DE HAES & SMETS 2011: 227-41) is subject to ambivalences. At least three sources of ambivalences can be assumed: First, there are specific role expectations the society has towards the physician. The physician's role includes technical competence, universalism, affective neutrality, functional specificity, and collectivity-orientation (PARSONS 1951). Being affectively neutral implies that the physician treats patients equally and does not become emotionally aroused during professional activities. Second, the translation into every day routine is constricted by obstacles such as lack of time to explain complex information, lack of tools to facilitate treatment planning, or insensitivity to patients' needs (BALOGH, GANZ, MURPHY, NASS, FERRELL & STOVALL 2011: 1800-1805). Prior research within the WIN ON study based on the interview data revealed that a stressed oncologist has difficulties in showing empathy and patient-centredness (GROSS, ERNSTMANN, JUNG, KARBACH, ANSMANN, GLOEDE, PFAFF, WIRTZ, BAUMANN, SCHMITZ, OSBURG & NEUMANN 2014: 594-606). Third, building a partnership with the patient in oncology is a personal challenge (MAGUIRE 1985: 1711-1713, 1999: 2058-2065). It has been shown that oncologists find patient loss particularly difficult for relational reasons, e.g. in instances where they feel close to patients and their families, when they have long-term patients, and when deaths are unexpected (GRANEK, KRZYZANOWSKA, TOZER & MAZZOTTA 2012a: 1254-1260; GRANEK, MAZZOTTA, TOZER & KRZYZANOWSKA 2012b: 2627-2632; SHANAFELT, ADJEI & MEYSKENS 2003: 2616-2619). Oncologists find sharing a bad prognosis, especially when they care deeply for their patients, to be stressful (ABERNETHY, CAMPBELL & PENTZ 2019: 1163-1165). These findings might explain that oncologists' professional strategies to cope with patients' death include focusing on work, withdrawing from patients at end of life, and compartmentalization, i.e. drawing boundaries between home and work life (GRANEK, ARIAD, SHAPIRA, BAR-SELA & BEN-DAVID 2016: 4219-4227).

Theory and empirical evidence

Why should oncologists bear this personal and professional challenge of building a trustful relationship with their patients? Is there a goal that helps overcoming the ambivalences? Is there evidence that communicating well with patients makes any difference to health outcomes? The "effect model of empathic communication in the clinical encounter" (NEUMANN, WIRTZ, BOLLSCHWEILER, MERCER, WARM, WOLF & PFAFF 2007: 63-75) explains how empathy can lead to improved patient outcomes. As consolidation and extension of former models, this model describes an affective pathway of empathic communication leading to patients' emotion of feeling understood (SQUIER 1990: 325-339; SUCHMAN, MARKAKIS, BECKMAN & FRANKEL 1997: 678-682), and a cognitive pathway of empathic communication (SQUIER 1990: 325-339). The cognitive pathway postulates that patients, when experiencing physician's empathy, are supposed to tell more about their symptoms and concerns, facilitating the physician to collect more detailed medical and psychosocial information. This in turn leads to a diagnosis that is more accurate and helps the physician to understand and respond to the individual needs of the patients which may result in a better communication with regard to its informative, participative, and educative components (NEUMANN, WIRTZ, BOLLSCHWEILER, MERCER, WARM, WOLF & PFAFF 2007: 63–75) and to stronger adherence to treatment regimens and preventative strategies (SQUIER 1990: 325–339). Thus, patients may experience improved long-term health outcomes.

When looking at empirical evidence, many studies have revealed associations between a caring and educating communication, trust in physician, control of treatment and side effects, patients' satisfaction, perceived quality of care, reduced hopelessness, distress, and health outcomes (COULEHAN, PLATT, EGENER, FRANKEL, LIN, LOWN & SALAZAR 2001: 221–227; ERNSTMANN, WEISSBACH, HERDEN, WINTER & ANSMANN 2016: 396–405; ERNSTMANN, HERDEN, WEISSBACH, KARGER, HOWER & ANSMANN 2019: 2114–2121; FARIN & NAGL 2013: 283–294; FRANCO, JOSEPH, FEI & BICKELL 2009; HINNEN, POOL, HOLWERDA, SPRANGERS, SANDERMAN & HAGEDOORN 2014; LIN, CHAO, BICKELL & WISNIVESKY 2016: 976–989; MALY, LIU, LIANG & GANZ 2015: 916–926; ROBINSON, HOOVER, VENETIS, KEARNEY & STREET 2013: 351–358; SQUIER 1990: 325–339; STEWART 1995: 1423–1433). However, so far little is known as to how oncologists judge the importance of a trusting patient-physician-relationship. Do they believe that the partnership with their patients has the potential to impact health outcomes in a discipline dominated by seriously, chronically or terminally ill patients and invasive therapies such as surgical treatment, chemotherapy and radiation? Do they perceive conflicting aims, role conflicts or ambivalences in establishing trustful patient-physician-relationships? So far, there is one qualitative study addressing parts of the issues raised, showing that oncologists have a limited understanding of the value, implications, and motivation for improving patient-centred care in general (NGUYEN, BAUMAN, WATLING & HAHN 2017: 213–219).

Aims and methods

The present qualitative study was conducted 1) to improve our knowledge of oncologists' perceptions and experiences of the relevance of a trusting relationship between cancer patients and physicians for treatment process and patients' outcomes and 2) to examine sources of ambivalences in establishing a trustful patient-physician-relationship in cancer care.

The following analysis is part of the WIN ON study (Working conditions in oncology) (DFG Grant #: PF 407/4-1, WI 3210/5-1). WIN ON is an interdisciplinary prospective multicenter study examining the effects of working conditions of private practice oncologists on patient-physician-communication and patient reported outcomes. The ethics review committee of the University hospital of Cologne approved the research protocol. All participating physicians gave written informed consent to be interviewed or surveyed for the study.

The qualitative study part included semi-structured interviews with 11 oncologists (7 male, 4 female; 42–59 years of age; 1–18 years in private practice) selected by purposeful sampling according to sex, size and type of private practice and years in private practice. The interviews were conducted by two trained interviewers. The oncologists were recruited as members of the Professional Association of Office-based Hematologists and Oncologists in Germany (BNHO) via mailing. The interviews took place in oncologists' offices and had a mean duration of 60 minutes. The semi-structured questionnaire covered aspects of work organization, working conditions and patient-physician-communication in oncology practices. The interviews were audiotaped and transcribed according to transcription guidelines (FUSS & KARBACH 2014). The authors analyzed the interviews by combining inductive and deductive coding and categorization techniques of content analysis for research aim 1 (MAYRING 2010: 601–613): Deductive coding was based on the interview guiding questions as a priori codes. Inductive coding has expanded the coding tree by adding new aspects and allowing to reduce the material to new categories. For research aim 2 both content analysis and contrasting thematic coding techniques (FLICK 2010) were used. The sources of ambivalence were deductively coded based on the a priori assumptions. Contrasting the codes then helped to gain a deeper understanding of the positive and negative elements of each source of ambivalence.

Results

1) Relevance of the patient-physician-relationship in cancer care

General meaning and quality of the patient-physician relationship
The interviewed oncologists unanimously felt that the patient-physician relationship is of great significance in oncology. Feeling comfortable in the practice and having trust in the physician and the physician's therapeutic decisions were seen as an important basis and a main prerequisite for such a therapeutic alliance. Trust was considered fundamental to the patient-physician relationship – if there is distrust between the physician and the patient, the relationship is fundamentally destroyed. While a loss of trust can lead a patient to change the physician, the oncologists also believed that it is possible to regain that trust during treatment through conversations with the patient and therapeutic successes. All of the oncologists talked about trust in one direction only – the trust of the patient in the treating oncologist. Patients' trust in oncologists and their treatment is the goal of oncologists. The impact that physicians' trust in their patients has in the course of treatment was not mentioned during the interviews.

The first consultation with a physician was primarily seen as the cornerstone for a trusting patient-physician relationship since it determines whether the patient can develop trust in the physician. According to the majority of the oncologists, it is of vital importance that physicians take time to build such trust in their patients, provide them with sufficient information and plan therapy together with them. Several of the oncologists felt that the patient-physician relationship is particularly important in oncology. Unlike in other medical specialties, in oncology patients find themselves at "crossroads in their lives," a time when they are faced with existential questions and decisions. Trust is regarded as essential for getting patients to accept therapy suggestions and put themselves in the hands of their oncologists. It is therefore not seen as something voluntary since the patients have no other choice.

IP: Um, because I think that you do have to have trust in order to let yourself be treated the way patients here let themselves be treated. I think that in this case though, the patients are often at a, uh, crossroads in their lives—mm, not like with therapy for blood pressure or blood sugar—but a situation where they have to go into it with even more trust and, uh, also just have to have trust in the ones doing it and somehow tell themselves, 'these are the right ones for me right now.' They're making the right decisions for me or the right decisions with me.

In addition to the patient-physician relationship, some physicians emphasized the importance of the interprofessional practice team. These physicians placed less value on the personal relationship with the oncologist and more value on the overall atmosphere in the practice, which they defined as the sum of the personal relationships with the reception staff, nursing staff and oncologists. Conversations between a patient and the practice staff after the patient's first consultation with the physician, for example, could make up for the consultation not going well and instill trust in the patient.

I: In your opinion, how important really is the personal relationship between you and your patients for the success of treatment [...]?

IP: Very, very important. Although, um, I wouldn't necessarily say the personal relationship with just ME, but the relationship with WHOMEVER the patient encounters. (I: mm-hmm) That includes me, the receptionists, and the nurses. (I: okay) I think it's extremely important.

However, not all of the oncologists found the atmosphere in a practice to be of key importance. One oncologist made a clear distinction between the importance of the personal conversation between a patient and a physician and the influence of the practice team. To him, it is the patient-physician conversation that determines whether the patient will develop trust in the physician. If the conversation goes well, even a rather poor practice atmosphere can be tolerated. This oncologist also considered practice facilities and decor to be of secondary importance.

IP: Even unfriendly nurses in the reception area, diagnostic shortcomings, etc. can all be put up with if the, if it works, if the conversation goes well. [...] So, that's the only way, it's only through the conversation that trust can be gained (I: mm-hmm), that it can develop. Other things then, like the way things look here, whether we still have old wallpaper or whether the rose bush, uh, the bouquet of roses has wilted, aren't important, you know? (I: mm-hmm) It's the: conversation that is the most important.

Most of the oncologists described their relationship with their patients as being a close and stable relationship, which some of the oncologists believe can definitely come to take on a friendship-like nature. When caring for their patients, they often take the patients' environment into consideration. For some oncologists, providing patients with care and support beyond the actual treatment of cancer (sometimes over many years) can and should result in the development of a new form of bond where the boundaries between a professional and personal relationship become blurred.

Effects on patient-physician communication
Having trust in their oncologists encourages patients to ask critical questions about therapy and to express their needs and how they see things. According to some of the oncologists interviewed, a personal relationship must be present in order for the patient to feel confident enough to point out errors or to ask questions about anything that is unclear. Only then the patient can serve as a "second set of eyes" during care. The personal relationship between a patient and a physician is therefore considered a resource which helps to better adjust therapy to the individual patient.

IP: [...] The patient should have the feeling [...], mm, should be able to say, uh, something like 'Doctor is it possible something's been forgotten?' So, I need the patient as a second set of eyes [uh-huh okay] and he has to have the feeling that that's also, uh, what I would like from him.

IP: But, the question is whether I always ask: 'So, how are you doing?' and 'Are you doing okay?' [mm-hmm] or 'Do you have a fever?' mm, or [I: okay] so I can then see if all complications are now out of the way and I can now administer chemo. [I: mm-hmm yeah] That's why it's also good to, um, to get to know the patient personally. He knows he can tell me and, uh, I'll look into it, which is also good for me because then I can take care of it.

If, however, the relationship between a patient and an oncologist is a poor one, there is a great risk that messages will go unnoticed or will be misunderstood.

IP: WHEN THE PERSONAL RELATIONSHIP (.) IS POOR—it's possible, [I: mm-hmm] for a physician and patient not to be a good fit at all—um, I think that that threatens the success of treatment [uh-huh] because then, mm, messages don't get through: or go unnoticed.

Effects on compliance and long-term treatment
Some of the interviewed oncologists stressed how important a stable and personal patient-physician relationship is for the long-term treatment and follow-up care of their patients. Having a close relationship with their patients leads the patients to go in for regular check-ups, which make it possible to provide them with optimum care and support. One perceived benefit of a close relationship with the oncologist is that it can also lead the oncologist to take the role of the primary care physician in providing follow-up care or to supplement the follow-up care provided by the primary care physician with specialist care. This was considered particularly beneficial since an oncologist may be more likely than a primary care practitioner to recognize cancer-specific symptoms indicating relapse or deterioration in a patient's condition and can take countermeasures.

I: [...] if the relationship is a good one [yes] yes.

IP: Then they come here. The thing is that these special diseases aren't monitored as well by primary care physicians. [I: okay, mm-hmm] In other words, when these patients have a problem, I think that we detect it a bit earlier than primary care physicians do (.) yeah. [okay] Although we always discuss it with the primary care physicians first to see whether they want to send the patients to us [I: mm-hmm] when they're in a chronic stage.

A close patient-physician relationship was also seen as beneficial for patient compliance with acute therapy. If the patient tells the physician about side effects and symptoms they are experiencing as a result of chemotherapy, the physician can then better adjust the therapy based on the side effects experienced by the individual patient. Moreover, when there is a close relationship, the physician can somewhat explain these side effects and motivate their patients to continue with therapy despite the side effects by getting them to focus on relief or healing. This then results in better compliance, which also increases the chances that therapy will be more successful.

> IP: [...] if, um, we spot side effects early enough, counteract them and EXPLAIN WHY, why they should stick with it [I: uh-huh], why it's worth it to take this or that measure to counteract the side effects, then there is MUCH better compliance, MUCH better adherence and, OF COURSE, greater therapy success.

Effects on coping with the disease

A personal patient-physician relationship is considered to have numerous positive effects on the ability to cope with disease. Although the oncologists interviewed did not explicitly talk about the coping of cancer patients, it seems to be a latent construct which can be found in their statements and the positive experiences they have had in their practices. One example of coping found in the oncologists' statements is the activation of personal resources. A personal patient-physician relationship can help patients get back the strength they need to reestablish social contacts or to start doing things with renewed interest. Another example of coping can be found in a discussion of patient fears. As one oncologist expressed, he hopes that a personal relationship will also help alleviate fears that may be crippling and inhibiting patients. His statement primarily refers to patients with chronic diseases and includes the hope that the patients will be empowered to make the most of the time they have left.

> I: And, um, what effect do you think your relationship with the patient has [...]?

> IP: Well, what I hope is that he will get something out of the time we dedicate to him during therapy [mm-hmm], that he'll stop sitting there like a deer caught in the headlights and say, 'Okay, I have a bit of time now and a bit of strength. I'm either going to go, um, visit relatives or go to the opera' [...], that he'll keep living.

Once a personal and trusting relationship between the patient and physician has been established, it is then possible to discuss issues involving death and grief in the family. According to some of the oncologists, they can come to serve as a mediator between patients and their family members or as an adviser. The relationship also allows physicians to approach family members about existential issues. A long-term relationship can lead the oncologist to be consulted on private or spiritual matters as well. Such a stable relationship can also help with the acceptance of death and coming to terms with having lost the battle against cancer. Although a close relationship cannot be formed with every patient, if it is, some of the oncologists believe that it can lead to a blurring of professional and role boundaries.

> IP: [...] after a certain amount of time of trusting, they actually start asking questions that they feel moved to ask. They just let them out and that's what makes the difference, so to say. All of a sudden, they actually become their own life coaches [I: uh-huh] and I would say that we physicians are sometimes something like modern-day priests.

Effects on patient-reported outcomes

In terms of the effects a close patient-physician relationship has on the success of treatment, the oncologists credited the relationship as having a positive impact on patient satisfaction, well-being and quality of life. Interestingly, however, several of them made a distinction between treatment success and psychological (or subjective) outcomes. Whereas the concept of quality of life, for example, was considered to be limited to patients' psychological state, the construct of treatment success tended to be associated with physical parameters, especially survival time. These oncologists tended to deny that there is a connection between the patient-physician relationship and treatment success.

> I: In your opinion, how important really is the personal relationship between you and your patients for the success of treatment?

IP: For TREATMENT SUCCESS, mm, I don't think it's that: important. [I: uh-huh] For patient SATISFACTION [I: uh-huh] for their QUALITY OF LIFE, it's EXTREMELY important.

Some of the other oncologists, however, did consider a personal patient-physician relationship to affect the physical outcome of oncological treatment by helping patients handle the side effects to improve the course and result of treatment.

IP: Whether the tumor becomes five centimeters bigger or smaller in response to the chemotherapy probably can't be influenced by the conversation. But, uh, as far as how the patient feels, it's very important; it's also very important for how he gets through the many side effects of the therapy.

IP: [...] it has a SUBSTANTIAL impact, mm, on how patients handle the side effects [I: uh-huh]. THAT'S a big thing and then considering, mm, if you consider that as part of the outcome, uh [I: mm-hmm], the outcome of treatment, then, of course, it is of GREAT importance.

The significance of patients' motivation to continue with therapy was also mentioned during the interviews, with a connection being drawn between the motivation of the physician and the practice team on one side and the motivation of the patients on the other. If the physician and practice team demonstrate a high motivation to treat the patient, this motivation can then impact the patient's own confidence and motivation, making it possible to continue with therapy longer. In a best-case scenario, this can then have an impact on the individual survival rates of patients.

IP: [...] despite the fact that they have a chronic disease, how long patients with metastasized cancer live how long they SURVIVE depends greatly on how much motivation WE have [I: mm-hmm] and how much we are also able to communicate to patients [I: mm-hmm] that life keeps on going [I: mm-hmm], a bit more, and a bit more despite their disease and that has an impact on patient survival times.

2.) Sources of ambivalences

Ambivalences in building partnerships with their patients are not being reflected upon by most of the oncologists though possible sources of ambivalences are often mentioned. Organizational factors, e.g. working hours, time pressure, documentation or interruptions, were seen as obstacles for a patient-centred communication; however, oncologists did not attribute these factors to the quality of their patient-physician-relationships. They admitted disturbing effects of organizational factors on the quality of the encounters though the quality of the patient-physician-relationship was not associated with these factors.

The thematic coding revealed that for those oncologists who integrate death and dying into their daily practice, the patient-physician-relationship is a central aspect of their values and routines and might even get closer in the last period of patients' lives.

IP: [...] We have a glass with petals, [...] when one of our patients dies, um, a yellow rose is dried. [...] Of course, there are already many who have been cared for very intensively over the years and often with several contacts a week at the end. Um, that is not just demanding [...] You get a lot back. So many patients give you the feeling, 'It was good what you did.' It's nice.

The same oncologist states later:

IP: There is this way downhill. And yet there is a good relationship and a relationship in which, wherever I notice it, they rely on us to do what is possible [...], um, where there really is a basis of trust. And over a long time there often grows a personal relationship, where you just laughed a lot with each other, even in spite of difficult situations, or just some crap that you have gone through together, um, where really [..]a real relationship arises.

Another oncologist who lost her husband to cancer even shares her private experience with cancer and dying with her patients:

I: [...] How do you deal with the issues of emotional stress or dying and death if you are caring for a palliative patient?

> IP: Of course, I'm trying to talk to the patient about it. [...]. Then I sometimes say to the patients [...] 'When you get up there, tell my husband, he can get in touch with me'.

Another oncologist perceives close relationships to her patients, or "being involved", as a burden. Later in the interview when asked for the meaning of the patient-physician-relationship, she depicts the following situations, indicating that for her the quality of the relationship – or the potential of the relationship to cause inconvenience – is associated with the hope for cure.

> IP: [...] They come once a quarter or half a year and then, um, I am told half a life and what has happened in the last six months [hm] and uh they are so happy and satisfied when they are back. Even if it's just a routine check, they don't want to stop coming here. So, these are very, very strong ties [I: hm] yes. And that's the positive thing. It's not just seriously ill patients with whom we have to talk about dying now, but we also have a very large number of chronic patients [hm] who are doing well. We can care for them for many years and that is highly satisfactory [...].

> IP: [...] They [physicians in cancer centers] do everything possible and then you can no longer help him and then he is sent to the oncologist. Now he should go on [I: hmhm]. And then, these relationships are extremely difficult [I: hm okay], you don't have much that you can offer as treatment options.

Another oncologist reports similar experiences of relationships being associated with the illness trajectory. Here, patients are described as distancing from physicians when their hope for cure is not fulfilled.

> IP: [...]There are sometimes alienations. So, one starts hopefully therapies and they do NOT lead to the desired outcomes, [...] then it comes to depreciations because we can't make it, [I: mhm] also times of disappointment, unmet expectations, [I: mhm] blame, depreciations, that also happens.

Some oncologists report strategies of professional distance and intellectualization as coping mechanism in situations when they are affected by the patient's fate.

> IP: [...] This is, um, that is, this is more difficult. Breaking bad news is difficult, when there are no treatment options at all. It is one of the most difficult things.

> IP: [...] You do learn how to abstract things, how to ignore them. There are always individual, individual fates that of course affect you and touch you, but not in such a way that this, um, that this bothers you at the end of the day, no.

One oncologist describes ambivalences in terms of religious doubts and in terms of putting everything into perspective in his personal life as consequence of close relationships in late stage and end-of-life care.

> IP: [...] Working in oncology, especially in the continuous care of patients [...] until their death, of course, has a significant impact on our own lives. [I: mhm] You can't avoid thinking about the meaning of life and [...] draw your own conclusions from it. [I: mhm] So oncology and religiosity are [...] a very difficult field. [I: mhm] I know [...] that uh, uh, it is very difficult as an oncologist not to [...] develop doubts about your own religious belief. [I: mhm] Um, for me personally, that's what happened.

> IP: [...] It is a tremendous enrichment if you understand early what is important in life. Um, it is a disadvantage because sometimes you can no longer get upset in real life. [I: mhm] Yes, you can no longer get upset about your accountings [...] because it is actually not so important after all. That's a typical discrepancy yes. [I: yes] [...] I mostly experience it as positive. [...]

His positive conclusion in terms of personal and professional growth is reflected in the following quote:

> IP: [...] Establishing a relationship, [...] keeping the emotionality [I: mhm] [...], maybe that is what makes the work really interesting after so many years. If you pass the master's exam [I: mhm] and suddenly can open the gate to a completely different level.

Summary

The qualitative analysis suggests that a trusting patient-physician-relationship is an important aspect in cancer care for oncologists. Trusting the physician and the physician's therapeutic decisions is seen as an important basis for a therapeutic alliance by the oncologists. However, some oncologists acknowledge the importance of themselves as central person more than others who emphasize the importance of a team of physicians or a multiprofessional team in private practice. An impact of a trusting patient-physician-relationship on treatment success is rather associated with psychological adjustment than with clinical outcomes, e.g. morbidity or mortality. Some oncologists perceive positive effects of a trusting patient-physician-relationship on treatment outcomes following the described cognitive pathway of empathic communication. For oncologists, close relationships to their patients might be a burden as well as a satisfying aspect of their work.

Discussion

The aim of this study was to explore the oncologists' perspective on the relevance of the patient-physician-relationship and sources of ambivalences in establishing trustful patient-physician-relationships in cancer care. The interviews are rich; we were able to discuss the topic of patient-physician-relationship with all interviewees. The oncologists have different approaches to the subject of relationships, which they are aware of or became aware of during the conversation. These approaches are describable and stable for them and prove functional for their respective medical practices despite occasional ambivalences. The findings show that for oncologists, a trusting patient-physician-relationship is an important prerequisite for successful cancer treatment in terms of open communication, adjustment of treatment to patients' needs, compliance, control of adverse events, activation of patient's resources, patients' treatment confidence, reduction of patients' anxiety, meeting family and caregiver needs and patients' coping efforts. These positive effects are attributed to the oncologists themselves, to a team of oncologists, or to a multiprofessional team in private practice.

Some oncologists consider a personal patient-physician relationship to affect the treatment outcome whereas others feel doubtful about such an association. Different opinions might partly arise from divergent definitions of the concept of treatment or treatment outcome, from quality of life to physical parameters or survival. Some of the variance might result from different experiences with the effects of a partnership or due to a different willingness to build close relationships. The willingness might depend upon aspects of physicians' personality, bonding styles, communication styles, or communication skills. These associations cannot be examined in our data and could be subject to future studies. Another explanation for doubts concerning the association between partnership and treatment outcomes might be the fact that some oncologists are not aware of the cognitive pathway linking communication to treatment outcome. This would be in line with the findings of Nguyen, Bauman, Watling & Hahn (2017: 213–219), who reported a limited understanding of the value, implications, and motivation for patient-centred care in oncologists. The methodologic approach of our study does not allow to test these assumptions; the interviews might be biased by social desirability. The affective pathway of empathic communication leading to patients' emotion of feeling understood is recognized by the oncologists. However, the pathway postulating that patients are supposed to tell more about their symptoms and concerns, facilitating the physician to collect more detailed information which in turn leads to a diagnosis that is more accurate and helps the physician to respond to the individual needs of the patients, is only partially realized by the oncologists. Remarkably enough, some oncologists describe different pathways in terms of indirect effects of trust, but direct psycho-neuroimmunological effects of trust such as anxiolytic or antidepressant effects of oxytocin are not considered at all. However, the interview guideline did not include any specific follow-up questions on this topic, which might partly explain this finding.

The major impact of the health status and the course of treatment becomes evident in several respects. A deterioration of health condition or the possibility of cancer treatment not working has a significant impact, both for the trusting relationship from the patient's perspective and for the burden of a trustful therapeutic alliance for the oncologists. Suspicion and mistrust could arise, and oncologists might distance themselves for their protection. Most oncologists feel more comfortable in close relationships as long as the therapy works, as long as the "arrangement of hope" (Hermann 2005) holds.

Supporting critically ill patients can be both enriching and stressful for some respondents. The effects on one's own life are substantial and are sometimes perceived as ambivalences. Life perspectives change, even religious doubts may arise. The principle of partnership and a therapeutic alliance is perceived as both fascinating and strenuous and might lead to personal maturation. Being rejected by patients in case the therapy does not work could be a painful experience for oncologists in close relationships having to process their unfulfilled expectations as well as the frustration of their patient.

The role expectation of affective neutrality was not mentioned in the interviews; those oncologists placing more emphasis on relationship building even reported dyadic expectations of building a therapeutic alliance with the cancer as enemy both patient and physician are fighting against. Organizational aspects were not regarded as barriers for a trustful patient-physician-relationship; however, contextual factors in private practice were perceived as disturbing factors during the medical encounter. Hence, the consequences of a disturbed communication for patient-physician-relationship (GROSS, ERNSTMANN, JUNG, KARBACH, ANSMANN, GLOEDE, PFAFF, WIRTZ, BAUMANN, SCHMITZ, OSBURG & NEUMANN 2014: 594–606) are ignored or perceived as reducible by oncologists' communication skills.

Considering the integrative model of patient-centeredness (SCHOLL, ZILL, HÄRTER & DIRMAIER 2014) our results underline oncologists' recognition of a trustful and caring patient-physician-relationship as central principle of patient-centeredness. Aspects of communication, teamwork and continuity of care are mentioned in the context of patient-centred care. Whether these aspects are perceived as enabling or associated factors of patient-centeredness remains unclear. Patient information, patient involvement in care, patient empowerment in terms of supporting self-management and emotional support are seen as important activities and as closely related to trustful patient-physician-relationships. Active involvement of and support for the patient's relatives and friends tend to be less of a topic.

Limitations

There are limitations to our research that should be considered when interpreting the results. Due to the exploratory character of our study, our results should be considered indicatory. This is one of the first studies qualitatively examining the oncologists' perspective on the relevance of patient-physician-relationships. The interview sample size is small; however, maximum variation of the sampling criteria was achieved. Nevertheless, there may be self-selection bias due to the interviewees' interest in the study. The interviewees' responses regarding the relevance and ambivalences of relationships to their patients might be subject to self-consistency as well a self-serving and belief bias. Our results suggest different patterns or types of relationship preferences. We are not able to build such types based on our data collected to explore all aspects of the relevance of trustful relationships and sources of ambivalence in our sample. Type-building should be subject to future research.

Implications

Contemporary oncology practice acknowledges more and more the importance of partnering with the patient and family in dealing with the illness (BAILE & AARON 2005: 331–335). Even renewed interest in promoting compassion as desired professional attitude did arise (CAMERON, MAZER, DELUCA, MOHILE & EPSTEIN 2015: 1672–1685; GELHAUS 2012: 397–410). However, when thinking about patient-physician-relationships in oncology, differences between acute care in cancer centers and follow-up care in private practices of oncologists have to be considered. Physicians in hospitals will in most cases not have the chance to establish and maintain a close relationship to their cancer patients during a short hospital stay of a few days. In large cancer centers with multiprofessional care teams cancer patients might not even know who is their primary contact person.

However, in long term follow up care, the relationship is an important resource and central aspect of the quality of care. In private practice oncology, the oncologist is the central contact person and expert, and – following our results – might even be consulted on private or spiritual matters. This seems particularly relevant since patients are offered less psycho-oncological or psychosocial support from other sources in long-term and follow-up treatment than in cancer centers during acute care.

What kind of support do oncologists need to fulfill this important task? The support will have to address contextual factors as well as the communication skills and the attitude needed to establish trustful patient-physician-relationships. However, the keys for establishing trusting relationships, e.g. the role of authenticity, remain to be identified (STIEFEL & BOURQUIN 2019). Earlier analyses of the WIN ON survey and interview data has shown that the working conditions play a central role – emotionally exhausted oncologists might not have the personal and organizational resources to build and maintain close relationships to their patients (GROSS, ERNSTMANN, JUNG, KARBACH, ANSMANN, GLOEDE, PFAFF, WIRTZ, BAUMANN, SCHMITZ, OSBURG & NEUMANN 2014: 594–606 ; NITZSCHE, NEUMANN, GROSS, ANSMANN, PFAFF, BAUMANN, WIRTZ, SCHMITZ & ERNSTMANN 2017: 462–473). The same effect has been shown in cancer centers (ANSMANN, WIRTZ, KOWALSKI, PFAFF, VISSER & ERNSTMANN 2014: 352–360).

Existing communication skills trainings address aspects of communication such as breaking bad news and discussing unanticipated adverse events, discussing prognosis, reaching a shared treatment decision, responding to difficult emotions, coping with survivorship, running a family meeting, and transitioning to palliative care and end of life (KISSANE, BYLUND, BANERJEE, BIALER, LEVIN, MALONEY & D'AGOSTINO 2012: 1242–1247; MERCKAERT, LIBERT & RAZAVI 2005: 319–330); however, aspects of building and maintaining a trustful alliance to cancer patients over a long period are rarely addressed. Moreover, existent trainings rather address skills and techniques instead of values or reflexivity (STIEFEL & BOURQUIN 2016: 1660–1663). Private practice oncologists are often working in group practice, but are not involved in a large multiprofessional care team in their daily routine as it is standard practice in cancer centers. There might be a need to make use of Balint groups, also in private practice oncology (BAR-SELA, LULAV-GRINWALD & MITNIK 2012: 786–789), where defence mechanisms, emotional exhaustion, loss, grief, disappointment or anxiety could be addressed. Even the offer of psycho-oncological support for all medical professions who are dealing with cancer patients (TAN-RIVERDI 2013: 530) or trainings addressing death competence (DRAPER 2019: 266–274) have been recently discussed. An interprofessional discussion of support needs of oncologists working in private practice and joint efforts to develop targeted interventions addressing individual and contextual factors of individual relationship-building needs might be helpful in the future.

Acknowledgments

The study was funded by the German Research Foundation (DFG) (PF 407/4-1; WI 3210/5). The authors wish to thank the participating oncologists for their trustful collaboration. Special thanks go to Dr. Christian Schulz-Quach for his inspiring keynote lecture at the 2019 Annual Conference of the PSO (Arbeitsgemeinschaft für Psychoonkologie in der Deutschen Krebsgesellschaft) in Düsseldorf; Germany, that broadened our perspective on ambivalent relationships in oncology and palliative care.

References

ABERNETHY, ELI ROWE; CAMPBELL, GAVIN PAUL & PENTZ, REBECCA 2019. Why many oncologists fail to share accurate prognoses: They care deeply for their patients. *Cancer* 15: 1163–1165.

ANSMANN, LENA; WIRTZ, MARKUS A.; KOWALSKI, CHRISTOPH; PFAFF, HOLGER; VISSER, ADRIAAN & ERNSTMANN, NICOLE 2014. The impact of the hospital work environment on social support from physicians in breast cancer care. *Patient Education and Counseling* 96: 352–360.

BAILE, WALTER F. & AARON, JOANN 2005. Patient-physician communication in oncology: past, present, and future. *Current Opinion in Oncology* 17: 331–335.

BAR-SELA, GIL; LULAV-GRINWALD, DORON & MITNIK, INBAL 2012. "Balint group" meetings for oncology residents as a tool to improve therapeutic communication skills and reduce burnout level. *Journal of Cancer Education* 27: 786–789.

Balogh, Erin P.; Ganz, Patricia A.; Murphy, Sharon B.; Nass, Sharyl J.; Ferrell, Betty R. & E. Stovall 2011. Patient-centered cancer treatment planning: improving the quality of oncology care. Summary of an Institute of Medicine workshop. *The Oncologist* 16: 1800–1805.

Begenau, Jutta; Schubert, Cornelius & Vogd, Werner (eds) 2010. Die Arzt-Patient-Beziehung aus soziologischer Sicht. In Vogd, Werner (ed) *Die Arzt-Patient-Beziehung*. Stuttgart: Kohlhammer: 7–33.

Cameron, Rachel A.; Mazer, Benjamin L.; DeLuca, Jane M.; Mohile, Supriya G. & Epstein, Ronald M. 2015. Search of compassion: a new taxonomy of compassionate physician behaviours. *Health Expectations* 18: 1672–1685.

Coulehan, Jack L.; Platt, Frederic W.; Egener, Barry; Frankel, Richard; Lin, Cheng-Tang; Lown, Beth & Salazar, William H. 2001. "Let me see if i have this right…": words that help build empathy. *Annals of Internal Medicine* 135: 221–227.

Committee on Quality of Health Care in America, Institute of Medicine 2001. *Crossing the Quality Chasm: A New Health System for the 21st Century*. Washington, DC: The National Academies Press.

Draper, Emma J.; Hillen, Marij A.; Moors, Marleen; Ket, Johannes C. F.; van Laarhoven, Hanneke W M & Henselmans, Inge 2019. Relationship between physicians' death anxiety and medical communication and decision-making: A systematic review. *Patient Education and Counseling* 102: 266–274.

Ernstmann, Nicole; Herden, Jan; Weissbach, Lothar; Karger, André; Hower, Kira & Ansmann, Lena 2019. Prostate-specific health-related quality of life and patient-physician communication. A 3.5-year follow-up. *Patient Education and Counseling* 102: 2114–2121.

Ernstmann, Nicole; Weissbach, Lothar; Herden, Jan; Winter, Nicola & Ansmann, Lena 2016. Patient-physician communication and health-related quality of life of patients with localised prostate cancer undergoing radical prostatectomy. A longitudinal multilevel analysis. *BJU International* 119: 396–405.

Farin, Erik & Nagl, Michaela 2013. The patient-physician relationship in patients with breast cancer: influence on changes in quality of life after rehabilitation. *Quality of Life Research* 22: 283–294.

Flick, Uwe 2010. *An introduction to qualitative research (4. ed.)*. Los Angeles, California: SAGE.

Franco, Rebeca; Joseph, Kathie-Ann; Fei, Kezhen & Bickell, Nina A. 2009. Breast cancer patients' perceived quality of care: The importance of trust and communication. *Journal of Clinical Oncology* 27: 15_suppl, 6554–6554.

Fuss, Susanne & Karbach, Ute 2014. *Grundlagen der Transkription. Eine praktische Einführung*. Opladen: Budrich.

Gelhaus, Petra 2012. The desired moral attitude of the physician: (II) compassion. *Medicine, Health Care, and Philosophy* 15: 397–410.

Granek, Leeat; Ariad, Samuel; Shapira, Shahar; Bar-Sela, Gil & Ben-David, Merav 2016. Barriers and facilitators in coping with patient death in clinical oncology. *Supportive Care in Cancer* 24: 4219–4227.

Granek, Leeat; Krzyzanowska, Monika K.; Tozer, Richard & Mazzotta, Paolo 2012a. Difficult patient loss and physician culture for oncologists grieving patient loss. *Journal of Palliative Medicine* 15: 1254–1260.

Granek, Leeat; Mazzotta, Paolo; Tozer, Richard & Krzyzanowska, Monika K. 2012b. What do oncologists want? Suggestions from oncologists on how their institutions can support them in dealing with patient loss. *Supportive Care in Cancer* 20: 2627–2632.

Gross, Sophie E.; Ernstmann, Nicole; Jung, Jonghwan; Karbach, Ute; Ansmann, Lena; Gloede, Tristan; Pfaff, Holger; Wirtz, Markus A.; Baumann, Walter; Schmitz, S.; Osburg, Sandra & Neumann, Magdalena 2014. Can a stressed oncologist be good in a consultation? A qualitative study on the oncologists' perception. *European Journal of Cancer Care* 23: 594–606.

De Haes, Hanneke & Bensing, Jozien 2009. Endpoints in medical communication research, proposing a framework of functions and outcomes. *Patient Education and Counseling* 74: 287–294.

Hermann, Anja 2005. *Das Arrangement der Hoffnung. Kommunikation und Interaktion in einer onkologischen Spezialklinik während der chirurgischen Behandlung von Knochen- und Weichgewebesarkomen*. Frankfurt am Main: Mabuse-Verlag.

Hillen, Marij; de Haes, Hanneke C J M & Smets, Ellen M A 2011. Cancer patients' trust in their physician-a review. *Psychooncology* 20: 227–241.

Hinnen, Chris; Pool, Grieteke; Holwerda, Nynke; Sprangers, Mirjam; Sanderman, Robbert & Hagedoorn, Mariet 2014. Lower levels of trust in one's physician is associated with more distress over time in more anxiously attached individuals with cancer. *General Hospital Psychiatry* 36: 382–387.

Kissane, David; Bylund, Carma L; Banerjee, Smita C; Bialer, Philip A; Levin, Tomer T; Maloney, Erin K & D'Agostino, Thomas A 2012. Communication skills training for oncology professionals. *Journal of Clinical Oncology* 30: 1242–1247.

Lin, Jenny; Chao, Jennifer; Bickell, Nina A & Wisnivesky, Juan P. 2016. Patient-provider communication and hormonal therapy side effects in breast cancer survivors. *Women & Health* 57: 976–989.

Maguire, Peter 1985. Barriers to psychological care of the dying. *British Medical Journal* 291: 1711–1713.

Maguire, Peter 1999. Improving communication with cancer patients. *European Journal of Cancer* 35: 2058–2065.

Maly, Rose C.; Liu, Yihang; Liang, Li-Jung & Ganz, Patricia A 2015. Quality of life over 5 years after a breast cancer diagnosis among low-income women: effects of race/ethnicity and patient-physician communication. *Cancer* 121: 916–926.

Mayring, Philipp 2010. Qualitative Inhaltsanalyse. In Mey, Günter & Mruck, Katja (eds) *Handbuch qualitative Forschung in der Psychologie*. Wiesbaden: Springer VS: 601–613.

Merckaert, Isabelle; Libert, Yves & Razavi, Darius 2005. Communication skills training in cancer care: where are

we and where are we going? *Current Opinion in Oncology* 17: 319–330.
NEUMANN, MELANIE; WIRTZ, MARKUS; BOLLSCHWEILER, MARKUS; MERCER, STEWART W.; WARM, MATHIAS; WOLF, JÜRGEN & PFAFF, HOLGER 2007. Determinants and patient-reported long-term outcomes of physician empathy in oncology: a structural equation modelling approach. *Patient Education and Counseling* 69: 63–75.
NGUYEN, TIMOTHY K; BAUMAN, GLENN S; WATLING, CHRISTOPHER J & HAHN, KARIN 2017. Patient- and family-centered care: a qualitative exploration of oncologist perspectives. *Supportive Care in Cancer* 25: 213–219.
NITZSCHE, ANIKA; NEUMANN, MELANIE; GROSS, SOPHIE E; ANSMANN, LENA; PFAFF, HOLGER; BAUMANN, WALTER; WIRTZ, MARKUS; SCHMITZ, STEPHAN & ERNSTMANN, NICOLE 2017. Recovery opportunities, work-home conflict, and emotional exhaustion among hematologists and oncologists in private practice. *Psychology, Health & Medicine* 22: 462–473.
PARSONS, TALCOTT 1951. *The social system* New York: The Free Press.
ROBINSON, JEFFREY D.; HOOVER, DONALD R; VENETIS, MARIA K; KEARNEY, THOMAS J & STREET, RICHARD L JR 2013. Consultations between patients with breast cancer and surgeons: a pathway from patient-centered communication to reduced hopelessness. *Journal of Clinical Oncology* 31: 351–358.
SCHOLL, ISABELLE; ZILL, JÖRDIS M; HÄRTER, MARTIN & DIRMAIER, JÖRG 2014. An Integrative Model of Patient-Centeredness. A Systematic Review and Concept Analysis. *PLOS ONE* 9 (9): e107828.
SHANAFELT, TAIT; ADJEI, ALEX & MEYSKENS, FRANK L. 2003. When your favorite patient relapses: physician grief and well-being in the practice of oncology. *Journal of Clinical Oncology* 21: 2616–2619.
SIEGRIST, JOHANNES. 2005. *Medizinische Soziologie*. München, Jena: Elsevier Urban & Fischer.
SQUIER, ROGER W. 1990. A model of empathic understanding and adherence to treatment regimens in practitioner-patient relationships. *Social Science & Medicine* 30: 325–339.
STEWART, MOIRA A. 1995. Effective physician-patient communication and health outcomes: a review. *Canadian Medical Association Journal* 152: 1423–1433.
STIEFEL, FRIEDRICH K. & BOURQUIN, CÉLINE 2016. Communication in oncology: now we train - but how well? *Annals of Oncology* 27: 1660–1663.
STIEFEL, FRIEDRICH K. & BOURQUIN, CÉLINE 2019. Moving toward the next generation of communication training in oncology: The relevance of findings from qualitative research. *European Journal of Cancer Care* 28:e13149.
SUCHMAN, ANTHONY L.; MARKAKIS, KATHRYN; BECKMAN, HOWARD B. & FRANKEL, R. 1997. A model of empathic communication in the medical interview. *Journal of the American Medical Association* 277: 678–682.
TANRIVERDI, ÖZGÜR 2013. A medical oncologist's perspective on communication skills and burnout syndrome with psycho-oncological approach (to die with each patient one more time: the fate of the oncologists). *Medical Oncology* 30: 530.
TRAVADO, LUIZA; GRASSI, LUIGI; GIL, FRANCISCO; VENTURA, CIDÁLIA & MARTINS, CRISTINA 2005. Physician-patient communication among Southern European cancer physicians: the influence of psychosocial orientation and burnout. *Psycho-Oncology* 14: 661–670.
WEBER, MAX 1921. *Soziologische Grundbegriffe*. Wirtschaft und Gesellschaft. Tübingen: Mohr.
ZILL, JÖRDIS M.; SCHOLL, ISABELLE; HÄRTER, MARTIN & DIRMAIER, JÖRG 2015. Which Dimensions of Patient-Centeredness Matter? Results of a Web-Based Expert Delphi Survey. *PLOS ONE* 10 (11): e0141978.

This article has been subjected to a double blind peer review process prior to publication.

Nicole Ernstmann, Prof. Dr. rer. medic., is a health services researcher with a background in psychology and nursing. She is head of the Chair of Health Services Research at the Institute of Medical Sociology, Health Services Research and Rehabilitation Science at the University of Cologne and heads the master's program in Health Services Research. Her research focuses on medical communication and patient-provider-relationship, health literacy, and patient- and family-centered care.

University of Cologne
Faculty of Medicine and University Hospital Cologne
Institute of Medical Sociology
Health Services Research and Rehabilitation Science
Chair of Health Services Research
e-mail: nicole.ernstmann1@uk-koeln.de

Sophie Elisabeth Groß, Dr. rer. medic., studied social sciences at the University of Cologne and Utrecht, NL. At the Institute for Medical Sociology, Health Services Research and Rehabilitation Science (IMVR), she focussed on the field of oncological health services research. Since 2018, she has been working for the Institute for Health Services Research at the Rhineland Regional Hospital Association in Cologne. Within her work at this institut, she focuses on healthcare research for psychiatric and somatic-psychiatric comorbid patients as well as healthcare research for people with disabilities.

LVR Institute for Research and Education & LVR Institute for Health Services Research
LVR Clinic Cologne
e-mail: sophie.gross@lvr.de

Ute Karbach, PD Dr. rer. pol., heads the "inCare" working group at the Institute of Medical Sociology, Health Services Research and Rehabilitation Science (IMVR). She is concerned with the analysis of care concepts, e.g. integrated care models, but also with the possibilities of inclusive care. Another focus is the investigation of digital innovations in care. She is also interested in the extent to which organizational development measures can support the implementation and dissemination of innovations. A particular concern of the "inCare" working group is to realize the possibilities of participatory research as far as possible.

University of Cologne
Faculty of Human Sciences & Faculty of Medicine and University Hospital Cologne
Institute of Medical Sociology
Health Services Research and Rehabilitation Science
Chair of Quality Development and Evaluation in Rehabilitation
e-mail: ute.karbach@uk-koeln.de

Lena Ansmann, Prof. Dr. rer. medic., is professor for medical sociology at the Medical Faculty of the University of Cologne. Her Chair is part of the Institute of Medical Sociology, Health Services Research and Rehabilitation Science (IMVR). Her research is located at the interface between Medical Sociology and Health Services Research. Her research focuses on the one hand on the wider context of healthcare, particularly on the organizational context in e.g. hospitals and private practices. On the other hand, she researches under which conditions patient-centered care can be realized and contributes to the development, evaluation and implementation of complex interventions in equally complex healthcare organizations. Lena Ansmann is lecturing predominantly in the Human Medicine study program, where she is representing the field of Medical Sociology.

University of Cologne
Faculty of Medicine and University Hospital Cologne
Institute of Medical Sociology
Health Services Research and Rehabilitation Science
Chair of Medical Sociology
e-mail: lena.ansmann1@uk-koeln.de

André Karger, Dr. med., MME, is physician for psychosomatic medicine, psychotherapy and psychiatry. He is vice-director of the Institute for Psychosomatic Medicine and Psychotherapy and head of psycho-oncology at the University Hospital Düsseldorf, Germany. He is interested in communication in healthcare and was PI of the recently completed KommRhein Interpro-Study (German Cancer Aid).

Heinrich-Heine University Düsseldorf
Institute for Psychosomatic Medicine and Psychotherapy
Medical Faculty and University Hospital
e-mail: andre.karger@med.uni-duesseldorf.de

Holger Pfaff, Prof. Dr., Managing Director of the Center for Health Services Research Cologne and the Institute for Medical Sociology, Health Services Research and Rehabilitation Science at the University of Cologne. He has been an honorary professor at Macquarie University (Sydney) since 2019. He was a Visiting Scholar and Visiting Research Fellow at the University of Michigan, Case Western Reserve University, the University of Aberdeen and the Universitat Autònoma de Barcelona.

University of Cologne
Faculty of Human Sciences & Faculty of Medicine and University Hospital Cologne
Institute of Medical Sociology
Health Services Research and Rehabilitation Science
Chair of Quality Development and Evaluation in Rehabilitation
e-mail: holger.pfaff@uk-koeln.de

Markus Wirtz, PD Dr. phil., is Professor of Educational Psychology (Focus Research Methods) at the University of Education in Freiburg. He studied psychology and and obtained his doctorate at the University of Münster. His research focuses on assessment and evaluation in the areas of chronic diseases, health services research, educational school research, health psychology and health education. He is currently PI in the project "Structural modelling and assessment of health literacy in allergy prevention of new parents' in the DFG research group 'Health Literacy in Early Childhood Allergy prevention".

University of Education Freiburg
Research Methods in Health Sciences
e-mail: markus.wirtz@ph-freiburg.de

Walter Baumann, Dr. rer. med, is a medical sociologist, with professional experiences in the German social insurance system. He has been the executive director of the Scientific Institute of Office-Based Hematologists and Oncologists in Germany (WINHO) which is oriented on health services research and quality assurance in outpatient oncology care in collaboration with private practices and academic research institutions. His current scientific interests are directed towards theories in health services research.

Former affiliation Scientific Institute of Office-Based Hematologists and Oncologists in Germany
e-mail: drwbaumann@t-online.de

Melanie Neumann, Priv.-Doz. Dr. rer. med., is senior researcher at the University of Witten/Herdecke. She studied sociology at the University of Bielefeld and conducted her doctoral thesis at the University of Cologne, Center for Health Services Research, on empathy in patient-physician relationship with focus on patient-reported outcomes. At the University of Witten/Herdecke, Institute for Integrative Medicine, she did research on educating medical students in empathy resulting in her Habilitation. Meanwhile, Melanie was also a lecturer for Qualitative Methods at the Department of Psychology, University Witten/Herdecke. After this research time, she took a break from it for several years to work as an art and body therapist. Few years ago, she started research in parts again at the University of Witten/Herdecke on issues like e.g. placebo effects in nutrition, psychosocial effects of vegan diet and on evaluating medical students' education in Integrative Medicine. Currently, Melanie examines the issue of finding meaning in (your own) life by conducting health services studies with psychotherapists, psychotherapy and chronic/acute somatic patients, spiritual/religious persons and those with near-death experiences.

University of Witten/Herdecke
Department of Health
Chair for Psychosomatic Medicine and Psychotherapy
Gemeinschaftskrankenhaus Herdecke
e-mail: melanie.neumann@uni-wh.de

Digital Healing? Digital Capitalism?
Neoliberalism, Digital Health Technologies, and Citizen Health

NICK J. FOX

Abstract The emergence of digital health and illness technologies and the digitisation of capitalist economic production reflect the increasing cyborgisation of organic matter within current economic and social relations. In this paper I employ a materialist and posthuman approach to 'digital health', investigating micropolitically what digital technologies and apps actually do, within the contexts of contemporary social relations and the emergence of digital capitalism. This enables new insights into the impacts of the digital upon social production, making sense of the contribution of both human and non-human matter both to digital health and to the wider economics and politics of neoliberal health care. The paper evaluates four digital health technologies to consider what capacities they produce in bodies and the micropolitical impact of the technology in terms of power, resistance and social order. I then consider how these micropolitics might be changed by altering the contexts or other forces, and argue that this opens up ways for digital technologies to be used to promote radical and transgressive possibilities, by re-engineering the interactions between technologies and other materialities. I conclude by discussing 'digital activism'. I examine how technologies and apps may be engineered to democratise data: to enable collective responses to health issues, to challenge health policy and to organise against health corporations, environmental polluters, and purveyors of fast and processed foods. This collective, bottom-up model of 'citizen health' (RIMAL et al. 1997) counters both the marketisation of health and the paternalism of health care.

Keywords capitalism – citizen health – digital health – micropolitics – new materialism

Introduction

The medical device market was estimated to be worth $512bn in 2022, with an annual growth of six per cent (FORTUNE BUSINESS INSIGHTS 2023). Medical devices range from CAT scanner to hospital bed; surgical instrument to hearing aid (TOPHAM 2003). Personal medical devices (PMDs) are a defined sub-category, comprising near-body devices or technologies designed for use by a single individual, primarily outside healthcare facilities (REN & BATRA 2013). Many PMDs enable monitoring of body functions or performance, and are used either for self-care purposes or with medical oversight; some have capacities for an associated therapeutic intervention.

Personal or 'near-body' medical devices are nothing new: early examples include false teeth from Roman times (CRUBÉZY & GIRARD 1998) and spectacles from the medieval period (CASHELL 1971). Later devices included artificial limbs and wheelchairs, and more recently, contact lenses, cardiac pacemakers and joint prostheses. Since the 1980s, however, a new range of near-body devices have emerged that build in some kind of connectivity using wireless internet or radio-frequency (RF) technology (PANTELOPOULOS & BOURBAKIS 2010), Internet of Things (IoT) technologies (KARTHICK, RAMKUMAR, AKRAM & KUMAR 2021) or other information or communication technology (ICT) affordances (LUPTON 2021). For example, a monitoring device may link to a remote health care facility and transmit clinical data on blood pressure or blood sugar, to be collected and aggregated remotely by biomedical personnel. Alternatively, devices may process this data themselves and respond – for instance to deliver medication or actuate a heart pacemaker. This new generation of PMDs will be described here as *digital health technologies* (DHTs).

Many of these DHTs monitor body parameters, from blood pressure and chemistry, to food intake or hours slept per night, while others sense body motion or activity (KAPLAN & STONE 2013: 478; LUPTON 2013: 393–394). Longitudinal monitoring can be used to manage diet or exercise regimes (TILL 2014), to identify rare or irregular events and syndromes that develop slowly over time (RODGERS et al. 2012: 936), to monitor food intake, or to alert emergency services, for example in the event of a fall or loss of consciousness (PATEL, PARK & BONATO 2012: 2). Infusion pumps automatically deliver therapeutic doses of drugs such as insulin or analgesics, according to medically pre-designated schedules, while implantable devices both monitor and intervene, for example to provide heart pacing or – if needed – more dramatic interventions such as cardiac defibrillation (GOLDENBERG, GILLESPIE & MOSS 2010).

The claimed benefits associated with the clinical DHTs are improvements in health care delivery to an ageing population that requires more frequent health monitoring (SILICON LABS, n.d.: 1). Networking devices via digital mobile technology can reduce costs in care delivery by connecting people to their health care providers, while improving access by patients and providers to reference materials, lab tests, and medical records (WEST 2013: 1). However, warnings have been raised concerning security risks – in particular for those implanted in patients – from both malicious attacks and accidental breaches (MAISEL & KOHNO: 2010).

Devices with a specific medical application are subject to regulatory authority – for example by the Food and Drug Administration (FDA) in the US and Medical and Healthcare Regulatory Authority (MHRA) in the UK. However, others – such as the *Fitbit* and Apple Watch, or apps for mobile phones such as *WellnessConnected* or *Map My Fitness* that monitor body activity are marketed commercially. Some of these devices have become part of a 'Quantified Self' self-tracking movement (LEE 2013, LUPTON 2014; LUPTON 2019: 2004–2006) that encourage people to evaluate their fitness and health indicators, their time use or hours of sleep, with the aim of enhancing wellbeing and personal efficiency (PADDOCK 2013; THOMAS LUPTON & PEDERSEN 2018). The digital data gathered by these devices can either be retained for private use, or uploaded to servers provided by their manufacturers, enabling data analysis and data sharing with other users (LUPTON 2013: 394). In 2015, 63 per cent of US citizens wished to monitor their health using connected devices (SALESFORCE 2015), while the market for self-care monitors was $18b in 2016, with projected growth of almost 20 per cent per annum to 2023 (LOOMBA & KHAIRNAR 2018).

Critiques of these DHTs argue that they are part of a neoliberal trend towards 'digital capitalism' (FUCHS 2018; SCHILLER 2000; STAAB 2017). This has been defined as the facilitation of capitalist social relations such as free trade, globalisation, privatisation and individualism by digital technologies (BARASSI 2015). It reflects both the emergence of a capitalist knowledge economy, and the development of web-enabled digital technologies for commerce and marketing, and as a platform for consumerism. The growing digitisation of capitalist economic production (SCHILLER 2000) has facilitated not only the development of DHTs but also the emergence of a wide range of digitally-enabled commerce and services, from Amazon to Uber (GRABHER & VAN TUIJL 2020). These opportunities have accelerated the move toward the privatisation and marketisation of health care and other personal services (FAULKNER-GURSTEIN & WYATT 2023), and have consequently made the digital technology sector a growth area for investment and take-overs (SCHILLER 2011), while undermining traditional modes of retailer/consumer or provider/client interactions (STAAB 2017: 289). In relation to healing, digital capitalism supplies opportunities to replace conventional professional/client models with market- and data-driven care (FOX 2017: 144–145).

In this paper, I shall consider the social, economic and political implications of these developments for care and healing, by examining the micropolitics inherent in the networks/assemblages surrounding DHTs. I will explore 'digital health' via a materialist and posthuman approach (fully described in the next section), investigating micropolitically what digital technologies and apps actually *do*, within the contexts of contemporary social relations. This enables new insights into the impacts of the digital upon social production, making sense of the contribution of both human and non-human matter both to digital health and to the wider economics and politics of neoliberal health care (MACGREGOR 2001; MOONEY 2012). However, I also consider how DHTs may be re-engineered to counter digital capitalism and foster new forms of collective activism around health and well-being.

A new materialist framework for analysing digital health

To assist in analysis of the micropolitics of digital health technologies, I apply a new materialist framing (BARAD 1996; COOLE & FROST 2010; FOX & ALLDRED 2017. The new materialisms focus upon the interplay of material forces within the unstable assemblages that emerge around bodies and technologies such as DHTs. They have been informed by a disparate skein of social theories including actor-network theory (LATOUR 2005), biophilosophy (ANSELL PEARSON 1997; MASSUMI 1996), feminism and queer theory (BRAIDOTTI 2006; GROSZ 1994; HARAWAY 1997), philosophical posthumanism (BRAIDOTTI 2013), quantum physics (BARAD 1996) and Spinozist monism (DELANDA 2006; DELEUZE 1988). Like post-structuralism, this 'new' materialism is concerned fundamentally with the workings of power within physical and social spaces, but is focused firmly upon social production rather than social construction (COOLE & FROST 2010: 7), and emphasises matter rather than textuality.

As an approach to studying social and natural phenomena, new materialism steps back from an anthropocentric emphasis upon the consequences of human social processes (in the current case, DHTs and their application) for human health and human subjectivities. In place of this anthropocentric focus, the new materialisms adopt a posthuman or 'more-than-human' breadth, acknowledging the capacities of all matter to affect. This more-than-human breadth shifts the ontological focus of social inquiry from entities to relationality: from what humans, their bodies and their identities *are*. Instead it explores what relational networks or *assemblages* of animate and inanimate entities *do*. The aim of such an inquiry is consequently to examine how bodies and non-human matter affect and are affected (DELANDA 2006: 4),

and what capacities to do, think and feel are thereby produced in bodies, collectivities of bodies, and in other matter. Significantly, this shift from a privileged and agentic human to 'flows of affect' in assemblages acknowledges that things, organisations, social formations and concepts contribute to social production as much as – if not more than – human bodies/subjects.

However, this ontology also extends materialism beyond traditional concerns with structural and 'macro' level social phenomena. Power is explored not by positing 'causal' or 'explanatory' social structures such as 'capitalism' or 'biomedicine', but by unpicking the play of forces or 'affect economy' (CLOUGH 2004: 15) that assemble around the actions and events that produce and reproduce the world and human history. These forces may be physical, psychological or cultural, and – importantly, include the material products of thoughts, desires, feelings and abstract concepts (BRAIDOTTI 2000: 159; DELANDA 2006: 5), thereby cutting across both the nature/culture and mind/matter dualisms that invest much social theory (VAN DER TUIN & DOLPHIJN 2010: 155).

Applied to empirical research, an ontology of assemblages and affects requires an approach to data that can reveal the web of material relations surrounding DHTs and their use (FOX & ALLDRED, 2015). These materialities range from the manufacturers and retailers that market these devices, the science, engineering and design that makes them work, the medical and information technology professionals that develop DHTs or assess data they produce, through to the domestic and other spaces where these technologies are used, the physiological and biomedical processes that they monitor or manage, and the desires, expectations and concerns of users. As such, new materialist analysis dissolves boundaries between what are conventionally regarded as the 'macro' level of institutions and social organisation and the 'micro' level of human desires and experiences, recognising that what these aspects of the social have in common is an ability to affect or be affected.

The task of analysis will therefore be to document the assemblages of bodies, technologies and other relations that accrete around DHT use; to explore how these relations affect and are affected during DHT use; and to assess the micropolitics of these assemblages and the consequences for DHT users and others involved with them. The first step in this analysis is to examine four different DHTs – selected to present a range of devices, from those with a biomedical objective to those intended for use by individuals or organisations independently of clinical oversight. For each of these DHTs, the analysis will examine the relational assemblage surrounding its development and use, consider what this assemblage does, and evaluate the micropolitics that link the particular device to bodies, organisations, ideas and desires. These micropolitical analyses will then be used to explore the different interests that may be served by DHTs, and what these suggest for the future development of such devices.

The micropolitics of digital health technologies

The four DHTs to be analysed in this section range from a monitoring app to support clinical decision-making through to an app that links consumers to virtual health and fitness coaches. Based on the available literature and manufacturers' online marketing materials, I will first describe the DHT, and then analyse it micropolitically to understand what it does, not only functionally, but also in terms of the capacities it produces: in users and in other interested parties (for example, health professionals and/or commercial or corporate interests).

MS Mosaic: A multiple sclerosis management app

MS Mosaic is an iPhone app developed by researchers at North Carolina's Duke University, US.[1] It aims to enable multiple sclerosis sufferers to monitor their condition on a daily basis, but also provide clinicians with data on their patients' disease between check-up consultations to assist in disease management and medication prescribing.

The app incorporates a range of different data collection techniques, including a daily survey of changes to sufferers' symptoms, a battery of performance tests to assess hand coordination and walking speed, and tests of memory and attention. It also gathers data from the iPhone's built-in sensors, such as steps taken or hours slept per day. Users can send a report to their doctor summarising trends since their last check-up. The developers suggest that such additional data will assist clinicians to more successfully manage this progressive but unpredictable disease via medication and other therapies (LEWIS 2017).

This summary allows identification of the key material elements within the *MS Mosaic* assemblage. These can be summarised as comprising at least:

body; disease; symptoms; iPhone; sensors; app; clinicians; researchers; pharmaceutical industry

In addition to the stated functions, a range of other micropolitical effects can also be identified. While the app supplies users with a capacity to monitor their disease on a daily basis, the principal beneficiaries are clinicians, however. By gathering a range of data, *MS Mosaic* provides the clinicians with a capacity to assess disease progression 'objectively': they can now interrogate the disease directly, without recourse to patients' memories and subjective reports of their symptoms. Consequently, patients are disempowered during check-ups, with their accounts of disease progression sidelined in favour of data gathered by the app.

Fitbit: A self-tracking DHT

The *Fitbit* is one of a number of commercial devices (similar devices include the *Nike+ Fuelband*, the *Apple Watch* and *Garmin Vivofit*) that can be worn or carried on the body. The device monitors various body parameters including heart rate, and incorporates an accelerometer to monitor and record motion and posture, hours slept and so forth. Data is sent wirelessly to a computer or mobile phone where it can be displayed graphically and can calculate calories burned and other functions; this also enables data to be shared.

The *Fitbit*-user assemblage comprises at least the following relations:

body movements; terrain; device; wearer; manufacturer; associates

The key affect driving this assemblage is the *Fitbit*'s capacity to gather data on posture, movement and heart rate and turn these into quantifiable outputs that can be displayed, analysed and interpreted. However, the affect economy that links assembled relations produces not only the device's specific functionalities but also new capacities in the user (including motivations towards certain behaviours such as exercise or sleep), new opportunities to share and compare behaviours with peers. At the same time, this affect economy also provides the device's manufacturers with the capacity to exploit the data gathered for commercial purposes.

These complex affective flows generate a specific micropolitics that has the outcome of responsibilising the user, but at the same time – by quantifying and making explicit certain aspects of daily life, and enabling comparisons with other users – encouraging certain normative behaviours around fitness, sleep, weight etc, creating new body routines and regimens, and producing competitiveness with self/others. By drawing users into an assemblage with commercial interests, private aspects of a user's life are commodified and commercialised (TILL 2014).

Splendid project

Splendid is a European Union-funded project still in its pilot stage that aims to reduce obesity among adolescents and young adults by providing personalised services to guide users toward healthy eating and encourage exercise.[2] It uses an interactive system to accurately track eating and physical activity, and provides goal-oriented feedback to the user. The programme uses a range of body sensors (a mandometer to monitor eating behaviour, an accelerometer to assess physical activity, and a chewing sensor). Outputs from these devices link by smart-phone to clinicians, who provide advice on nutrition and exercise to participants.

The *Splendid*-assemblage comprises at least the following elements:

> body; food; terrain; sensors;
> phone; clinicians; population

The DHT serves its stated aims by gathering detailed data on eating and exercise and crunching this data using algorithms to process and evaluate the behaviour of participants. More broadly, *Splendid* creates capacities for public health professionals to obtain detailed data on users' eating and exercise behaviour, allowing them to personalise their advice and diet plans.

This has a number of micropolitical effects. First it biomedicalises eating and exercise and locates them as elements at a population level that contribute to 'problem' categories such as overweight and obese. Second, it places assessment of these in the hands of the technology, disempowering users from assessing their own food consumption and health needs. Finally, it aggregates its target users (who may be profoundly different on many variables) as an 'at risk' population.

Vida: Virtual health and wellness coaching

Vida is a digital platform developed by Vida Health. This is one of a small number of US commercial start-ups that provides virtual coaching: to address 'unhealthy' behaviours associated with chronic conditions such as obesity, hypertension and diabetes, as well as a range of mental health issues.[3] At the core of *Vida* is a mobile phone app, which can be linked to a wide range of trackers and monitors, including pedometers and wireless scales. These enable needs for behaviour change to be identified, and progress towards targets assessed. Participants can select a coaching style such as 'cheerleader' or 'drill sergeant' to suit their own preferences; they are then matched by the app with a list of virtual coaches recommended by Vida. Coaches include nutritionists, physical therapists, cognitive behavioural therapists and social workers (MAO et al. 2017: 3). Participants enter into a commercial subscription to Vida that covers the costs of the app and the health coaching. The app is marketed to individuals, but primarily to US employers who wish to introduce a tailored health programme for their staff.

The Vida-assemblage comprises at least the following relations:

> body; app; monitors; coach;
> health programme; employer;
> Vida Health; shareholders; profit

According to its website, the stated objective of the Vida app is to 'support individuals with evidence-based programs that address their behaviors and underlying health conditions'. Analysing the app micropolitically, the approach replaces a conventional patient/professional relationship with a consumerist and privatised model, in which individuals (or their employers) pay for coaching to achieve health promotional and public health objectives. The app serves as an intermediary between consumers and health coaches, providing users with the capacity to access a wide range of health coaches suited to their individual needs. However, the main outcome of the app's business model is to supply Vida Health with a capacity to monetise the data gathered by its body-monitors by putting clients and coaches together. In addition, by marketing directly to employers, the company gains a capacity to enrol organisations as a third party in their business.

This materialist and micropolitical analysis of these four DHTs provides the basis for the following discussion of contemporary moves towards digital health and digital capitalism as drivers in healing relationships.

From digital health to digital capitalism

The four DHTs assessed in the previous section, while having in common similar technical functions (variously linking body sensors or monitors to phone or internet platforms), diverge significantly once analysed micropolitically. At one end, *MS Mosiac* supplies a digital solution to support a conventional interaction between patient and health professional. As such it may be considered as medico-centric, serving principally to enhance clinical decision-making. At the other, *Vida* replaces this patient/professional model with a consumer relationship, in which paid-for commercial services assist individuals to achieve behavioural changes.[4] Between these extremes, the *Splendid* project uses digital monitoring to address public health objectives, targeting at-risk individuals and this improve population-level health, while *Fitbit* and similar platforms offer means for individuals to track aspect of their daily activities and fitness, and their parent company's to gather a wide range of health data from users, with potential commercial uses.

These four case studies together summarise the contemporary spectrum of DHTs, supplying a snapshot of the ways in which digital health technologies and apps are currently being used. This spectrum ranges from supporting traditional clinical activities through to a full-blown digital capitalism that privatises and individualises many features of health care. The issues around patient/professional interactions and recent trends towards self-care have been very well addressed by social scientists researching health. However, it is the emergence of 'digital health capitalism' upon which I wish now to focus in this chapter, before then offering an alternative perspective: 'citizen health' (cf. RIMAL et al. 1997).

In the introduction I outlined the main features of digital capitalism, and it is worth summarising these briefly once again. Specifically, digital capitalism may be understood as the enabling of marketised, privatised and individualised social relations via digital technologies (BARASSI 2015). These technologies increase efficiency by reducing overheads associated with physical business infrastructure such as offices or retail outlets; they bring together a wide range of providers and consumers; they remove geography as a factor in providing goods or services; they mirror or mimic many aspects of conventional markets. These features enable digital commerce to reduce margins and hence increase competitiveness, at the expense of traditional providers. *Amazon*, *AirBnB*, *Uber* and *Asos* are well-known examples of digital capitalist enterprises.

The *Vida* app described earlier reflects all these aspects of digital capitalism. It overcomes a need for premises such as gyms to deliver fitness coaching; it connects clients to a wide range of potential coaches independent of physical location, increasing the likelihood of achieving a 'good fit' and hence continued purchase of services; it mimics the conventional relations between client and coach without physical co-presence. Finally, by providing a 'one-stop shop' for coaching across both physical and mental health it drives down cost margins for purchasers of services (both individual consumers and employers), undercutting other non-virtual providers of health and wellness therapies.

The critique offered earlier of *Vida* serves to offer a more generalised commentary on what might be termed 'digital health capitalism'. First, it substitutes social relations between 'patient' and 'health professional' with market relations, in which health and fitness are commodities to be purchased alongside other goods. These marketised relations privatise health care, replacing both clinical care and public health with monetised services. In this way, they consolidate and potentially extend globally a neoliberalised and marketised model of care, in which consumers (or in the case of the *Vida* model, employers) have both moral and financial responsibility for health and fitness, rather than communities or governments. Digital health capitalism consequently undermines conventional health and welfare service delivery, potentially disadvantaging those least able to afford privatised care, and consequently increasing health inequalities.

While this critique of *Vida*'s business model does not diverge notably from a standard political economy assessment, the materialist and micropolitical perspective offered in the previous section provides a further twist to the analysis. The *Vida*-assemblage engages client bodies at the level of their behaviour, with the objective (via coaching) of establishing new health and fitness capacities, while removing capacities deemed unhealthy or negative. The micropolitics of this DHT excludes any acknowledgment of extraneous or underlying causes that may be producing such 'unhealthy' behaviours. These may include poverty or lack of access to resources or health care; natural or sociocultural environmental causes; problems or issues in home or work lives; and inequalities or discrimination deriving from an individual's social identity or social position. *Vida*'s business model thus implicitly individualises and de-socialises health. This model of health care gains a further twist, given Vida Health's main customer target (US employers responsible for staff health through insurance schemes), such that employee health emphasises personal responsibility for ceasing 'unhealthy' behaviours.

This analysis reveals digital health capitalism not simply as the most recent development in contemporary health care, but as also reflecting features of neoliberal marketisation of services. The importation of privatised and individualised social relations into health care undermines social and public health models of health and illness, and contributes to the current dismantling of socialised health and welfare systems in many jurisdictions. However, a micropolitical perspective enables not only the analysis of DHTs, but also potentially the re-engineering of such technologies to meet alternative micropolitical objectives. It is to this task that I turn in the final section of this chapter.

Digital health activism and citizen health

I have shown, with recourse to four case studies, that digital health technologies have been used to support health care models, including a clinician-focused approach, self-care, and the commercial endeavours that I have labelled as 'digital health capitalism'. In the previous section I focused on the last of these, identifying the affective movements that this approach to health care mediates. However, I now wish to suggest that – just as commercial interests may seek to establish marketised and neoliberal DHTs – there is an alternative and diametrically-opposed model of care possible. DHTs may be used to foster what might variously but described as 'digital health activism' or 'citizen health'.

Underpinning this approach is resistance and refusal of models of health care that constrain action to promote health and wellbeing, not only individually, but also collectively. Hence, in opposition to a top-down public health model, health activism resists surveillance and responsibilisation of individuals for their health and wellness, and re-emphasises a range of forces beyond individual control. Against a biomedical approach to health care, it rejects medicocentric emphases on disease entities in favour of positive understandings of health and wellness. And in opposition to commercial or corporate interests, it counters marketised approaches to health and wellness, while also identifying the negative consequences of markets for both human health and environmental sustainability (FOX & ALLDRED 2020).

My proposition here is that DHTs may be co-opted as part of this resistance: to establish some very different capacities in their users. DHTs developed according to a health activism agenda would:

• Promote health and illness not in terms of a biomedical model – linking health not to individual biology or psychology, but to the capacities of people and collectivities to engage productively with their social, economic, political and cultural milieux.

• Provide a means for collective and intersectional responses to health and illness issues – enhancing capacities for people and communities to address health and illness threats and opportunities together and across sectional (social class, gender, sexuality, race etc.) divides, rather than as individuals.

• Counter marketised health care initiatives that turn users of services into consumers, and monetise health and wellness services.

• Challenge and develop health policy – providing data and analytical capacities and resources that can inform health policy development or campaigns for health-related improvements to a locale or sector.

• Organise against health corporate interests – offering a means to challenge the power of corporations such as environmental polluters, purveyors of fast and processed foods, and against corporate health care providers.

• Synchronise health and environmental sustainability – rejecting policy initiatives that seek human health or development gains at the expense of the environment and sustainability.

Elsewhere (FOX 2017) I have outlined an example of a DHT that could deliver on some or all of these objectives, based on existing digital technology solutions. A network of health devices could be used by users to gather and crunch relevant health data (physiological, social, environmental) in order to assess health status and risks to health across a locality (or a specific sub-community such as LGBT citizens or teenage parents). This DHT would be based on different communication architecture from a many-to-one or 'hub-and-spoke' model underpinning apps such as those described earlier in this chapter that link bodies individually to health professionals or to corporate databanks. Instead, it would use a many-to-many communication protocol to build networks of connected bodies and social formations that may challenge biomedical health care, neo-liberalism and individualising DHTs.

For example, air quality monitors could be installed across a neighbourhood to assess risks to health from traffic pollution, and crunch data into statistics that may be disseminated to local media and social media, and sharing knowledge resources via local libraries and universities. Data on health-related problems suffered by members of a community as a consequence of housing defects in social or rented accommodation (such as damp, poor loft or wall insulation, or costly energy sources) can be collated and sent to local government housing and public health departments. Evidence from such digitally-enabled networks may be used by community groups to co-ordinate action and build coalitions with health professionals, politicians, researchers and others, to engage local and national media, and to support local policy development.

A DHT such as this can contribute to what has been called a 'citizen health' agenda (RIMAL et al. 1997), which rejects an individualised approach to health, and opposes biomedical or corporate interests, including the neo-liberalisation and privatisation of health care and the monetisation of health and wellness. Health activism may be regarded as 'a challenge to the existing order and power relationships that are perceived to influence some aspects of health negatively or impede health' (ZOLLER 2005: 344), often focusing on inequality or inequity, or facilitating collective mobilisation (PARKER et al. 2012: 100). DHTs can be radically re-engineered to serve different, radical and critical, agendas. It is not hard to envisage producing apps for networked devices that can subvert the principles underpinning commercially-developed monitoring devices; indeed, some platform providers such as *Apple* apparently welcome app developers to contribute to their health-related app portfolio. It is not fanciful to see possibilities for DHTs that may deliver to collectivities some of the capacities suggested under the rubric of citizen health, or even transform the micropolitics of technologies such as *Splendid* or *Vida* that were discussed earlier.

Concluding remarks

The materialist and micropolitical analysis conducted here has considered DHTs not as pre-existing, stand-alone entities, but in terms of what they do, in the widest sense, within the assemblages of human and non-human relations that enable them work. By exploring different DHTs in this way, it has been possible to reveal the specific affect economies that mediate the relations between bodies and technology in each case, and by assessing these economies also to identify the micropolitics that these various DHTs manifest and sustain. This approach thereby enables a materialist reading of any specific DHT, and an opportunity to offer a critical assessment of how devices contribute to different agendas, for instance, of biomedicine, public health or digital capitalism.

The materialist approach offers the potential to design device assemblages with specific micropolitics and affect economies that can further such objectives, and the paper has offered the possibility of a 'resisting' device-assemblage that might achieve certain capacities to address community-level health needs or counter threats to health, for instance, from local polluters or developers. In part, such a resisting assemblage works because of the affects designed into the technology (for example, enabling many-to-many sharing of data and community information, and providing access to resources), but it also inheres in the affectivity of its users, which in the example articulated earlier within this resisting perspective included a collective rather than individualised orientation and an antagonism to top-down power associated with both biomedicine and digital capitalism.

If the last century saw the rise of industrialised medicine, and the dominance of a biomedical model of health, I would suggest that we are now living in an era in which digital technologies open the door to the colonisation of health care by digital capitalism, undermining those jurisdictions in which socialised medicine and not-for-profit welfare systems have until now resisted the full-blown marketisation of health. As such, DHTs pose a clear and present danger. However, I have argued here that they also supply opportunities for community, public health and activist groups to contribute to an agenda for health activism and citizen health. In this alternative future, a new generation of DHTs that resist and subvert the consumerisation, biomedicalisation and individualisation of health can play their part.

Notes

1 See https://analogrepublic.com/work/ms-mosaic.
2 See https://splendid-program.eu/.
3 See http://www.voda.com.
4 Vida Health's business model also establishes employee health as a core concern for business and public sector organisations, introducing a neo-paternalist (SCHRAM et al. 2010) element into workplace relations.

References

ANSELL PEARSON, K. 1999. *Germinal Life*. London: Routledge.
BARAD, K. 1996. Meeting the universe halfway; realism and social constructivism without contradiction. In Nelson, L.H. & Nelson, J. (eds) *Feminism, Science and the Philosophy of Science*. Dordrecht: Kluwer: 161–194.
BARASSI, V. 2015. *Activism on the Web: Everyday Struggles Against Digital Capitalism*. London: Routledge.
BRAIDOTTI, R. 2000. Teratologies. In Buchanan, I. & Colebrook, C. (eds.) *Deleuze and Feminist Theory*. Edinburgh: Edinburgh University Press: 156–172.
BRAIDOTTI, R. 2013. *The Posthuman*. Cambridge: Polity.
CLOUGH, P.T. 2004. Future matters: technoscience, global politics, and cultural criticism. *Social Text* 22(3): 1–23.
COOLE, D.H. & FROST, S. 2010. Introducing the new materialisms. In COOLE, D.H. & FROST, S. (eds) *New Materialisms: Ontology, Agency, and Politics*. Durham, NC: Duke University Press: 1–43.
CRUBÉZY, E.; MURAIL, P. & L. GIRARD et al. 1998. False teeth of the Roman world. *Nature* 391 (1 Jan 1998): 29.
DELANDA, M. 2006. *A New Philosophy of Society*. London: Continuum.
DELEUZE, G. 1988. *Spinoza. Practical Philosophy*. San Francisco CA: City Lights.
FAULKNER-GURSTEIN, R. & WYATT, D. 2023. Platform NHS: reconfiguring a public service in the age of digital capitalism. *Science, Technology & Human Values* 48(4): 888–908.
FORTUNE BUSINESS INSIGHTS 2023. Medical Devices. Global Market Analysis, Insights and Forecast, 2023-2030. *Fortune Business Insights* (online summary). https://www.fortunebusinessinsights.com/industry-reports/medical-devices-market-100085 [08.09.2023].
FOX, N.J. 2017. Personal health technologies, micropolitics and resistance: A new materialist analysis. *Health* 21(2): 136–153.
––– & Alldred, P. 2015. Inside the research-assemblage: new materialism and the micropolitics of social inquiry. *Sociological Research Online* 20(2): 6. http://www.socresonline.org.uk/20/2/6.html [08.02.2020].
––– 2017. *Sociology and the New Materialism*. London: Sage.
––– 2020. Re-assembling climate change policy: Materialism, posthumanism, and the policy assemblage. *British Journal of Sociology* 71(2), 269–283. https://on-

Fuchs, C. 2018. Capitalism, patriarchy, slavery, and racism in the age of digital capitalism and digital labour. *Critical Sociology* 44(4-5): 677–702.

Goldenberg, I.; J. Gillespie & Moss, A.J. et al. 2010. Long-term benefit of primary prevention with an implantable cardioverter-defibrillator. *Circulation* 12(2): 1265–1271.

Grabher, G. & van Tuijl, E. 2020. Uber-production: From global networks to digital platforms. *Environment and Planning A: Economy and Space* 52, 1005–1016.

Kaplan, R.M. & Stone, A.A. 2013. Bringing the laboratory and clinic to the community: mobile technologies for health promotion and disease prevention. *Annual Review of Psychology* 64: 471–498.

Karthick, R.; Ramkumar, R.; Akram, M. & Kumar, M.V. 2021. Overcome the challenges in bio-medical instruments using IOT-A review. *Materials Today: Proceedings* 45: 1614–1619.

Latour, B. 2005. *Reassembling the Social*. Oxford: Oxford University Press.

Lee, VR. 2013. The Quantified Self QS. movement and some emerging opportunities for the educational technology field. *Educational Technology* (Nov/Dec 2013): 39–42. http://digitalcommons.usu.edu/itls_facpub/480 [08.02.2020].

Lewis, C. 2017. Duke researchers launch app to monitor MS symptoms. *Duke Health*. https://physicians.dukehealth.org/articles/duke-researchers-launch-app-monitor-ms-symptoms [08.02.2020].

Loomba, S. & Khairnar A. 2018. Fitness Trackers Market by Device Type. Allied Market Research. https://www.alliedmarketresearch.com/fitness-tracker-market [11.01.2020].

Lupton, D. 2013. Quantifying the body: monitoring and measuring health in the age of mHealth technologies. *Critical Public Health* 23(4): 393–403.

— 2014. Self-tracking modes: reflexive self-monitoring and data practices. In *Imminent Citizenships: Personhood and Identity Politics in the Informatic Age workshop*, Australian National University, Canberra, 27 August 2014. https://papers.ssrn.com/sol3/papers.cfm?abstract_id=2483549 [08.02.2020].

— 2019. Toward a more-than-human analysis of digital health: inspirations from feminist new materialism. *Qualitative Health Research* 29(14): 1998–2009.

— 2021. Young people's use of digital health technologies in the global north: narrative review. *Journal of Medical Internet Research* 23(1): e18286.

Maisel, W.H. & Kohno, T. 2010. Improving the security and privacy of implantable medical devices. *New England Journal of Medicine* 362(13): 1164–1166.

Mao, A.Y.; Chen, C.; Magana, C.; Barajas, K.C. & Olayiwola, J.N. 2017. A mobile phone-based health coaching intervention for weight loss and blood pressure reduction in a national payer population: a retrospective study. *JMIR mHealth and uHealth* 5(6): e80.

Massumi, B. 1996. The autonomy of affect. In Patton, P. (ed) *Deleuze: a Critical Reader*. Oxford: Blackwell: 217–239.

McGregor, S. 2001. Neoliberalism and health care. *International Journal of Consumer Studies* 25(2): 82–89.

Mooney, G. 2012. Neoliberalism is bad for our health. *International Journal of Health Services* 42(3): 383–401.

Paddock, C. 2013. How self-monitoring is transforming health. *Medical News Today* (15 August 2013) http://www.medicalnewstoday.com/articles/264784.php [08.02.2020]:

Pantelopoulos, A. & Bourbakis, N.G. 2010. A survey on wearable sensor-based systems for health monitoring and prognosis. *IEEE Transactions on Systems, Man and Cybernetics – Part C: Applications and Reviews* 40(1): 1–12.

Parker, A.G.; Kantroo, V. & Lee, H.R. et al. 2012. Health promotion as activism: building community capacity to effect social change. *Proceedings of the SIGCHI Conference on Human Factors in Computing Systems*, 99-108. https://dl.acm.org/doi/abs/10.1145/2207676.2207692 [08.02.2020].

Patel, S.; Park, H. & Bonato, P. et al. 2012. A review of wearable sensors and systems with application in rehabilitation. *Journal of NeuroEngineering and Rehabilitation* 9: 21. https://jneuroengrehab.biomedcentral.com/articles/10.1186/1743-0003-9-21 [08.02.2020].

Ren, J. & Batra, J. 2013. *Personal Medical Device Technology-as-a-Service*. Sunnyvale, CA: MQ Identity Inc.

Rimal, R.N.; Ratzan, S.C. & Arnston, P. et al. 1997. Reconceptualizing the 'patient': health care promotion as increasing citizens' decision-making competencies. *Health Communication* 9(1): 61–74.

Rodgers, M.M.; Cohen, Z.A. & Joseph, L. et al. 2012. Workshop on personal motion technologies for healthy independent living: executive summary. *Archives of Physical Medicine and Rehabilitation* 93(6): 935–939.

Salesforce 2015. State of the Connected Patient. https://www.salesforce.com/form/conf/2015-state-connected-patient/ [08.02.2020].

Schiller, D. 2000. *Digital Capitalism: Networking the Global Market System*. Cambridge MA: MIT Press.

Schiller, D. 2011. Power under pressure: digital capitalism in crisis. *International Journal of Communication* 5: 924–941.

Schram, S.F.; Soss, J.; Houser, L. & Fording, R.C. 2010. The third level of US welfare reform: Governmentality under neoliberal paternalism. *Citizenship Studies* 14(6): 739–754.

Silicon Laboratories. n.d. The Heartbeat Behind Portable Medical Devices: Ultra-Low-Power Mixed-Signal Microcontrollers. http://www.silabs.com/Support%20Documents/TechnicalDocs/Personal-medical-device-market-white-paper.pdf [08.02.2020].

Staab, P. 2017. The consumption dilemma of digital capitalism. *Transfer: European Review of Labour and Research*, 23(3): 281–294.

Thomas, G.M.; Lupton, D. & Pedersen, S. 2018. 'The appy for a happy pappy': expectant fatherhood and pregnancy apps. *Journal of Gender Studies* 27(7): 759–770.

Till, C. 2014. Exercise as labour: quantified self and the transformation of exercise into labour. *Societies* 4: 446–462.

TOPHAM, D. 2003. *Medical Devices: The UK Industry and its Technology Development*. Loughborough: Prime Faraday Partnership, University of Loughborough.

VAN DER TUIN, I. & DOLPHIJN, R. 2010. The transversality of new materialism. *Women: A Cultural Review* 21(2): 153-171.

WEST, D.M. 2013. Improving Health Care through Mobile Medical Devices and Sensors. *Brookings Brief* (22 October 2013). http://www.brookings.edu/research/papers/2013/10/22-improving-health-care-mobile-medical-devices-apps-sensors-west [08.02.2020].

ZOLLER, H.M. 2005. Health activism: communication theory and action for social change. *Communication Theory* 15(4): 341-364.

This article has been subjected to a double blind peer review process prior to publication.

Nick J. Fox is one of the UK's leading proponents of new materialist and posthuman social theory. He has written widely on new materialist theory, sexualities, health, environment, research methods and political sociology, with over 100 peer-reviewed papers and books including *The Body* (Polity, 2012) and the groundbreaking *Sociology and the New Materialism* (Sage, 2017; with Pam Alldred, Nottingham Trent University London). Nick has held appointments at the Universities of Bristol and Sheffield, and is currently professor of sociology at the University of Huddersfield, UK. He is co-convenor of the British Sociological Association study group on new materialisms.

University of Huddersfield
Department of Behavioural and Social Sciences
School of Human and Health Sciences
Queensgate
Huddersfield HD1 3DH
e-mail: N.J.Fox@hud.ac.uk

Feeling Out of the Box

Ambivalences of Unexpected Amelioration among Sickened Health Professionals through Displacing Cooperations in Brazil

MÁRCIO VILAR

Abstract How do people with diagnosed autoimmune diseases feel, and what they do and think when they unexpectedly encounter an unregistered drug that may help them to heal, instead of palliatively controlling symptoms of autoimmune reactions through conventional immunosuppressants? What then if they are health professionals who became patients? How does such an encounter affect their lives, their perceptions and attitudes towards their respective medico-legal environments? In this article, I analyse letters exchanged between a physician in Brazil and eight of his patients, who are also health professionals, mainly between 1997 and 2000, concerning their experiencing of using an unregistered medicine, the "anti-brucellic vaccine" (VAB), to treat different immunopathologies such as rheumatoid arthritis. Considering VAB users as capable of systematically evaluating and communicating their experiences of illness and recovery, I seek to understand and discuss the tensions surrounding the repositionings and attitudes of affected health professionals within the co-production of medical evidence in the context of disruptive biotechnological innovation in Brazil. Apparently, their own experience with VAB seemed to have enabled them to re-ground their medical knowledge, experience, and skills in relation to their own and someone else's health in anticipation of the mediation regularly played out by conventional medical knowledge, technologies and procedures. Furthermore, when VAB-using physicians self-analyse and dialogue with others, writing and exchanging evaluative reports about their own and others' health and therapeutic experiences of using VAB, they seemed to implicitly co-produce medical evidence that can be taken into consideration by potential users.

Keywords immunotherapies – displacing cooperation – therapeutic narratives – evidence making – Brazil

> "In me what feels is always thinking."
> Fernando Pessoa (1969 [1914]: 144)

Introduction

In September 1997, physician GENÉSIO P. DA VEIGA received a letter from Luís asking him about the possibility of gaining treatment for his 55-year-old wife Fernanda, who was constantly suffering from joint pain in her knees, mostly in colder weather. Luís wrote that "according to medical orientation" (letter from 1997), Fernanda presented with symptoms of rheumatoid arthritis, a typical autoimmune disease characterized by joint inflammation that established rheumatology considers to be incurable and, therefore, chronic. Since her diagnosis, she had carried out conventional treatment with palliative drugs based on immunosuppression to relieve the symptoms. However, Luís was not sure "whether the medication is correct [...] or whether she has not been conducting the prescribed treatment adequately". He only knew that in the course of Fernanda's treatment, "the results [of using conventional drugs], in fact, have not been favourable until this moment". After being encouraged by one of his close friends, a physician living in a neighbouring city, whose respective wife considered herself "cured from arthritis" through VEIGA's treatment, Luís decided to contact Veiga directly, stating: "I would like to obtain your orientation to know how to proceed".

The therapy Luís was looking for was called "anti-brucellic vaccine" (VAB), a drug produced in Brazil by VEIGA and also used by other physicians and patients against several immunopathologies for many years. Nevertheless, following the rationale of vaccinotherapy as one of the biotherapies, which medico-scientists developed in the first half of the 20th century (LÖWY 2005; 2008; also COPE 1966: 39–61), and based on a colloidal understanding of immunopathologies as complex multifactorial metabolic disturbs sometimes referred to as *collagenosis* (e.g. SCHOR 1974), VAB has rather unspecific immunostimulating effects and is used for curative purposes. This approach is the opposite of that of immunosuppressants. The latter increasingly became the standard therapeutic approach to palliatively treat symptoms of immunopathologies worldwide concomitantly with the rise and acceptance of "autoimmunity" as a new biomedical paradigm (KUHN 2012[1962]), after which stimulation of one's immune system in the context of "autoimmune diseases" would worsen one's symptoms (ANDERSON & MACKAY 2014). Keeping up with this trend, even the newest and most technologically sophisticated pharmaceuticals offered in rheumatologic offices, such as the biologicals (e.g., monoclonal antibody drugs like adalimumab, etanercept, and rituximab), were designed to function in accordance with this same rationale. In 2005, the *Brazilian Health Regulatory Agency* (ANVISA) officially prohibited the production, commercialisation and distribution of VAB. Officially, for it was unregistered. After a period of approximately ten years circulating irregularly, VAB became available again through another medicinal product (VILAR 2024), just a few years before VEIGA's death at the age of 102 in early 2018.

A series of questions arise from this briefly resumed figuration, which entwines lay people, scientists and health professionals; chronicity and the witnessing of unexpected healing, globally established pharmaceuticals and a competing locally unregistered version of a Brucella-based immunostimulant drug to treat immunopathologies. For instance, how do physicians, caregivers and patients with diagnosed autoimmune diseases feel, think and act when they unanticipatedly encounter a therapy that helps them to heal, instead of palliatively controlling symptoms through conventional treatments? Which role do trust, medical knowledge, the senses and antigenic power play in the evaluation of people in adopting or refusing a novel therapy? What kinds of evidence, and means to produce evidence, meet the criteria to evaluate a new drug in the context of autoimmunity in Brazil and for whom?

In this article, I seek to understand some tensions surrounding the positioning of VAB users within the co-production of medical evidence in the face of disruptive biotechnological innovation and co-regulation in Brazil *before* VAB prohibition. My intention is to know how some of the conditions of possibility for physicians, patients and caregivers enabled these players to cooperate or not with each other in liminal contexts in Brazil. I particularly pay attention to different sorts of displacements that are implied when some among them cooperate to promote an off-label biotechnology that they see as innovative and promising. With this in mind, I here focus on one question that condenses the abovementioned interlinked problematizations. Given that several physicians tended to ignore and/or be understandably sceptical towards VAB, for it was absent in their treatment protocols, what could explain the uptake by some of these allopathic health professionals of VAB, as users and promoters, cooperating with VEIGA and, in some cases, regularly prescribing and/or recommending VAB?

To address this question, I analyse health reports in form of letters written by health professionals educated at medical schools who themselves became chronic patients or caregivers and who, after having personally witnessed VAB healing effects through unconventional means, began to cooperate with VEIGA, and occasionally engaged in VAB's promotion as a promissory biotechnological innovation. My argument is that, by seriously addressing how VAB users systematically evaluate and communicate their therapeutic experiences, it becomes possible to observe ambivalences that emerge when, as one finds on Luís' letter, a physician recommends an unregistered drug, and therefore endorses a therapeutic possibility that is largely unknown within established biomedicine.

According to CIARA KIERANS & KIRSTEN BELL, ambivalences can be seen "as something produced by (and productive of) our orientation to the social world" (2017: 26–27); and here I would include dis- and reorientation as well. Like technologies in general, and as an unauthorized biotechnology in particular, VAB might be "intrinsically ambivalent in its effects" (ibid.; referring to DE LAET & MOL 2000). Simultaneously, VAB's effects upon the world depend on the attitudes of those who encounter it, who (re)position VAB and themselves amidst flows and forces "within which [VAB is] made to work or fail" (KIERANS & BELL: 27). Thus, delineating VAB-related ambivalences might contribute, on the one hand, to reveal whom and what are involved in the networks of power through which VAB is circulated and informally co-regulated; be it as an object of dispute and/or a way to improve health, evidence making, market competition, ethical and moral questioning etc. On the other, it can reveal how VAB users deal with the dynamics of such networks, which often unfold through biomedical interstices, before the judicialization of VAB.

Apart from introduction and conclusion, this article is divided into two main sections. In the first, I briefly contextualise VAB's development and evidence-making issues, and recall general aspects of becoming a health professional and of related expectations. I also highlight some implications of working with letters as a way to learn about the therapeutic experiences and attitudes of VAB-related health professionals who deviated from standard treatments. In the second section, I approach central moments in the letters' authors' therapeutic trajectories, and consider the ways through which these sick health professionals became involved in the co-production of medical evidence as they moved from being immunosuppressant users to being VAB users. Mainly, I explore how they directly experience immunopathologies, conventional treatments and VAB, and how they re-assess their trained senses and ontoepistemological commitments before amelioration as standing between divergent biomedical therapeutic models, and respective orientations and expectations.

Contextualisation and analytical framing

Brucella, Brucellosis and VAB

"The vaccine", as many users referred to VAB, was indeed a lysate of dead Brucella, a bacterium that might cause an anthropozoonosis called brucellosis and has a multifaceted trajectory.

Since its identification by microbiologist DAVID BRUCE in Malta in 1886/1887 as responsible for the *Malta fever* (later called *undulant fever*), variations of the gram-negative bacteria genus Brucella have been extensively researched, mainly through the examination of host animals such as *brucella abortus* in cattle, *suis* in pigs, *melitensis* in goats and sheep, etc. (AKPINAR 2016). As several other microorganisms, Brucella – named after BRUCE – has an intriguing relationship with symptoms of immunopathologies in humans. However, the signs of its presence and agency in human bodies are hardly recognisable as its history of involvements with multiple scientific endeavours suggests, including the set of multidisciplinary apparatuses, practices and mindsets through which scientists could learn to perceive, conceptualize and work with it. For instance, Brucella has also been used as a material in the development of different biotechnologies ranging from vaccines (DE MELLO 1979) to bioweapons (PAPPAS et al. 2006). More recently, it also has become the object of proteomic and genomic analyses with paleontological and archaeological goals, which also investigate how brucella and animals have mutually adapted to each other in the long durée (GRECO et al. 2018; SUÁREZ-ESQUIVEL et al. 2020; ROTHSCHILD & HAEUSLER 2021).

In 1956, microbiologist GENÉSIO PACHECO, then president of the World Health Organization's "International Commission on Brucellosis", and primatologist MILTON THIAGO DE MELLO, later president of the Brazilian Academy of Veterinarian Medicine, both based at the Institute Oswaldo Cruz in Brazil, published a treatise on brucellosis in Portuguese (PACHECO & DE MELLO 1956). Pacheco also worked with VEIGA, who was his homonymous nephew and a recently graduated physician working as a laboratory technician at the National Plague Service. Yet, opposition from other physicians was common at that time, who contended that brucellosis was irrelevant in Brazil.

For decades, PACHECO and his team argued that the increasing number of cases of brucellosis among animals reflects its correspondent increase among humans. Its incidence "[...] in Brazil is huge [and] knowledge about its existence is too small, therefore its diffusion takes place freely" (PACHECO et al. 1969: 747). As VEIGA told me, this controversy arose partly on account of the symptomatology of brucellosis taught at the medical schools in the country, which had been based on its most common European variant, the *melitensis*. The problem being that in Brazil brucellosis was and still is predominantly provoked by the types *abortus* and *suis*, which present different symptoms. In addition, brucellosis is highly contagious. Known as a "disease of a thousand symptoms" (PACHECO et al. 1969: 752), it is difficult to diagnose, which has contributed to making brucellosis almost invisible as a health problem. Experts have therefore mostly ignored it, whilst local non-professionals have managed to identify the symptoms by comparing similar cases.

It was only in 2001 that the *Brazilian Federal Government* initiated the *National Program of Control and Eradication of Animal Brucellosis and Tuberculosis*, officially recognising brucellosis as a national epidemic. Although most medical professionals remain unacquainted with its spread among humans and continue to see it mainly as a zoonosis, recent studies corroborate the claims made by PACHECO and VEIGA that human brucellosis in Brazil is endemic, and its effects are multiple, and still largely misunderstood, and underestimated (e.g. MAURELIO et al. 2022; NOGUEIRA & DE CASTRO 2022; BOURDETTE & SANO 2023).

In 1979, DE MELLO called attention to a forty-year-long associated controversy around the best treatment for brucellosis. Several attempts had been made to develop vaccines that could substitute for the standard antibiotic-therapy. Among those vying for vaccine development, a further discussion arose as to whether to use living, attenuated or dead brucella (DE MELLO 1979: 676). PACHECO and his team had their own breakthrough in the 1960s with a "curative vaccine" named Bruvac (PACHECO et al. 1969), which they designed mainly to cure already contaminated patients. Whilst PACHECO used Bruvac, VEIGA used another similar registered drug called Brulise, which he had developed earlier. Both drugs were approved and registered by the then *Brazilian National Medicine and Pharmacy Inspection Service*. Nevertheless, the debate around best treatment rages on in Brazil and elsewhere (WARETH et al. 2020).

In the 1980s, after his retirement, VEIGA compared his own observations of VAB on arthritis-affected patients with brucellosis, with the results of a 1950s experiment (MEISELAS et al. 1961; VEIGA 1969). After finding evidence that VAB had the potential to treat arthritis, he adapted it to treat people with this and other immunopathologies off-label. Despite having been successfully applied in several cases, as the results of a small-scale study with 377 patients suggest, the treatment was not recognized in the established field of rheumatology and it did not figure in public health policies. With it, VEIGA's continued use of VAB entered a grey area.

Health professionals, medical competence and institutional reproduction

Some of VEIGA's patients were themselves also health professionals. To understand the impact of their VAB therapeutic experiences on their perceptions and attitudes regarding their personal, professional and institutional environments, and their approaches to drug evaluation, it is useful to first consider what it means to become and live as a health professional.

In general, the medical profession track includes a long education process that implies multiple changes related to, among others, personal knowledge, worldview, ethical posture, lifestyle, self-presentation, public and corporate commitments, social status, as well as perceptual, emotional and sensorial (pre)dispositions. As ethnographies of medical schools and physicians' education show (e.g. BECKER et al. 1992 [1961], ATKINSON 1976), this learning process tends to deeply affect their perception of their environments and how they pursue the goal of identifying and treating diseases in distinct ways.

On the one hand, medical students have to learn through a series of predefined exercises how to identify symptoms and relate them to a growing catalogue of described ailments. For that, neophytes should develop a receptiveness for what patients narrate about what they feel, and do not feel, in their bodies. Likewise, they should develop the skill, knowledge and practical capacity to "categorize and rank" (CARR 2010: 18) both whom utters and the uttered (FOUCAULT 1989 [1963]). That includes becoming able to (de)codify symptoms that sometimes remain invisible for the untutored eye. To remain functional when confronted with potentially stressful and overwhelming situations, they also learn to constrain their empathy through protective mechanisms such as by treating patients during surgical operations or emergencies (GOFFMAN 1961).

On the other hand, they are instructed about existing authorised technologies that aim to produce accurate, numeric views about the patients' vital signs, which their own human senses may not precisely ascertain, such as imaging occurrences under the skin, listening to air currents through the lungs, or gauging accurate body temperature readings. An important task for medicine and nursery students, thus, is to familiarise themselves with and learn to use such monitoring-intervening devices, from the most cutting-edge to the simplest ones (FAULKNER 2009).

Part of the training therefore consists of internalising the idea that medical technologies are more reliable than human feelings and perceptions, even though medical technologies function mostly as inorganic extensions of the physicians' bodies by helping them to sense, perceive and do things they could not do otherwise. Concomitantly, their users not only delegate much of their sensory capacities and judgments to these instruments but also are affected by them in several ways. Put differently, in tandem with the development of their professional skills, neophytes learn to commit to and co-operate with technologies, and the premises upon which they were designed, which sometimes may even take over their tasks, and reframe their techno-scientific, sensorial and intuitive calculations.

Likewise, prospective health professionals must learn which drug one should prescribe from those authorised by legal-scientific institutions responsible for separating what works from what does not, what belongs to Medicine and what does not. As part of scientific and health institutions, physicians and bioscientists have to know what they come to know through reliable sources of information and truth (e.g. BEISEL, CALKINS & ROTTENBURG 2018). These comprise institutionalized means to which they commit and which they reproduce in order to reproduce themselves as recognisable legitimate health professionals and, despite internal differences and contradictions, to take part in medical and life sciences as if these were a single unified body. I.e. at least as a façade that stands before and is continually re-introduced as such to uninitiated audiences.

That is why the use of devices and substances designed or converted for medical purpose is regulated by legitimate institutions that establish the standards of what counts as evidence, proof, and truth through conventions. These same conventions produce official documents in which the elements that constitute and reproduce biomedicine are framed, filtered, stabilised, and actualised, such as curricula, legislation, treatment protocols, techno-regulatory and ethics guidelines, and research agendas (CAMBROSIO 2010). Thus, entering the biomedical world as a health professional who co-constitutes it, and who is also co-produced by it, also unfolds as a displacement from an ordinary life. This displacement simultaneously generates a distinctive consciousness which is co-formative of a particular epistemic culture, and therefore of a way of being in the world (KNORR-CETINA 2007: 363).

This does not mean that health professionals live in a parallel reality. Far to the contrary, the efforts of differentiation that make up biomedicine take place amidst contingent alliances and conflicts between sociocultural, politico-economic, scientific-religious and other-than-human forces that affect and are affected by them (FLECK 2019 [1935]). Biomedical realities express, co-constitute and are co-constituted by the geopolitical and historical circumstances under which they emerge. In other words, the distinct consciousness, recurrent practices and affective predispositions normally associated with the formation of health professionals are *installed* within the broader society in which they act as institutional actors who "play critical roles in stabilizing and maintaining institutional arrangements, as well as power structures within them" (CHURCHER et al. 2023: 11). In this sense, for instance, health professionals (re) produce distinctive marks that help them preserve their recognisability as authoritative and legitimate professional medical practitioners.

Yet, what happens to this distinct consciousness and the behaviour associated to it when health professionals become chronically ill, go through conventional treatments without positive results, and then try an unconventional therapy, to which they attribute a substantial amelioration of their condition?

Letters as research material and as sensorial mediums

To sketch a picture of the therapeutic journeys of health professionals who used VAB to treat rheumatoid arthritis, I explore eight letters sent to Veiga. These were mostly written between 1997 and 2000 by a cardiologist, a veterinarian, a nurse, a psychologist, a general surgeon, a dentist, a clinician, and a health insurance agent. I selected them from hundreds of letters that are part of the vast personal archive of Veiga, which grew over the decades since the 1980s, and to which I obtained access, for these are the ones which reveal a singular perspectival conjunction. I.e., their authors were (or still are) health professionals, chronic patients, users of conventional and then unconventional treatment, and finally patients in recovery process, or healed ones. I did not find negative self-reports written by these or other health professionals within any of my research materials that I could use here to counterbalance the positive ones.

On two occasions after Veiga's passing, a close relative and guardian of his letters, as well as a central interlocutor in my research since 2018, granted me access to the originals and allowed me to copy those of almost 300 authors, in 2019 and 2021. As I explain elsewhere (Vilar 2024), my access to them and further research empirical materials was facilitated, among other reasons, by my status as a former VAB user. Some of these letters were with a collaborating physician who was initially unsure about bringing the letters to one of our meetings, but changed his mind after having talked to their guardian. In principle, these were all letters that Veiga's relative-guardian and their collaborators keep with them. The rest remain scattered.

As parts of an archive that can no longer be found in a single place, many letters were lost through residence changes in the last years. Besides, Veiga discretely had forwarded some to medical scientists and health professionals to draw their attention to VAB's efficacy and to potentially initiate medico-scientific cooperation. For instance, in a private letter written in 1988 to Veiga, a scientific collaborator and professor of biomedicine at a public university reported the results of tests that he conducted with VAB in animals:

I did an experiment where I induced arthritis in rats using collagen II and, during the induction time, I vaccinated two groups of rats with the [Brucella] endotoxin in the dilutions of 1/100 and 1/500 against another group that received physiological saline. In 15 days, all animals that received saline presented symptoms of arthritis in the joints of the hind legs and those that received the vaccine, in both groups, had nothing.

In another experiment, three groups of animals received, with an interval of three days, for 30 days, the vaccine in dilutions of 1/50, 1/100 and 1/500 each group. After this period, all animals and a control group that had received saline were treated with collagen II to induce arthritis. After 28 days, we obtained the following result: All animals in the control group [...] had arthritic symptoms. Those who received vaccine diluted 1/100 and 1/500 did not show symptoms. This experiment is being repeated.

Apart from this cooperation at laboratory level, the great majority of the letters consists of partial health reports written by lay VAB users, at different moments of their therapy, in response to Veiga's request for evaluation of his treatment. The identities of the letters' authors are diverse and include not only diagnosed people but also caregivers, patients' relatives, and accompanying physicians. Many wrote messages on the back of the self-evaluation form that was sent to them by Veiga, and some attached the results of their laboratory exams. Some letters point to how health professionals worked in cooperation with patients to decide frequency and dosages at the clinical and ambulatory contexts.

These correspondences generally unfolded at the same time as phone conversations between Veiga and his patients which aimed to monitor and eventually modify the dosages in the course of the therapy. In their narratives, VAB users frequently describe early attempts to get better by using conventional treatments, and sometimes explain their emotional states and living conditions before, after and during their shift from immunosuppressants to VAB. Extrapolating Veiga's request for therapeutic feedback, the letters not only communicate the change of symptoms and substantial improvement or cure, but also gratitude, good wishes, indignation, hope, fear, anger, relief, encouragement, frustration, thoughts about conventional pharmaceuticals, medical institutions and the value of living. I therefore use this rich content to analyse these letters as textual narratives.

As ANNE BYRNE states, "the importance of narrative for framing, understanding, and interpreting experience and organizing knowledge of the world is now widely recognized by scholars and researchers […]" (2017: 44; see also CORTAZZI 2001; STANLEY 2004). While acknowledging the limitations of letters (for example, that they represent only one side of a conversation, which is only partially available, and that there is little biographical knowledge of their authors), one can understand and explore them as dialogical and reciprocal textual narratives that are part of ongoing correspondences in at least two ways.

Firstly, as a "discourse with a clear sequential order that connects events in a meaningful way for a definite audience and thus offers insights about the world and/or people's experiences of it" (BYRNE 2017: 44; referring to HINCHMAN & HINCHMAN 1997: xvi). These insights, presented from the perspective of letters' authors as insiders, include matters of "private, personal, or familial interests [and] a situation or professional occupation, proffering a public profile to fit the human qualities of personal or professional practices" (BYRNE 2017: 45). Secondly, the letters can be attended to as "a story with a plot involving a change in the situations of fortunes of a main character" (ibid.: 44). Letters are registers of key moments of the authors' ongoing and contingent interpretative processes, providing researchers with the opportunity to focus "on the roles of narrative participants in constructing accounts and in negotiating perspectives and meanings" (ibid.), as well as to know "the techniques and strategies that writers use to tell their story" (ibid.).

Given the heterogeneity of the papers, such as the ink used, markers of the passage of time, diverse calligraphies, attached documents, disclosed personal information of their authors, quantity and diversity of accompanying stamped letter envelopes etc., I had no doubt of the authenticity of the letters that I analyse here; a conviction reinforced by other aspects. In principle, as letters addressed privately to a health professional, most of their authors did not have the pretension to turn them into public documents. Even though many writers were clearly willing to contribute to VEIGA's efforts to demonstrate VAB's efficacy and legitimacy to the biomedical establishment, and seemed aware that someone else could read their messages later (SIMMEL 1992[1908]: 429–432), the letters, as sensorial mediums, are primarily situated within the domain of physician-patients relationships, and therefore subjected, in principle, to concealment and discretion.

Furthermore, in contrast to the private exchange of letters and phone calls of VEIGA's era, nowadays most cooperation work between scientists and non-scientists to underpin biotechnological innovations, in general, take place via the internet (e.g. SLEEBOOM-FAULKNER 2014; SONG 2017; PETERSEN et al 2019). Social networks became popular in Brazil from the 2000s and the internet became an ideal public platform through which strangers can share therapeutic stories, and get together. Instead, the private letters to VEIGA were generally not aimed at influencing public opinion or at pressuring medico-regulatory institutions. Not least, the letters that I use here, with one exception, were written and exchanged before ANVISA prohibited VAB.

Self-reports as medical evidence

To my knowledge, VEIGA never publicly revealed the letters that he received from his patients and collaborators. When he was formally prosecuted, he included 34 letters in his legal defence, but only the judge and the involved parties could access these. However, it is clear that he aimed to use them to enrich a broader corpus of medical evidence that could help improve VAB's status. Hence, he privately shared and discussed some of them as medical cases with medical partners and potential scientific collaborators.

Yet, a major ambivalence arose during such cooperations given that a progressive dismissal of patients' narratives and testimonies in the standard process of evaluating the therapeutic effects of substances was concomitantly taking place. While personal therapeutic experiences and respective narratives are vital in producing diagnoses, they do not always play a role in the evaluation of the effects of substances that are proposed as potential pharmaceuticals. Reverberating an axiom of modern medical science after which a "*cure proves nothing*" (STENGERS 2003: 14), one of the main arguments used to justify this dismissal is the view that human senses, perceptions and feelings, being apprehended as subjectivity, would contaminate neutral and/or objective assessments of antigenic power (e.g. GREENHALGH 2001: 301; BALAJ 2022).

In the context of efforts to overcome related limitations, practices such as randomised clinical trials (RCTs) have increased and gained legitimacy worldwide. This particular set of standard scientific criteria for the discovery of universal truths has since the 1990s had a decisive impact on the approval or refusal of any drug by regulatory institutions, including VAB. To illustrate this, I now make a short comparative digression by setting out the way in which a central legal institution in Brazil argued against the liberalisation of another contested drug, which had been presented as an unspecific immunostimulant.

In contrast to VAB, which remained a silent controversy, the case involving the synthetic phosphoethanolamine (or "Fosfo") as a promissory cure for cancer gained worldwide resonance (CASTRO 2017; FERRANTE 2019; VILAR 2020). By stating that the law 13.269, of 13 April 2016, which facilitated access to Fosfo in exceptional circumstances and without being registered at ANVISA, was not based on "rational justification", the then Prosecutor General of the Republic of Brazil (PGR) echoed further similar explanations argued by medico-scientific regulatory institutions (PGR 2018, 22 October: 8). Emphasizing that evidence-based medicine (EBM), as a "systematic process of discovering, evaluating and using findings as a base for clinic decisions", is the established model for the production of scientific evidence in Brazil, the PGR argued that the use of published "scientific articles of partial research results" and of "unsystematic patients reports" are inadequate evidence of a substance's capacity to heal (ibid.: 7–9).

In disqualifying involved scientists and stakeholders, it seems that here too, as ISABELLE STENGERS observes elsewhere, *"irrationality"* (2003: 15, emphasis in original) is mobilized "to condemn not only charlatans who use cures as proof of some kind of snakes oil's effectiveness, but also the public that lets itself be taken in by this proof" (ibid.: 16). Nevertheless, in principle, in imagining and seeking to practice rational measurements of health realities exclusively through vehicles that circumnavigate human affects, established biomedicine and regulatory science run the risk of producing knowledge that is detached from lived experience (INGOLD 2010). Not for nothing, EBM and its component RCTs have been regularly criticised by members of medical communities, social scientists and humanities scholars (e.g. EPSTEIN 1995; MCKEVITT 2013; ADAMS 2016; AHUJA 2019; RATNANI et al. 2023). Some of EBM's limitations might reproduce and deepen the discrepancy between biomedicine as part of a modern science's longing to apprehend reality from outside it and this same reality as though scientists would not inhabit it and participate in it (MERLEAU-PONTY 2007 [1961]; TAMBIAH 1990).

In VAB's case, sick health professionals searching for further therapeutic possibilities are among several actors who "navigate contemporary medical, humanitarian, and governmental regimes in search of rights and resources" (ADAMS & BIEHL 2016: 124), including healing ones, and expose themselves to the unknown.

> Experiences, often unpredictable, of the social, political, and medical effects of interventions also give rise to new claims of efficacy, new regimes of truth and falsity, and new political and epistemological engagements with outcomes that matter to people. These cumulative experiences form alternative, practice-based forms of evidence that can challenge orthodoxies and perceptual deficits of all kinds and are, in our view, the very fabric of alternative theorizing in global health and beyond. (ibid.)

Indeed, VEIGA and his collaborators did nothing to oppose an EBM approach. To the contrary, they were willing to combine EBM with further modes of knowledge production that included patients' narratives about their own therapeutic experiences, laboratory tests and bibliographic research. They also used methods of comparison with conventional drugs, by integrating data from the accumulated therapeutic experiences. VEIGA also sought to co-organise a clinical trial in the early 1990s with rheumatologists in the city of São Paulo that were recommended to him by the *Health Municipal Secretary*. He contacted them for this purpose. However, as he argued in his defence, they simply did not answer.

Mutual affects between sick health professionals, conventional drugs and VAB

Feeling and communicating pain and following standard treatment

In his letter from 1998, veterinarian Juarez, from Paraguay, stated that his problem "started with severe pain in my left arm one night in April 1990". Although the pain apparently vanished after he took "some anti-inflammatory drugs, muscle relaxants, etc. [...] as the days went by, there were pains in the joints of the fingers, wrists, wristbands, which forced me to consult with a rheumatologist". Similarly, surgeon Xavier explained that in "1990, I was affected by an inflammatory process in all joints of my body, having all the evidences of positive rheumatic activities". As in JUAREZ's case, XAVIER also sought a rheumatologist who conducted laboratory tests, which confirmed his prediction. Not all health professionals treated by VEIGA had arthritis. Navy doctor Kalil, for instance, explained that in his case it is "another immunological disorder – *pemphigus vulgaris* – confirmed by histopathological examination".

Usually, as soon as a physician, as an institutional actor, produces a diagnosis attesting an immunopathology, palliative therapy begins. "We immediately started conventional treatment based on ASA [acetylsalicylic acid] (6 g. x day), indomethacin (50 g. x day) and chloroquine diphosphate", wrote XAVIER. In Juarez's case, the rheumatologist gave him "a series of possibilities to start the treatment, which in the end were based on diclofenac, methotrexate, chloroquine, plus 5 mg of cortisone". Routine laboratory tests continued as part of medical monitoring. Despite that, JUAREZ stated: "My general condition remained the same if no improvement, with mild to severe pain, and the perception I had about the disease was that it increasingly compromised more joints, hands, elbows, soles etc." Like others who undergo palliative treatment, Juarez sought further physicians and medical possibilities, switching "from doctor to doctor", as another VAB user wrote. Indeed, Xavier's experience of recurrent inflammations is emblematic of what many chronic patients go through:

After a long period of use of drugs with changes in anti-inflammatory drugs to piroxicam, sodium diclofenac, always used with analgesics such as dipyrone and protectors of the gastric mucosa such as cimetidine, there was no improvement in the condition. I could even say that there was a worsening. (Letter from 1997)

Juarez's experience with conventional treatment echoes that of Xavier with the difference that the first more explicitly expressed his fear that the excessive and regular use of palliative drugs was causing his malaise.

A year later and with three years or so since the beginning of the disease [...], I started to have a new pain crisis more intense than usual. I then went to another rheumatologist who advised me on applications with gold salts, diclofenac, cortisone 5 mg, after a while chloroquine was added, the gold salts applied every 15 days. I can tell you that with this treatment or with this scheme, I stayed for almost five years, having the disease relatively controlled, but always in pain. At a certain time of the year with more pain than at others, but always taking medication, which has always worried me about the time I spend taking these medications. Until, on one occasion, in one of the many routine checks that I did every three months with the doctor, I realized that the disease was progressing and bothering me more each day. (Letter from 1998)

Further health professionals shared the concern that conventional treatment negatively affects the health of chronic patients. General practitioner ARTHUR, for instance, who reported on the health state and therapeutic experience of his wife, Catarina, who was diagnosed with polyarthralgia, verified long-term sequels occasioned by additional drugs that should relieve the side effects of primary drugs. According to him, for five years, Catarina "suffered from widespread pain, which periodically removed her from work, creating serious professional problems. She underwent all conventional treatments given by rheumatologists, such as anti-inflammatory drugs that ended up altering her gastric mucosa with pains that persist today" (letter from 2000). In the case of Luísa, an experienced nurse, it did not help to look for further treatment possibilities in Europe. As she wrote, "I went through several specialists and each one saturated me more with so many medications, which only caused me more pain, because I was already impregnated with so many drugs for pain and this only complicated me, [so much so that] even my human dignity was shaken" (letter from 2013).

As I could observe in public talks, rheumatologists ascertain that contemporary immunosuppressants have less side effects as the medication used in the 1990s (VILAR 2024). The fulfilment of the biomedical promise of a stabilised relief for autoimmune symptoms, i.e., of achieving "remission" (instead of searching for a "cure"), remains understood as being conditional on patients remaining on their palliative path. And yet, despite several technological changes, the standard treatment remains guided by the same immunosuppression-centred thought style and, consequently, palliative. Not surprisingly, as CHARLES E. ROSENBERG wrote not long ago, "For the clinician, [...] [autoimmune diseases] are a group of well-established, if frustratingly intractable, ailments to be diagnosed and treated. For sufferers and their families they are misfortunes to be experienced and endured" (ROSENBERG 2014: xi). This seems also valid for health professionals as patients.

Involuntary symmetrisation
According to some studies, when physicians become chronic patients, they may change their perception and actions towards their patients and colleagues as part of their pursuit of learning how to live as a permanently ill person (e.g. KLITZMAN 2008; KAY et al. 2008; OPRISAN et al. 2016). As doctors in patients' clothes and vice versa, sick physicians and other health professionals keep both roles while interacting ambiguously with the health care system, from receiving pharmaceutical treatment after diagnosis to regular check-ups. These interventions not only occasionally relativize their medical authorities by turning them into patients of other health professionals, but also co-shape their horizons of expectation, and their intimate and personal lives.

In contrast to people with curable diseases, people with chronic ones in general, and immunopathologies in particular, are regarded as (virtually) perpetually ill and likely to become increasingly unwell. By becoming artificially immunocompromised through immunosuppressants, which in addition to their often short-term effects and high costs normally provoke several side effects leading them to take additional drugs for their life time (DUMIT 2012), such chronically ill patients begin relationships with new actors and within new networks that characterise the world of disability which they join from the moment of diagnosis onwards. In this world, they actively recreate themselves as immunocompromised persons while seeking to achieve remission, retard the inevitable, control the unpredictable, and protect themselves from quackery.

Yet, their unintended initiation into the realm of chronic living seems to lead to at least two mutually implicated situations in their lives. Firstly, they become displaced from the position of figures symbolically immune against and/or above ailments, and now they occupy places of vulnerability. Secondly, by seeking to come to terms with their conditions, they are granted the possibility of diminishing the distance between themselves and their patients. In other words, having a first-hand understanding of how their patients feel in multiple situations in their daily lives, being affected by comparable *intensities* (FAVRET-SAADA 2012: 441–442), including unsignifiable ones and knowing unmeasurable pain that are hard to see, sick health professionals might recalibrate the usual differentiations between themselves and their patients, and the diseases which they seek to treat. They now unintentionally face a mutually understandable destiny.

Moreover, in reporting symptoms through their letters, sick health professionals did not only verbalize visible potential signs on the surface of their bodies to VEIGA but also those intensities that they could feel under their skin. As they shifted their sensorial attention between their bodily interior and exterior as interconnected environments, they articulated their feelings and perceptions with their vocabulary and knowledge in ways that render them intelligible. This includes regarding symptoms as discontinuities of an otherwise healthy state. While assessing changes in their health by paying attention to their exteroceptive and interoceptive senses, they interacted with a multitude of others. In so doing, they seemed to co-manipulate and describe their health state while discerning between different intensities at play in and through their bodies, particularly the impact of different medications.

Switching treatments

The feeling of not getting better after years of treatment, and the recognition that illness may only worsen, seem to be a key moment during the therapeutic journey of a chronic patient. A growing scepticism concerning the effects of existing conventional pharmaceuticals may provoke a fissure in the trust that keep their expectation attached to the palliative path, opening up patients' receptivity towards unknown therapies. Besides the possibility of skipping standard treatment altogether (e.g. DUMIT 2012: 174–179), the revelation that the biomedical expectation of a future cure will not be fulfilled within one's life span tend to reinforce the chronic patient's disposition to look for something outside the palliative path. This potential search is also partially encouraged by rheumatologists themselves, who often orient their clients to try to find out what might be good to control inflammation processes on a more individual level (such as physiotherapy, diet and psychological support). However, for them this should only be pursued *as long as it does not jeopardize the conventional treatment*, what is clearly not the case for many people who come across VAB.

"Already disillusioned and sad for not getting better with conventional treatment and physiotherapy, I heard about the vaccine", wrote XAVIER (letter from 1997). Given the emerging lack of prospects and the constant search for relief, dental surgeon Ana expressed her decision *to bet* on VAB:

> I use VAB as an alternative for the treatment of RSI [repetitive strain injury] since January 1996 on my own initiative. I received a referral from a friend and I myself sought treatment because I had already undergone many previous therapies without any results. I was not induced to use it, nor to believe it would be efficient. Due to the lack of alternative treatments, I read Dr Veiga's explanatory leaflets and decided to use VAB. (Letter from 1997)

Prospective VAB users had to evaluate the many potential risks of taking an unregistered substance that is little known amongst rheumatologists. They also had to evaluate the requirement to quit conventional treatments to allow VAB to work properly. As I stated in the introduction, while VAB works through a stimulation of one's immunity as a way to rehabilitate it, palliative treatments are engaged in suppressing the immune system's activities to prevent an increase of autoimmune symptoms. In principle, these therapeutic models are mutually exclusive. To adopt one means to have to give up the other.

The experiences of people abandoning conventional treatment as a condition for using VAB vary. Being a health professional makes the decision more difficult. An eventual adoption of VAB automatically re-positions those health professionals who opted to try it, as their decision puts them *en route* to collision with not only authorized pharmaceuticals, but also with the authorisers (i.e., the medico-legal institutions themselves to which they are committed as licensed medical experts), including their own colleagues.

Arthur described his dilemma when he heard about VAB for the first time and resisted his wife Catarina's decision to use it:

> In 1997, a friend of the family, a non-rheumatologist, ordered VAB and presented it to my wife based on results she had already seen. I confess that, at that time, I did not believe in this vaccine unknown in the medical field and I even advised my wife not to use it for fear of the side effects that could arise. (Letter from 2000)

However, Catarina chose *to bet* on a close friend's favourable testimony of VAB as a guarantee in the face of the potential risks of adopting an off-label drug, rather than on her physician-husband's suspicion who did not know about VAB. As Arthur explains, "Despite my advice and driven by the hope of being without the pain, my wife took the vaccine religiously for a year, with another year of maintenance dose, having finished the treatment in July 1999" (letter from 2000). In this case, it may appear at first that trust based on institutionalised expertise (i.e., vertical, hierarchic) was subsumed to trust based on friendship (i.e., horizontal, non-hierarchic). Yet, the positive experience of Catarina's close friend regarding VAB rather occupied a gap within her husband's medical education. After all, ARTHUR's suspicion concerning VAB was not based on homologated biomedical knowledge about VAB's effects but rather on its absence. Therefore, there was no institutionalised expertise to consult. In other words, Catarina was not standing between two truths but rather between her friend's shared hope based on personal experience with a specific thing and her husband's shared fear of the unknown based on an impersonal general caution.

Similarly, health professionals can discuss their decision on whether to adopt VAB with friends who sometimes belong to the medical field. In Juarez's case, a physician friend, knowing about his health state, informed him about VAB, as this friend had "a daughter who had the same problem" (letter from 1998).

Beyond the mobilisation of trust present in the dynamics of mutual identification and interpersonal relationships, several potential users travelled long distances to meet Veiga, to have their health state directly evaluated by him and learn more about VAB. Veiga administered VAB case by case, according to the individual medical history of each patient. Sometimes, people were advised to completely stop conventional treatments before starting VAB, whereas others would gradually decrease conventional drugs. According to Arthur's observations about Catarina's treatment, "already in the middle of the treatment, she started to feel pain relief and abandoned the use of anti-inflammatory drugs" (letter from 2000). Xavier stated, "I abandoned the use of conventional treatment and today I use only the vaccine and, when there is some worsening of the disease, I use some anti-inflammatory" (letter from 1997). Luísa explained that "three months after undergoing VAB treatment, [...] I no longer take the drugs I used to take. I only take the vaccines. [...] As I am a nurse, after starting the vaccine, I gradually weaned off the medications" (letter from 2013). Juarez also described coming off elements of his medication regime:

> I started treatment on July 11, 1998. At that time, I was taking 200 mg of chloroquine daily, plus fortnightly applications of gold salts (sodium aurothiosulfate 0.05 mg), plus 100 mg of daily backup, plus 5 mg of cortisone also daily. Today, almost 90 days after starting the first dose of the vaccine, I am taking 100 mg of voltaren and 5 mg of cortisone daily. The other drugs (gold salts, chloroquine) have been suspended since the vaccine started. (Letter from 1998)

Based on their specialities, I assume that most of the letters' authors worked more as technicians than as scientists searching for biotechnological innovations. They followed pre-established protocols and tended to use and reproduce therapeutic techniques, drugs and devices designed by someone else, without necessarily having to critically reflect on their own practices (as institutionalised ones), despite the tinkering that their professional praxis requires (LÖWY 2008: 172). Yet, when confronted with the option of adopting VAB they have to take a decision and think about it without having other previously elaborated biomedical thinking route to rely on.

Switching treatments would inevitably provoke attritions within their biomedical worlds by turning professional expectations upside-down, as some related acts of biomedical disobedience that I addressed elsewhere show (e.g. VILAR 2020; 2024). Nevertheless, not only their health, career and reputation might be put in risk. If, unexpectedly, the adopted unconventional drug positively works by doing exactly the opposite of what the conventional treatment does, then switching treatments might result in a mutual estrangement and potential decoupling between those health professionals who try it and the hegemonic immunosuppression paradigm.

Feeling and communicating amelioration and using VAB

Of the eight health professionals I foreground here who became patients and VAB users, Flávia was the only patient who stated that she could not cease conventional treatments. As she put it, "I would love to be able to reduce this medication, but I don't see how to get rid of the corticoid", yet she "felt a marked improvement, [...] and the crises are not so intense anymore" (letter from 1997). The other health professionals, on the contrary, reported relief when departing from conventional treatment. As Iara wrote, "What has bothered me a lot is the feet. [The right foot] hurts more than the left, but just being able to run out of cortisone and anti-inflammatory drugs is already great" (letter from 1997). She continued:

> I started the second glass [i.e. phial] on 14 July 1997, and I have a 90% improvement in my general condition, I have not felt any more reactions, neither allergic nor pain (reaction). I still feel pain,

except that my knees have improved a lot. [...] Foot pain is constant, but you can take it. [...] I have slept better and I am 70% more active (agile) in everything, the morning stiffness has decreased 70%, I am already exercising my activities in the clinic where I work almost normally. I can already lift weights above five kg (before I couldn't even do 500 g). (Letter from 1997)

Iara's "reactions" correspond to those that may eventually occur when one increases VAB dosage during the desensitization phase of VEIGA's therapy, which in total took two to three years on average. VAB users feel and perceive such reactions through a worsening, instead of a weakening, of the autoimmune symptoms few hours after a dosage change. In this case, VEIGA instructed the patient to repeat the previous dosage a couple of times before increasing it again some weeks later. In her letter, Iara's past reactions are overshadowed by her description of health improvements.

Also emphatically, Xavier wrote that his amelioration was not only physical but emotional as well.

I started using [VAB] according to [VEIGA's] orientation and, after the first bottles [i.e. phials], it started to get better oedema, pain, morning stiffness, walking improved and also the joy of life, because the irritability and depression caused by the disease disappeared. [...] More than three years after using the vaccine, without interruption, if I am still not cured, I had an improvement of 70% of the previous condition and, I must add that during all this period that I used the vaccine, I never had a side effect. [...] Therefore, it is worth mentioning that the vaccine was important in my recovery and, perhaps without it today, I would be in a wheelchair or inactive in a bed. (Letter from 1997)

There are VAB users who go as far as to speak about *cure*, as Kalil did:

I interrupted [i.e. concluded] my treatment after 198 injections according to the instructions given to me by [Veiga's] brochures and by [him] on some phone calls. [...] After the first stage, I started to show improvements [...]. I have never used corticosteroids, except in local applications. I also never had any reaction to the vaccine and since I stopped treatment, on 8 February 1997, I consider myself practically cured; which I attribute to the use of VAB. (Letter from 1998)

In their reports, VAB users firmly connected their corporeal and emotional well-being with improvements in other domains of life, such as the rehabilitation that allowed them to gradually return to work, and to take care of their ordinary affairs. Cristina wrote:

I have been on treatment with the vaccines for 9 months. When I started the process with Veiga's medicines, I was walking with a crutch, practically dragging myself. Today I am without support, walking without limping. I still cannot walk much, but the improvement was great. (Letter from 2000)

As Ana also enthusiastically wrote, following a recovery of her capacity to move, she throw herself back into the flow of collective daily life.

The great relief is that I find myself active in the exercise of the profession that caused me such an injury, when in other times there was a need to interrupt with great difficulty, my professional activity, this had profoundly negative consequences from a financial, family and emotional point of view. (Letter from 1997)

Likewise, in her letter from 2013, Luísa replies to VEIGA as the following:

For the past two years, I was already depressed with so much pain. And with my impending disability, as I hadn't been able to drive a car for more than two years. And these days, I even managed to drive a little: I feel that little by little my life is returning to normal. [...] I no longer need a wheelchair, and I manage to do my activities at home and I am gradually returning my quality of life. I am already able to move around alone, only with the help of a crutch when I have to leave the house and do some walking.

The feeling of musculoskeletal and emotional improvements, along with the possibility of rehabilitating to the point of resuming activities which had to be left aside, causing multiple losses, seem to mutually reinforce each other synergistically (e.g. BARAK 2006). Apparently, stop feeling pain refers not only to a growing absence of suffering but also to the re-achievement of homeostasis as VAB users may experience it through feelings of improvement and wellbeing.

It is noteworthy that VAB users, as health professionals, are quite aware of EBM as the standard evaluation criteria to attest the efficacy of any substance with pharmaceutical pretensions. Nevertheless, most of them tend to reposition the evidence-based aspect of RCTs as secondary in comparison to the primacy of their lived amelioration experience that they attribute to effects co-generated through VAB. ANA's statement illustrates this point straightforward:

> I have no means to prove the results scientifically, but I was able to observe that, in the six years in which I present the disease, those of 96 and 97 [during which Ana used VAB] were the best for me, without however having a total cure. (Letter from 1997)

Likewise, based on his direct observation of Catarina's therapeutic trajectory, her physician-husband Arthur provided a clinical verification with potential validity: "As a doctor I can attest to the vaccine's efficacy, since she has been pain-free for more than two years without the medication she used to take and six months without VAB."

In this sense, the authors of the letters that I exam here could help solve a core problem of biomedicine as a branch of modern science. As I mentioned in section 2.4, despite the crucial importance of an objective approach, the efficacy of EBM methods is sometimes criticised for its seemingly excessive analytical distancing from reality that, as part of contemporary biomedical attempts to pasteurize medical assessments, often exclude patients' reports that could be considered as co-constitutive of medical evidence. This distancing resembles MAURICE MERLEAU-PONTY's critical characterization of the methodological rationale of modern science as "surveying thought, thought of the object in general" (2007 [1961]: 352). For him, modern scientists paradoxically aim at producing knowledge empirically through experimental manipulation of indices and variables within closed abstract models that, in parallel, simulate the reality it tries to *grasp* (e.g. INGOLD 2010: 74–75) without touching or getting it. For this reason, according to him, modern scientific thinking should instead "be placed back in the 'there is' which precedes it, back in the site, back upon the soil of the sensible world and the soil of the worked-upon world such as they are in our lives and for our bodies" (ibid.; also INGOLD 2010, 2022). This seems to be the case at least for Iara, Flávia, Xavier, Kalil, Cristina, Ana, Luísa and Catarina, for whom the process of evaluating the efficacy of different medications cannot be separated from their own and others' lives' destinies.

By skipping conventional treatment, and exposing themselves to an opposite therapeutic model, while cooperating with peers and non-peers, the actions of these physicians show how they opportunely carry out this ontoepistemological re-grounding work, which implies a re-hierarchisation of sources that they can use to co-produce potential medical evidence. In so doing, they reinforce an understanding of evidence making as "[…] not only the domain of global experts, but an ethical and political proposition that knowledge can come in many forms and be distinctively mobilized" (ADAMS & BIEHL 2016: 124).

Dissemination and boundarization

Following their witnessing of VAB's therapeutic effects, some health professionals shared their positive experiences in ways that could engage potential users. As Arthur, for instance, wrote:

> I have already recommended the vaccine for a cousin who suffers from RSI and was even retired by a medical board due to professional incapacity. Despite being at the beginning of the treatment, she started driving and leaving the house again, which she had not done for some time. (Letter from 2000)

Such recommendations, as a part of the displacing cooperations that I explore in this article, held the potential to surreptitiously disseminate the effects of VAB and, with it, to prepare the conditions of possibility for its future medical acceptance, not only among potential patients but also among members of immunological and rheumatological communities and networks.

Nevertheless, an unregistered drug is assumed to be dangerous (and many surely are) while authorised therapies are supposed to work, and medicine is supposed to pursue ways of achieving a cure, or to at least attempt to heal patients. Broadly speaking, dissemination of a potentially dangerous drug is not only ethically unacceptable and subject to criminal codes. It is also unethical to stimulate hope among people in situations of vulnerability in order to make profit by selling false products. Yet, when the opposite of this seems to occur, i.e. when an unregistered drug seems to work, destabilizing the expectation of established biomedicine, then the authority of regulatory institutions, and their representatives and apparatuses, might become relativizable and be thrown into question. That seems to be the case especially from the perspective of those who quit the medication conventionally prescribed and embrace unconventional therapy in order to feel better and achieve amelioration.

In this sense, as part of the cascade of discontinuities propelled by their use of VAB as a biotechnology personally experienced as capable of challenging chronicity, some VAB-related health professionals also expressed a particular lament due to, as Arthur put it,

> the fact that the vaccine is not publicised in the medico-hospital milieu. I really think that we [as health professionals] are depriving a large number of patients of getting rid of joint pathologies and their painful consequences, not to mention the low cost that this [i.e. VAB] represents for public health... (Letter from 2000)

On the one hand, that is probably why several of VEIGA's correspondents, in tune with this lament, responsively expressed a correspondent wish, as Iara wrote, that VEIGA, whose name became to some extend inseparable from VAB, could "bring to others relief, joy, life and cure" (Letter from 1997). On the other, as Arthur ends his letter to VEIGA with "Congratulations" accompanied by the imperative "and keep up this beautiful and extremely important work, which only true doctors can do" (Letter from 2000), he anticipatedly rehabilitate VEIGA, few years before VAB's ban, by evoking the core and self-defining biomedical differentiation between true and false physicians, doctors and charlatans.

Such displacements seem to provide a clue about how the encounters of letters' authors with VAB co-generated further ambivalences that affected their health, perception and attitudes towards themselves and their respective private and professional environments.

Concluding remarks

Most scholarship on chronic pain and disability seems to focus on the suffering subject and on how people manage to live as chronic patients (e.g. MILES 2013; GONZALEZ-POLLEDO & TARR 2018). There appears to be a limited scholarship on people's experiences of improvement from chronic illness, particularly on how biomedical actors themselves improve through unconventional means and related implications. Contributing to fill this gap, I have analysed eight self-reports of sick health professionals who, after unsuccessful experiences with conventional immunosuppressive therapy, successfully tried VAB as an unknown off-label drug based on the opposite principle of unspecific immunostimulation. My primary aim has been to try to understand how health professionals cooperate with each other in unpredictable and risky circumstances in order to practice their profession, and to improve from immunopathologies that most of their peers regard as chronic. For it, I presented and discussed aspects of how sick physicians, conventional treatments and VAB as a disruptive biotechnological innovation mutually affect each other. In so doing, I have considered their reported experiences in terms of repositionings that took place through displacing cooperations as parts of the co-production of medical evidence in Brazil.

Overall, the letters show aspects of how their authors mobilised different resources, as part of their evidence-making efforts, to evaluate the efficacy of conventional and unconventional drugs, such as clinical information, trustworthy relationships and testimonies, and their own sensorial and experiential knowledge (e.g. LAMBERT 2009; MCKEVITT 2013; SONG 2017; BALAJ 2020). The descriptions of the letters' authors of how palliative treatment, following short-term relief, mostly worsened their health in the middle and long-term reinforce the liminal and ambiguous character of immunosuppressants as authorized drugs, which are only used because there would be nothing else available to treat immunopathologies that are regarded as chronic. Paradoxically, the expressed therapeutic frustration with immunosuppressants, which could be linked to a neoliberal politics of resignation (BENSON & STUART 2010), seems to have played an important role in the elaboration of a political economy of hope (NOVAS 2006) towards VAB as a promising biotechnological innovation, despite its risks as an unregistered drug.

As health professionals trained and educated to believe in the efficacy of registered drugs, the personal therapeutic experiences of the authors challenge not only the chronicity of their immunopathologies, but also immunosuppression as the guiding paradigm of contemporary rheumatology. Emerging ambivalences found expression in frictions, tensions and uncertainties, but also in realignments between them and constituents of their multiple environments. VAB users recount their potential resolutions as having unfolded alongside two basic life-changing displacements that they underwent. The first displacement took place when they shifted from the state of living as healthy persons to the state of living as chronic patients following the conventional immunosuppressing palliative path. The second took place when they shifted from the state of living as immunocompromised chronic patients without expectations of health improvement (or, as one says in Brazil, as *desenganados*; i.e. after having been "undeceived" by their colleagues) to a state of unexpected amelioration informally achieved through a then unknown immunostimulating curative path. Throughout their passages from one state to another, health professionals intercalated experiences of exposing themselves and of being vulnerable with those of making use of what was on their ways, including biotechnologies, medico-scientific explanations, their own expertise, others' witnesses, emotional support, personal bonds, contacts etc. (INGOLD 2022: 58).

Backed by displacing medical mindsets and practices, and informed by the health changes in daily life that they experience through biotechnologies based on opposite principles, health professionals transfiguratively re-evaluated the pharmaceutical landscape they are taught to reproduce. Their participation both in established biomedicine and in cooperative networks that circumvent the later contributed to this. In particular, their own experience with VAB seems to have enabled them to re-ground their medical knowledge, experience and skills in relation to their own and someone else's health in anticipation to the mediation regularly played out by conventional medical knowledge, technologies and procedures. Furthermore, when VAB-using physicians self-analyse and dialogue with others, writing and exchanging evaluative reports about their own and others' health and therapeutic experiences of using VAB, they seemed to implicitly co-produce medical evidence that might be taken into consideration by potential users.

Acknowledgements

I would like to thank all colleagues who shared their thoughts, critics and suggestions concerning parts of this article that I presented, in 2020, at the EASST/4S meeting and at the Colloquium of the Research Group 'Biotechnologies, Nature and Society' at the Goethe University Frankfurt, especially Thomas Lemke. I also thank Harriet Gardner and Lesley Branagan who respectively proofread and copy-edited different drafts of this manuscript, and for their remarks. I am especially in debt with Ehler Voss and Cornelius Schubert for their invitation to submit this article to *Curare*'s special issue "Ambivalences of Healing Cooperations in Biomedical Settings", and to the anonymous reviewers. The research work, from which this article is an output, was funded by the Deutsche Forschungsgemeinschaft (DFG, German Research Foundation); project number 419940268. I do not have any conflict of interests to declare.

Notes

All translations of source material reproduced in this article originally written in Portuguese and Spanish were translated by myself into English. I anonymized all letters' authors but not the names of historical persons and/or the dead. Finally, I herewith state that I am not a health professional and I am not authorized to confirm the efficacy or inefficacy of any drug.

References

ADAMS, VINCANNE 2016. What is critical global health? *Medicine Anthropology Theory* 3, 2: 187–197. https://doi.org/10.17157/mat.3.2.429

ADAMS, VINCANNE & BIEHL, JOÃO 2016. The work of evidence in critical global health. *Medicine Anthropology Theory* 3, 2: 123–126. https://doi.org/10.17157/mat.3.2.432

AHUJA, ABHIMANYU S. 2019. Should RCT's be used as the gold standard for evidence based medicine? *Integrative Medicine Research* 8, 1: 31-32. https://doi.org/10.1016/j.imr.2019.01.001

AKPINAR, ORHAN 2016. Historical perspective of brucellosis: A microbiological and epidemiological overview. *Le Infezioni in Medicina* 24, 1: 77-86. https://www.infezmed.it/media/journal/Vol_24_1_2016_14.pdf

ANDERSON, WARWICK & MACKAY, IAN R. 2014. *Intolerant bodies: A short history of autoimmunity*. Baltimore: University of John Hopkins Press.

ATKINSON, PAUL 1976. The Clinical Experience: An Ethnography of Medical Education. PhD thesis, Department of Educational Sciences, University of Edinburgh.

BALAJ, MIRZA 2022. Self-reported health and the social body. *Social Theory & Health* 20: 71-89. https://doi.org/10.1057/s41285-020-00150-0

BARAK, YORAM 2006. The immune system and happiness. *Autoimmunity Reviews* 5, 8: 523-527. https://doi.org/10.1016/j.autrev.2006.02.010

BECKER, HOWARD S.; GEER, BLANCHE; HUGHES, EVERETT C. & STRAUSS, ANSELM L. 1992 [1961]. *Boys in White: Student Culture in Medical School*. New Brunswick (US) & London: Transactions.

BEISEL, ULI; CALKINS, SANDRA & ROTTENBURG, RICHARD 2018. Divining, testing, and the problem of accountability. *HAU: Journal of Ethnographic Theory* 8, 1/2: 109-113. http://dx.doi.org/10.1086/698360

BENSON, PETER & KIRSCH, STUART 2010. Capitalism and the politics of resignation. *Current Anthropology* 51, 4: 459-486. https://doi.org/10.1086/653091

BOURDETTE, MARCELO D.S. & SANO, EDSON S. 2023. Características epidemiológicas da brucelose humana no brasil no período de 2014-2018. *Revista Cereus* 15, 2: 27-40. https://doi.org/10.18605/2175-7275/cereus.v15n2p27-40

BYRNE, ANNE 2017. Epistolary research relations: Correspondences in anthropological research: Arensberg, Kimball, and the Harvard-Irish Survey, 1930-1936. In Ó GIOLLÁIN, DIARMUID (ed) *Irish Ethnologies*. Indiana: University of Notre Dame Press: 36-59. https://doi.org/10.2307/j.ctvpj782n.6

CAMBROSIO, ALBERTO 2010. Standardization before biomedicine: On early forms of regulatory objectivity. In GRADMANN, CHRISTOPH & SIMON, JONATHAN (eds.) *Evaluating and standardizing therapeutic agents, 1890-1950*. London: Palgrave Macmillan: 252-261.

CARR, E. SUMMERSON 2010. Enactments of expertise. *Annual Review of Anthropology* 39: 17-32. https://doi.org/10.1146/annurev.anthro.012809.104948

CASTRO, ROSANA 2017. Testemunho, evidência e risco: Reflexões sobre o caso da fosfoetanolamina sintética. *Anuário Antropológico* 42, 1: 37-60. https://doi.org/10.4000/aa.1637

Churcher, Millicent; Calkins, Sandra; Böttger, Jandra & Slaby, Jan. 2023. The many lives of institutions: A framework for studying institutional affect. In Churcher, Millicent; Calkins, Sandra; Böttger, Jandra & Slaby, Jan (2023) (eds.) *Affect, Power, and Institutions*. Routledge: London & New York: 1-32.

COPE, ZACHARY 1966. *Almroth Wright: Founder of modern vaccine-therapy*. London & Edinburgh: Nelson.

CORTAZZI, MARTIN 2001. Narrative analysis in ethnography. In ATKINSON, PAUL; COFFEY, AMANDA; DELAMONT, SARA; LOFLAND, JOHN & LOFLAND, LYN (eds) *Handbook of Ethnography*. London: Sage: 384-94. https://doi.org/10.4135/9781848608337

DE LAET, MARIANNE & MOL, ANNEMARIE 2000. The Zimbabwe bush pump: Mechanics of a fluid technology. *Social Studies of Science* 30, 2: 225-63.

DE MELLO, MILTON T. 1979. Vacunas muertas y de extractos celulares contra la brucelosis. *Ciência e Cultura* 31, 6: 676-680.

DUMIT, JOSEPH 2012. *Drugs for life: How pharmaceutical companies define our health*. Durham and London: Duke University Press.

EPSTEIN, STEVEN 1995. The construction of lay expertise: AIDS activism and the forging of credibility in the reform of clinical trials. *Science, Technology, & Human Values* 20, 4: 408-437. https://doi.org/10.1177/016224399502000402

FAULKNER, ALEX 2009. *Medical technology into healthcare and society: A sociology of devices, innovation and governance*. Basingstoke: palgrave macmillan.

FAVRET-SAADA, JEANNE 2012. Being affected. *HAU: Journal of Ethnographic Theory* 2, 1: 435-445. Translated by Mylene Hengen and Matthew Carey. https://doi.org/10.14318/hau2.1.019

FERRANTE, MAURIZIO 2019. *A Saga da Fosfoetanolamina*. São Paulo: Primavera Editorial.

FLECK, LUDWIK 2019 [1935]. *Entstehung und Entwicklung einer wissenschaftlichen Tatsache: Einführung in die Lehre vom Denkstil und Denkkollektiv*. Frankfurt am Main: Suhrkamp.

FOUCAULT, MICHEL 1989 [1963]. *The Birth of the clinic: An archaeology of medical perception*. London & New York: Routledge.

GOFFMAN, ERVING 1961. *Encounters: Two studies in the sociology of interaction – Fun in games & role distance*. Indianapolis: Bobbs-Merrill.

GONZALEZ-POLLEDO, EJ & TARR, JEN (eds.) 2018. *Painscapes: Communicating pain*. London: Palgrave Macmillan.

GRECO, ENRICO; EL-AGUIZY, OLA; ALI, MONA F.; FOTI, SALVATORE; CUNSOLO, VINCENZO; SALETTI, ROSARIA & CILIBERTO, ENRICO 2018. Proteomic analyses on an ancient Egyptian cheese and biomolecular evidence of brucellosis. *Analytical Chemistry* 90, 16: 9673-9676. https://doi.org/10.1021/acs.analchem.8b02535

GREENHALGH, SUSAN 2001. *Under the medical gaze: Facts and fictions of chronic pain*. Berkeley, Los Angeles & London: University of California Press.

HINCHMAN, LEWIS P. & HINCHMAN, SANDRA K. (eds) 1997. *Memory, identity, community: The idea of narrative in the human sciences*. New York: SUNY Press.

INGOLD, TIM 2010. *Being alive: Essays on movement, knowledge and description*. London & New York: Routledge.

INGOLD, TIM 2022. Anthropological affordances. In Djebbara, Zakaria (eds) *Affordances in everyday life: A multi-*

disciplinary collection of essays. Springer, Cham: 51–60. https://doi.org/10.1007/978-3-031-08629-8_6

Kay, Margaret; Mitchell, Geoffrey & Clavarino, Alexandra 2008. Doctors as patients: A systematic review of doctors' health access and the barriers they experience. *British Journal of General Practice* 58, 552: 501–508. https://doi.org/10.3399/bjgp08X319486

Kierans, Ciara & Kirsten Bell 2017. Cultivating ambivalence: Some methodological considerations for anthropology. *Hau: Journal of Ethnographic Theory* 7, 2: 23–44.

Klitzman, Robert 2008. *When doctors become patients*. Oxford: Oxford University Press.

Kuhn, Thomas 2012[1962]. *The structure of scientific revolutions*. Chicago & London: The University of Chicago Press.

Lambert, Helen 2009. Evidentiary truths? The evidence of anthropology through the anthropology of medical evidence. *Anthropology Today* 25, 1: 16–20. https://doi.org/10.1111/j.1467-8322.2009.00642.x

Löwy, Ilana 2005. Biotherapies of chronic diseases in the inter-war period: From Witte's peptone to penicillium extract. *Studies in History and Philosophy of Biological and Biomedical Sciences* 36, 4: 675–95. https://doi.org/10.1016/j.shpsc.2005.09.002

Löwy, Ilana 2008. Immunology in the clinics: Reductionism, holism or both? In Kroker, Kenton; Keelan, Jennifer & Mazumdar, Pauline M.H. (eds) *Crafting Immunity: Working Histories of Clinical Immunology*. Cornwall: Ashgate: 165–76.

McKevitt, Christopher 2013. Experience, knowledge and evidence: A comparison of research relations in health and anthropology. *Evidence & Policy* 9, 1: 113–130. https://doi.org/10.1332/174426413X663751

Maurelio, Anna P.V.; Santarosa, Bianca P.; Ferreira, Danilo O.L.; Martins, Mayra T.A.; Paes, Antonio C. & Megid, Jane 2022. Situação epidemiológica mundial da brucelose humana. *Veterinária e Zootecnia* 23, 4: 597–60. https://rvz.emnuvens.com.br/rvz/article/view/838

Meiselas, Leonard E.; Zingale, Salvador B.; Lee, Stanley L.; Richman, Sidney & Siegel, Morris 1961. Antibody production in rheumatic diseases: The effect of brucella antigen. *The Journal of Clinical Investigation* 40, 10: 1872–1881. https://www.jci.org/articles/view/104411/pdf

Merleau-Ponty, Maurice 2007 [1961]. Eye and mind. In Toadvine, Ted & Lawlor, Leonard (eds) *The Merleau-Ponty reader*. Illinois: Northwestern University Press: 351–378.

Miles, Ann 2013. *Living with lupus: Women and chronic illness in Equador*. Austin: University of Texas Press.

Nerland, Monika 2012. Professions as knowledge cultures. In Jensen, Karen; Lahn, Leif C. & Nerland, Monika (eds) *Professional Learning in the Knowledge Society*. Rotterdam: SensePublishers: 27–48. https://doi.org/10.1007/978-94-6091-994-7_2

Nogueira, Carolina de C. & de Castro, Bruno G. 2022. Brucella abortus em humanos: Revisão da literatura. *Scientific Electronic Archives* 15, 1: 60–64. http://dx.doi.org/10.36560/15120221498

Novas, Carlos 2006. The political economy of hope: Patients' organizations, science and biovalue. *BioSocieties* 1, 289–305. https://doi.org/10.1017/S1745855206003024

Pacheco, Genésio & de Mello, Milton T. de 1956. *Brucelose*. Rio de Janeiro: Atheneu.

Pacheco, Genésio; da Silva, Dario S. & da Silva, José G. 1969. Nova vacina curativa contra a brucelose. *O Hospital* 76, 2: 747–753.

Pappas, Georgios; Paraskevi, Panagopoulou; Christou, Leonidas & Akritidis, Nikolaos 2006. Brucella as a biological weapon. *Cellular and Molecular Life Sciences* 63, 19-20: 2229–2236. https://doi.org/10.1007/s00018-006-6311-4

Pessoa, Fernando 1969. *Obra Poética*. Edited by Maria Aliete Galhoz. Rio de Janeiro: Aguilar.

Petersen, Alan, Schermuly, Alegra C. & Anderson, Alison 2019. The shifting politics of patient activism: From bio-sociality to bio-digital citizenship. *Health* 23, 4: 478–494. https://doi.org/10.1177/1363459318815944

PGR [Procuradoria Geral da República] 2018 (22 October). "Ação Direta de Inconstitucionalidade 5.501/DF". N.º 161/2018 – SFCONST/PGR (Sistema Único nº 303866 /2018). Ministério Público Federal. https://www.mpf.mp.br/pgr/documentos/ADI5501.pdf

Oprisan, Anca-Alexandra-Ioana; Vásquez-Costa, María & Costa-Alcaraz, Ana M. 2016. El médico como paciente: Una experiencia de aprendizaje transformativo. *Revista de la Fundación Educación Médica* 19, 1: 9–12. https://doi.org/10.33588/fem.191.826

Ratnani, Igbal; Fatima, Sahar; Abid, Muhammad M.; Surani, Zehra & Surani, Salim 2023. Evidence-based medicine: History, review, criticisms, and pitfalls. *Cureus* 15, 2: e35266. https://doi.org/10.7759/cureus.35266

Rosenberg, Charles E. 2014. Preface. In Anderson, Warwick & Mackay, Ian R. *Intolerant bodies: A short history of autoimmunity*. Baltimore: University of John Hopkins Press: ix-xii.

Rothschild, Bruce & Haeusler, Martin 2021. Possible vertebral brucellosis infection in a Neanderthal. *Scientific Reports* 11, 19846. https://doi.org/10.1038/s41598-021-99289-7

Schor, Gregório 1974. Artrite reumatóide e outras colagenoses. Distúrbios do metabolismo do colesterol. *Revista Brasileira de Medicina* 31, 5: 319–322.

Suárez-Esquivel, Marcela; Chaves-Olarte, Esteban; Moreno, Edgardo & Guzmán-Verri, Caterina 2020. Brucella genomics: Macro and micro evolution. *International Journal of Molecular Sciences* 21, 20: 7749. https://doi.org/10.3390/ijms21207749

Stanley, Liz 2004. The epistolarium: On theorising letters and correspondences. *Auto/Biography* 12, 201–35.

Stengers, Isabelle 2003. The doctor and the charlatan. *Cultural Studies Review* 9, 2: 11–36. https://doi.org/10.5130/csr.v9i2.3561

Sleeboom-Faulkner, Margaret 2014. *Global morality and life science practices in Asia: Assemblages of life*. Basingstoke: Palgrave Macmillan.

SONG, PRISCILLA 2017. *Biomedical odysseys: Fetal cell experiments from cyberspace to China*. Princeton & Oxford: Princeton University Press.

TAMBIAH, STANLEY J. 1990. *Magic, Science, Religion, and the Scope of Rationality*. Cambridge: Cambridge University Press.

VEIGA, GENÉSIO 1969. Artrite reumatóide e brucelose. *O Hospital* 76, 3: 1071-1076.

VILAR, MÁRCIO 2020. Following 'Fosfo': Synthetic phosphoethanolamine and the transfiguration of immunopolitics in Brazil. *Medicine Anthropology Theory* 7, 1: 87–116. https://doi.org/10.17157/mat.7.1.620

VILAR, MÁRCIO 2024. Tackling the unknown: Medical semiotics of inflammation and their legal-epistemological boundaries in Brazil. *Medical Anthropology* 43, 2: 130–145. https://doi.org/10.1080/01459740.2024.2324887

WARETH, GAMAL; PLETZ, MATHIAS W.; NEUBAUER, HEINRICH & MURUGAIYAN, JAYASEELAN 2020. Proteomics of *brucella*: Technologies and their applications for basic research and medical microbiology. *Microorganisms* 8, 5: 766. https://doi.org/10.3390/microorganisms8050766

This article has been subjected to a double blind peer review process prior to publication.

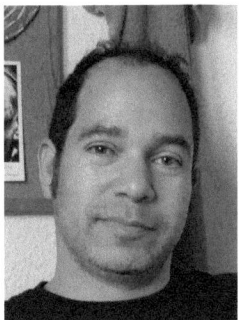

Márcio Vilar, Dr phil., is an anthropologist and researches the manifold effects of biotechnological innovations for the treatment of autoimmune diseases, especially in the field of life sciences. Since October 2023, he works as a contract teacher at the Institute of Social and Cultural Anthropology at the Freie Universität Berlin. Between 2019 and 2023, he conducted as PI his DFG research project on "Contested legitimacy of regenerative versus established biomedicine in Brazil: On the circulation and co-regulation of immunostimulating therapies for autoimmune diseases" (project 419940268) as a research associate in the research group "Biotechnologies, Nature and Society" at the Institute of Sociology at Goethe University Frankfurt.

Freie Universität Berlin
Institute of Social and Cultural Anthropology
Landoltweg 9–11, 4195 Berlin
e-mail: m.cunha.vilar@fu-berlin.de

UNABHÄNGIGE ARTIKEL
INDEPENDENT ARTICLES

Connected Epistemologies

A Fragmented Review of Post- and Decolonial Perspectives in Medical Anthropology

GIORGIO BROCCO

Abstract Over the last four decades, post- and decolonial ideas have gained prominence through the dissemination of influential works by renowned scholars and intellectuals in the humanities and social sciences. Pioneering voices such as Franz Fanon, Valentin-Yves Mudimbe, and Edward Said, along with scholars like Gayatri Spivak and advocates of Black feminism such as Sylvia Wynter and Françoise Vergès, have contributed to shaping this realm. Medical anthropology, critical medical anthropology and other related disciplines within the broad field of "medical/health humanities" have actively engaged with these critical theoretical impulses, refining epistemological and methodological approaches that align with post- and decolonial analyses. This article explores the intersections of post- and decolonial perspectives with current anthropological agenda, drawing attention to the manifold research avenues that have emerged from such entanglements. Specifically, the paper delves into three key research areas: (1) the examination of the influence of ideas about post- and decolonial subjectivities in connection to changing notions of health, disease, and disability; (2) the critical analysis of humanitarian and global health interventions; and (3) the exploration of indigenous systems of care and healing practices from the Global South. While acknowledging the fragmented, partial, situated nature of the selection of scholarly sources for this discussion, the article aims to shed light on the dynamic interplays between post- and decolonial theories and the multifold and complex medical anthropology landscapes.

Keywords decolonial theory – medical anthropology – disability anthropology – subjectivity – indigeneity

Introduction

The decolonial movements, the end of European colonization in Africa, the provincialization of Europe and other Global North countries (CHAKRABARTY 2000), along with the affirmation of new nation-states and political alliances at the global level, have been transformative social, economic, and historical events that have left an enduring impact on the history of the world at large. Over around the past 40 years, numerous empirical and analytical interventions have, in fact, emerged through the writings of figures like FANON (1963[1959]; 1965[1961]; 1986[1952]), MUDIMBE (1988) and SAID (2003[1978]), to name just a few scholars. These intellectuals have critically explored the dynamics of (neo)colonial power and its epistemological, political, and social ramifications in diverse regions of the Global North[1] and South (BHAMBRA 2014; MARZAGORA 2016). On a similar level, scholars within Subaltern Studies (SPIVAK 1988) and those associated with Black Feminism, such as Wynter (MAHMUD 2021) and VERGÈS (2021), have further pointed out issues like racial differentiations and discriminations based on physical attributes and geographic origins, gender disparities, xenophobia, and racism in many societies of both Global North and South. In a nutshell, the epistemological and analytical goals of such intellectual enterprises have been to deconstruct previous pervasive narratives and ideas centered around concept of the Global North, white, "Man" and redefine new ideals of humanism (WYNTER 2003: 260). Along these multifold historical and epistemological discussions, social and cultural anthropology, not without even very recent tensions and challenges (ALLEN & JOBSON 2016; JOBSON 2020), has gradually reevaluated some of its theoretical and methodological assumptions to adapt, embrace, and revitalize its research insights and analyses (SAVRANSKY 2017; FÚNEZ-FLORES 2022).

Merging political-economic approaches with culturally sensitive analyses of human health and well-being, scholars in medical anthropology and other sub-disciplines within medical humanities, such as critical medical anthropology[2], have been contributing significantly to discussions about the social and political economy of health, diseases and the body (SCHEPER-HUGHES & LOCK 1987). Since the early 1980s-1990s, the years in which it originated as a discipline in Anglo-American academia, critical medical anthropology has greatly developed these topics and raised various concerns with regard to how health and diseases have been constituted and responded to (SINGER 2004: 23–24). Following a strand of questions about the limits of biomedicine and biomedicalization (ILLICH 1974), critical medical anthropology has especially delved deeper into discussions about the political economy as well as the social determinants of health, diseases and ideas of the "body" not only in Global North contexts (SINGER 2004) but also in Global South academic spaces as in the case of Latin America (GAMLIN, GIBBON, SESIA, BERRIO 2020). In so doing, over the last two decades of the 20th century, these studies not only have laid the foundation for research that highlights the profit-making orientation of biomedicine and its hegemony but also the political role of international actors such as World Bank or the International Monetary Fund (IMF) in influencing national health policies and establishing unbalanced relations of power (BAER, SINGER, SUSSER 2004).

Along this strand of research, medical anthropologists and critical medical anthropologists have therefore begun examining the colonial and imperialist aspects of Global North science and medicine (ANDERSON 2009). Works by VAUGHAN (1991), ARNOLD (1993), and ANDERSON (2006) stand as noteworthy examples of how scholars focusing on health and healing have also started employing postcolonial and decolonial approaches and critiques to "provincialize" Global North systems of thought (CHAKRABARTY 2000), expose the colonial nature of medicine, and underscore the significance of Global South care practices and health perspectives. More precisely, such scholars have shed light on the role of colonial medicine in perpetuating global social biases and attitudes, including classism, racism, homophobia, sexism, ableism, and xenophobia.

More recently, a focus on how globalized medical practices, both historically and in the present, have imposed Global North perspectives on ontological and epistemological aspects related to health, illness, bodily normativity, morality and care in various Global South contexts has become prominent (ABADÍA-BARRERO 2022). Furthermore, scholarly attention to alternative discourses about Global North science and biomedicine from postcolonial local and national contexts, where these practices have been disseminated and/or enforced, has grown. Descriptions of how Global North biomedicine and science have undergone local processes of adaptation to cater to the needs of populations under imperial and colonial dominion and forms of neocoloniality have followed such interest. In fact, these adaptations entailed integrating and blending Global North medical and scientific practices and knowledge with "indigenous" systems of care and healing practices by local medical practitioners (GRABOYES 2018). However, such syncretic practices and the formation of "medical pluralism" as well as the "integration" of local healing systems within globalized biomedicine in Global South contexts have taken place within unbalanced power dynamics. Drawing on postcolonial and decolonial critics, various scholars have examined multiple economic, social, political and historical dis/junctures across various aspects of life in the post-colony (MBEMBE 2001), including health and medicine (GOOD, DELVECCHIO, HYDE & PINTO 2008). Others have endeavored to de-center Global North political and social influences (SPIVAK 1988; SAID 2003[1978]; CHAKRABARTY 2000), elucidating multiple and decentralized forms of modernity as well as outlining the development of theories from the Global South (COMAROFF & COMAROFF 2011; DEVISCH & NYAMNJOH 2011).

Due to the convergence of medical anthropology and critical medical anthropology with postcolonial and decolonial theories, numerous scholars have questioned the validity of the label "global" and highlight critical distinctions in the assessments and representations of health, well-being, illness, disability, and medicine. This emphasis has particularly concerned the unequal distribution of economic and political resources across various locations, whether in the Global North or South contexts (COMAROFF & COMAROFF 2003; STAPLES 2020). These critical intakes have effectively challenged the notion of a unified "global medicine and science model". Research emerging from the empirical and analytical entanglements between socio-cultural anthropology and post- and decolonial approaches have exposed the fallacious nature of certain epistemological approaches and critiqued assumptions that attempt to homogenize local variations within a global framework. For example, the interplay between Global North social, political, and medical categories, like race, genetics, and disease, has become far more complex and context-dependent than initially presumed (WHITMARSH 2009). The centrifugal forces generated by post- and decolonial approaches have thus offered insights into the "radical otherness" of practices and ideas related to ontologically distinct systems of care compared to Global North paradigms within shared histories of frictions, colonization and violence. In this regard, ANDERSON (2002) describes postcolonial realities and critical approaches in the following way:

> A postcolonial perspective suggests fresh ways to study the changing political economies of capitalism and science, the mutual reorganization of the global and the local, the increasing transnational traffic of people, practices, technologies, and contemporary contests over 'intellectual property'. The term 'postcolonial' thus refers both to new configurations of technoscience and to the critical modes of analysis that identify them. We hope that a closer engagement of science studies with postcolonial studies will allow us to question technoscience differently, find more heterogeneous sources, and reveal more fully the patterns of local transactions that give rise to global, or universalist, claims (ANDERSON 2002: 643).

These concepts once again underscore the capacity of post- and decolonial perspectives within medical anthropology and critical medical anthropology and STS (Science and Technology Studies) to illuminate post- and neo-colonial power structures and the epistemological mechanisms through which these configurations have manifested themselves in different regions and geographies outside the situated loci of production and diffusion.

Given the relevant role played by post- and decolonial critiques and strands of thought on socio-cultural anthropology, and medical anthropology at large, in Global North universities and places of knowledge production since the 1980s, similarities and difference between post- and decolonial approaches have constituted epistemological factors in their intertwinements with medical anthropology and other cognate disciplines within the realm of medical social sciences and humanities. In fact, both approaches have produced numerous debates and discussions about violent, and at the same time ambiguous, relationships of people with previous and existing regimes of coloniality. As aptly summarized by MARZAGORA (2016), some intellectuals advocate for a postcolonial approach that emphasizes the cosmopolitan and global nature of the world, where identities and practices are historically and socially constructed and situated within shared histories, forms of violence, dispossession and colonization. On the other hand, other scholars, within the realms of decolonial epistemologies and praxis, argue for the necessity of adopting a decolonial thinking (NDLOVU-GATSHENI 2013; MIGNOLO 2021) capable of fostering epistemic, social, and political disobedience against Global North hegemonies, rejecting them entirely (MARZAGORA 2016: 174–175).

In the case of the study of alternative and indigenous practices of care, well-being and health, a decolonial approach entails the rediscovery and affirmation of local healing systems in syncretic contrast with dominant Global North healing epistemologies. While a debate about the entanglements between social and cultural anthropology, sociology and other social sciences have already started (BHAMBRA 2014; ALLEN & JOBSON 2016; JOBSON 2020; FÚNEZ-FLORES 2022), the exploration of previous and ongoing intertwinements between medical anthropology at large (including critical medical anthropology) and post- and decolonial theories has been relatively understudied. Therefore, this article aims to explore - albeit incompletely and selectively - some of the developments in the discipline influenced by reflections generated within the intellectual and political discussions started by post- and decolonial thinkers and scholars. These influences, in turn, have shaped subsequent discussions and research within medical anthropology itself.

After briefly highlighting my positionality and addressing the reasons of the "fragmentation" of my review attempt, the paper will critically situate ongoing discussions and debates within post- and decolonial approaches and their existing influence to social and cultural anthropology. Subsequently, the text will shed light on three key epistemological dimensions through which post- and decolonial perspectives have intertwined with the diverse interests within contemporary medical anthropology. Given the finite space that could be dedicated to this vast topic as well as the myriad research insights arising from these intersections, the paper will particularly focus on exploring three dimensions of such interconnections. More precisely, it will elicit (1) how medical anthropologists have studied, grasped and interpreted subjectivities in post-colonial settings outside Global North contexts. Furthermore, the article will look at (2) the current critical perspectives about the "coloniality" of medical-humanitarian and global health interventions in various Global South geographies. Lastly, the text will critically elucidate (3) anthropological analysis of indigenous healing systems and their critiques against biomedical perspectives.

Limitations: A note on positionality and methodology

As a white European medical anthropologist who has previously worked on subjectivities and experiences of albinism in Tanzania and is currently researching health-related toxicity in Martinique (one of the overseas French departments in the Caribbean region), I find it important to acknowledge the intellectuals and scholars, within the domain of post- and decolonial thinking, who have influenced my ethnographic and anthropological endeavors so far. This acknowledgment becomes even more relevant considering the significant impact that these anlytical and empirical strands of ex-centric theorizing (HARRISON 2016) have had on social and cultural anthropology since the 1970s and 1980s (ASAD 1973; ABU-LUGHOD 1991). While writing and reflecting on the present review, I want to highlight not only my partial and "situated knowledge" (HARAWAY 1988) about the entanglements between medical anthropological and post- and decolonial approaches but also my incomplete understanding of the vast and diverse schools of thought within the post- and decolonial world. Therefore, I have decided to use the term "fragmented" to describe this review in order to emphasize that at least three layers of incompleteness have influenced the creation of this text.

The first layer concerns the potential misalignment of categories regarding scholars I have classified as post- and decolonial thinkers, who either do not define themselves as such or consider such a definition restrictive. Although they have influenced future research directions in various and complex ways, they often find it reductive to be solely classified as post- and decolonial scholars, as their research interests, works, and intellectual goals exceed this categorization. Similarly, there are scholars providing a decolonial critique of global health who do not necessarily classify themselves and their work within the disciplinary threshold of medical anthropology. Therefore, in approaching this review essay, I highlight these categorical limitations and potential misinterpretations to help readers contextualize this attempt.

The second layer of fragmentation in writing this text regards my own difficulties in analyzing and disentangling the vast and intertwined arrays of research lines and questions pertaining, on the one hand, to medical anthropology and its internal ramifications and, on the other hand, to post- and decolonial studies and perspectives. Departing from the reflections within a special issue on the field of medical anthropology in Europe (HSU & POTTER 2012), this issue is even more relevant if I consider the internal differences that exist between various medical anthropology schools, histories and genealogies. In fact, this limitation complicates my endeavor and presents an additional challenge in identifying the three ways through which the entanglements between medical anthropology and post- and decolonial approaches manifest. Rather than claiming completeness, which could misguide readers, I prefer to address mistakes, errors, and limitations upfront. I do this to invite readers, scholars, and intellectuals to ponder these intertwinements and continue ongoing research exploring these and other entanglements.

The third layer of fragmentation in this paper relates to the finitude and situatedness inherent in any review claiming to provide an exhaustive overview of a specific topic. Due to the limited space available here, I have chosen to document how various medical anthropologists, with their divergent approaches to ethnographic material, have interacted with post- and decolonial approaches. While acknowledging the mutual influences between empirical and theoretical data brought by these scholars and the critical perspectives produced by post- and decolonial intellectuals, I have opted to focus solely on one side of this interaction: the role played by post- and decolonial perspectives in generating new research directions in medical anthropology.

Finally, I want to emphasize that some scholars in medical anthropology, regardless of their positionality, may describe their work as either post- and/or decolonial without exclusively situating their studies within these approaches. For all these interconnected reasons, I chose to transform the limitations and incompleteness of my perspective, as well as my situated knowledge, into productive sites for sketching the entanglements between medical anthropology and post- and decolonial approaches. The intent of this review is thus epistemological, aiming to highlight the dialectical and productive interactions between scholars whose training and empirical viewpoints have been apparently divergent. This goal is particularly relevant today, as medical anthropology has germinated in various contexts around the world and has been influenced by the intersection of multiple scholarly traditions. Furthermore, my incomplete attempt aims to be useful to teach medical anthropology and its feminist decolonial critiques in class (WILLIAMS 2022).

Bearing in mind the strands of fragmentation in this review, I aim to shed light on the complex ways medical anthropologists have drawn inspiration from and engaged in dialogue with post- and decolonial thinkers while generating their epistemological and empirical interventions. Although it is extremely difficult to discern how scholars in this discipline and its related fields have interacted with this heterogeneous set of ideas and theories, I wish to highlight the theoretical and methodological divergences and similarities among post- and decolonial approaches. These approaches have described and made sense of intersectional matters such as class, race, and gender in both Global North and South contexts, as well as the complex knowledge of groups who have suffered from past and present forms of colonization, dispossession, and violence.

Before delving deeper into the three main fields through which post-colonial and decolonial approaches have been mobilized in medical anthropology, the following section attempts to identify the differences and similarities between post- and decolonial macro-approaches.

Framing post- and decolonial approaches in anthropology

In 2020, anthropologist Ryan Cecil Jobson published an article titled "The Case for Letting Anthropology Burn: Sociocultural Anthropology in 2019" (JOBSON 2020). The central argument of the text concerns the reasons why the theoretical and methodological foundations of anthropology should symbolically "burn out." Built on eurocentric epistemologies which constitute the base for present-day environmental and socio-economic issues, anthropology as discipline should rethink its analytical and empirical pivots and adopt decolonial positions (DERIDDER, EYEBIYI & NEWMAN 2021). Jobson explains his firm assessment about anthropology's current states by highlighting the discipline's association with neo-liberal perspectives along with the massive production of anthropological research and discourses characterized by moral perfectionism and ethnographic sentimentalism. These aspects, the author contends, do not align with the history of the discipline, which has been intertwined with and constructed around colonialism, slavery and the perpetuation of social inequalities all around the world. Advocating for anthropologists to reject neoliberal theoretical approaches, Jobson rather invites them to analyze and address pressing issues like: climate change on a global scale, contemporary forms of economic and political exploitation, the (re)emergence of repressive models of governance and the existing dynamics of power in an interconnected world. Furthermore, the author also outlines that decolonizing efforts both within and beyond the realm of academic anthropology are not enough to pursue novel ways to restructuring this discipline. In light of his arguments, the anthropologist therefore emphasizes that:

> Neither the colonial history of anthropology nor the insular character of the academic job market will be resolved by piecemeal revisions to a disciplinary canon or the diversification of the professoriate. [...], we are challenged to refuse a liberal settlement as the raison d'être of sociocultural anthropology. In 2019, anthropologists pointed the way forward in their refusal of convenient fixes to epistemological crises or a fixed object of the ethnographic imagination. [An] abolitionist anthropology demands that anthropology eschew an exceptionalism that places itself outside these histories of violence (JOBSON 2020: 267).

The arguments in this article delve into the influence of post- and decolonial thoughts in cultural and social anthropology (DEVISCH & NYAMNJOH 2011) and the ways they have been contributing for the renewal of the discipline's foundations. Although the difficulties in drawing linear and precise lines of demarcation between post- and decolonial approaches as well as the obstacles in generating any type of metaphors of genealogy (CHEN, KAFER, EUNJUNG & MINICH 2023: 12), it is relevant to outline the differences and similarities between these two epistemological approaches, praxes and perspectives in their own plurality, before showing how they have informed research in medical anthropology.

Post- and decolonial approaches emerged with the aim of destabilizing Global North modernity's foundations, challenging the hegemony of European-US political, economic and epistemological alliances and their associated power dynamics, and questioning notions of "otherness" as means to disrupt dominant understandings of reality and knowledge (FÚNEZ-FLORES 2022: 2). As remarked by BHABRA (2014: 15), the postcolonial perspective has mainly focused on the cultural, socio-economic, and material dimensions of social, cultural, political and economic realities after the end of historical colonization, mainly in the African continent. On the other hand, largely influenced by Anibal Quijano, María Lugones, and Walter Mignolo, the decolonial approach examines modernity and coloniality, tracing their origins back to the early European encounters with other continents and geographies (BHAMBRA 2014: 115). While both approaches share an interest in decolonization, they differ in their emphasis, epistemologies and praxes. Postcolonial thinkers point out the hybrid nature of socio-cultural and political realities resulting from periods of colonization and coloniality. At the same time, they also acknowlede the mutual influences between colonized and colonizing societies, although existing power unbalances, violent frictions, duress of dispossession between the two represent relevant differences (MBEMBE 2001; BHABHA 1994; DIAGNE & AMSELLE 2020). Conversely, decolonial scholars advocate for breaking free from the neo-colonial chains perpetuated by Global North countries and focus on reconstructing and regenerating social, cultural, political, gender and epistemological praxes and dimensions at the local level vis-à-vis Global North powers and existing regimes of coloniality (MIGNOLO & WALSH 2018; MIGNOLO 2021; LUGONES 2007; 2011; NDLOVU-GATSHENI 2013). In regard to decolonial thinkers and their perspectives, four key ideas have been introduced to comprehend how neoliberal and capitalist Global North-dominated-world-system has shaped modernity: the coloniality of power, the coloniality of knowledge, the coloniality of being (FÚNEZ-FLORES 2022: 6–7) as well as the lack of emphasis on the plurality of the epistemologies of the South and their consequent epistemological colonization (DE SOUSA SANTOS & MENESES 2019: 242–243). Scholars like SAVRASKY (2017) and FÚNEZ-FLORES (2022) emphasize that decolonial approaches should hinder the distinctions between ontology and epistemology typical of Global North epistemological and philosophical systems. Similarly, such reflections should abandon the differences between knowledge and reality, while adopting various epistemologies of the South in order to liberate decolonial imagination, methodologies and praxes for deciphering "modernity". Given the complexity of the debate around differences and similarities between post- and decolonial approaches and perspectives (MARZAGORA 2016; NDLOVU-GATSHENI 2013), the review article opts for a simplified reference to just both perspectives together in order to avoid excessive elaboration on their differences.

Returning to the broader influence of post- and decolonial perspectives on social and cultural anthropology, it is worth noting that well before the "institutionalized" emergence of these lines of research in the academic world and public arena, various thinkers and intellectuals had already criticized material and epistemological hegemony of Global North centers of power and show the internal contradictions and forms of violence produced by them (CESAIRE 2000; DU BOIS 1979; GLISSANT 1989; TROUILLOT 1991). For instance, the symbolic, cultural and social construction and perpetuation of "racial capitalism" (ROBINSON 2021) and consequent production of Global North hegemonic values are instances of these critiques. In fact, these scholars aimed to critically assess and disrupt Global North epistemic of modernity and its coloniality as both material and ideal enterprises able to generate colonial matrix of power (MIGNOLO & WALSH 2018: 114). Following such empirical and theoretical guidelines, socio-cultural anthropology, and medical anthropology, started interrogating the onto-epistemological foundations and historical roots of their disciplines which originated within the European imperialist and colonial framework (ARIF 2021).

ALLEN and JOBSON (2016) highlight that post- and decolonial ideas have been present in anthropological discourses since the inception of social and cultural anthropology. However, despite their circulation, many of these ideas and their proponents have been largely forgotten and banned from classical anthropological canon. For instance, the work of the Haitian anthropologist Anténor Firmin in his book *De l'égalité des races humaines* (FLUEHR-LOBBAN 2000) or the research and epistemological critiques by W. E. B. Du Bois (however, he has been highly influential in sociology and the field of social sciences at large), Zora Neale Hurston and Ela Cara Deloria (KING 2020) serve as striking examples of early attempts to problematize the essentialism surrounding the concept of race and the Eurocentrism inherent in the nascent discipline of anthropology – and the previous physical anthropology - during the early 20th century. Therefore, it becomes apparent that alongside the decentralization and decolonization of the anthropological gaze and the realignment of power structures, the project of decolonizing anthropology has always included a radical critique of the discipline and its knowledge production practices.

Since the latter half of the 1980s, however, post- and decolonial approaches have significantly influenced socio-cultural anthropology, particularly in the US, with crucial and critical perspectives on topics such as power dynamics, modes of representation, and anthropological writing (ALLEN & JOBSON 2016: 130; COMAROFF & COMAROFF 2011; Gupta and Ferguson 1992). For instance, Harrison's edited volume, "Decolonising anthropology: moving further toward an anthropology for liberation" (see also ALLEN & JOBSON 2016: 136-137), has offered a synthesis of the decolonial proposals and research praxes advanced by black liberation and feminist movements in the US and the ideas propagated by post-colonial and pan-Africanist intellectuals from the Global South. The concept of "decolonizing anthropology" has therefore sparked widespread discussions on decolonization and decolonizing intellectual practices in socio-cultural anthropology. Amid the emergence of postmodernism along with its associated epistemological limitations (MARZAGORA 2016), the decolonizing movement in anthropology has addressed needs for the epistemological liberation of theories and fieldwork practices, in so doing, emphasizing the hegemonic control exerted by many Global North countries over Global South societies and "minorities" living in Global North societies. Decolonial intellectuals like MIGNOLO (2021), WALSH (MIGNOLO & WALSH 2018) and QUIJANO (2000) have initiated an ongoing reflection and discussion around the "logic of coloniality" and its epistemics of "modernity" advanced by not only political entities but also intellectual endeavors and disciplines' commitments such as socio-cultural anthropology.

As far as it concerns us here, post- and decolonial approaches have furthermore prompted a renewal of the ethnographic gaze toward interconnected global realities (ALLEN & JOBSON 2016: 131). These approaches have challenge the notion that Global North political actors alone crafted modernity and its "savage slots" (TROUILLOT 1991) and shed light on how capitalist enterprises have facilitated the movement of bodies, commodities, and capital through the use of violence and power against populations in both the Global North and South over many years. Historical tragedies, such as the genocide of indigenous population in America and the enslavement and forced displacement of African peoples, stand as stark consequences of these phenomena (ALLEN & JOBSON 2016: 131). Currently, decolonial perspectives encompass various epistemological and empirical directions. Besides a deep critique of the logic and praxes of coloniality, scholars such as VIVEIROS DE CASTRO (2013) have also tried to shed lights on "radical otherness" and "perspectivism" as concepts useful to describe non-Global North ontological realities. These efforts have aimed to elicit that forms of reality conceived of by the subjects of anthropological research hold equal epistemological relevance as those produced by anthropological studies. Aligning with the ontological turn in anthropology, Viveiros de Castro and other proponents have chronicled the existence of diverse ontologies. In their attempt to dismantle Global North hegemonic ontology (FÚNEZ-FLORES 2022), there is, however, the risk to unintentionally reinforce reified and essentialized differential realities. Paradoxically, this could inadvertently strengthen the very Global North hegemony that decolonial scholars seek to combat, contributing to the invisibility of contemporary hegemonic forces that drive neoliberal exploitation and extractivism. To address these issues, SAVRANSKY (2017) advocates for modalities of reflection and research that cultivate imagination as the way to surpass the limitations of standard epistemological approaches. Hence, this scholar stresses on the fact that the focus should be on political and social movements that actively support the generation of alternative worlds. As Savransky eloquently states (SAVRANSKY 2017: 23):

> The task therefore is to take seriously, and think with, the differences that these movements have made, and still endeavor to make, in their attempts to possibilities of other worlds. [...] It is to exercise new decolonial, plural, alter-realisms that enable us to affirm not only the reality of the "West" [...] but also other realities in the making. A realism for which "reality" is, first and foremost, an ethical and political problem.

From this brief introduction to post- and decolonial approaches and their many facets, it is clear that social and cultural anthropology has developed a very close link with these new epistemological and empirical directions. Although I focused my attention on decolonial perspectives more than on postcolonial points of view, it appears clear that both approaches, in different ways, constitute a terrain of vehement debates and are producing an ongoing slow change in the theoretical and methodological apparatuses of the discipline. In regard to the ethnographic study of health, illness, disability, disease and the body, critical medical anthropology is one of the sub-disciplines that have firstly started to complexify these realms developing perspectives on health, disease, syndemics, sufferer experience, medicalization, medical hegemony and medical pluralism (SINGER 2004). Although the purposes of this sub-discipline, the intersections between post- and decolonial approaches to medical anthropology have not only endeavored to diversified the anthropological approach to these topics but also to decenter anthropological knowledge, praxes and epistemologies in regard to health and well-being by including decolonial critics to medicine and accounts of indigenous/local healing systems. Therefore, while this section has shown the influences and diatribes within the relations between socio-cultural anthropology and post- and decolonial reflections, the following parts of the paper will highlight how these approaches have brought about onto-epistemological changes within medical anthropology and its various aims.

Aporias of the subjects in health and well-being

Anthropological explorations of subjectivity have been shaped by various intellectual currents over the past century, including psychoanalysis, post-structuralism, and gender and feminist theories. Scholars like Foucault, Lacan, and Butler have provided valuable insights into the formation of the modern reflection on subject and subjectivity. Along these lines of inquiry, medical anthropologists have also dedicated their efforts to investigating subjectivity paying attention to psychological experiences, social conceptualizations of the self, and inner lives in diverse social, political, economic, and cultural contexts in various localities.

Building on Foucault's reflections, which trace subjectivities' formation and genealogies in relation to power networks, the post- and decolonial approach has brought attention to the significant role Global North colonialism and colonization, various forms of (neo)coloniality and unequal power distribution have played in shaping subjectivities in Global South contexts. One of the pivotal figures that has significantly influenced post- and decolonial thought within medical anthropology is FRANZ FANON (1963[1959]; 1965[1961]; 1986[1952]). The Franco-Martinican intellectual was among the first thinkers and scholars who described the ways colonial violence imposed forms of bodily and psychological domination on "colonized subjects". In his work, Fanon explored the psychological effects of colonial trauma, humiliation, and degradation on colonized individuals, revealing the onset of a range of psychic and bodily issues in these peoples (FANON 1963[1959]). Within post- and decolonial reflections on subjectivity, for instance, GILROY (1993) has also remarked that colonization, colonial regimes, and racial oppression have produced states of "double consciousness," where individuals' selves are not only influenced by colonial powers but also go through processes of identification with the subjectivity of colonizers. Following such analysis, a focus on hybridization and duality by BHABHA (1994) has also described the inner conflicting discourses in people who live under state of oppression. In this regard, GOOD, DELVECCHIO, HYDE and PINTO (2008: 13) suggest that this perspective encompasses a complex temporal interplay of various and multiple influences that have shaped and reshaped analysis of subjectivity in the postcolonies:

> the ambiguous, mixed identities common in the postcolonies are often elegized as spaces for creative subversion of master discourses. Remaining at the heart of this work, however, is the ongoing tension between modern, rational modes of subjectivity and selves and the "traditional," and the linking of this duality to colonial memories of power and humiliation.

In addition to these reflections, various decolonial scholars (QUIJANO 2000; MIGNOLO & WALSH 2018; MIGNOLO 2021) have emphasized that temporal and spatial dimensions of individuals and the self are characterized by praxes, regimes and epistemologies of coloniality which, in turn, determine their lived experiences as well as their subjectivities in relation to social, economic, political and health dimensions. Notwithstanding various empirical and analytical differences, FARMER (2005) and other medical anthropologists (DAS, KLEINMAN, RAMPHELE & REYNOLD 2000; GOOD, MARY-JO, HYDE & PINTO 2008; BIEHL, GOOD & KLEINMAN 2007) have addressed how pathologies and social suffering are caused by structural violence and poverty. While they pointed at these factors as main causes for the spread of diseases and suffering, they have not expressly referred to political and economic regimes of (neo)coloniality shaping lives and "local biologies" (NGUYEN & LOCK 2010) in Global South contexts.

The influence of post- and decolonial theories and approaches has led medical anthropologists to conduct investigations into the subjectivity of their interlocutors. This critical examination has explored various aspects, such as violence, forms of hierarchy, internalized modes of anxiety, and the intricate connections between global and national processes within postcolonial realities. These aspects have had profound spatial and temporal social, political, and economic implications for individuals, shaping their experiences in current contexts characterized by "economic crisis, state violence, exploited migrant communities, massive displacements, hegemonic gender politics, and postcolonial states." (BIEHL, GOOD & KLEINMAN 2007: 10)

By adopting the theoretical-epistemological perspective of post- and decolonial approaches, medical anthropologists have explored modes of subjectification determined by systems of governmentality and violence (DAS 2008) produced by states, social hierarchies, colonial powers and their traumas, biomedical information and the neoliberal market (BIEHL, GOOD & KLEINMAN 2007: 14; VAN WOLPUTTE 2004: 254). Following Bhabha's line of thought (BHABHA 1994) and the analysis of the postcolony and its continuous state of war by MBEMBE (2001), many medical anthropologists have emphasized the existence of not just one postcolonial condition, but multiple conditions, all intricately linked to the experiences of communities and individuals affected by historical events of colonialism and imperialism, both in the past and present. This viewpoint has paved the way for diverse examinations concerning various forms of citizenship and the development of postcolonial self and subjects. For instance, DAS (2008: 284; DAS, KLEINMAN, RAMPHELE & REYNOLDS 2000) highlights how the current "reality of violence", stemming from past events and frictions, has been able to make and unmake social words and gender as well as has linked processes of subject's formation and intersubjective relationships to emotions and social suffering connected to and caused by it (KLEINMAN, DAS & LOCK 1997). Particularly noteworthy are the entanglements between the use of post- and decolonial perspectives on the study of modern subjectivities in relation to multiple notions of health and ideas of symptoms. In fact, this focus sheds light on the profound connections between inner states of mind, psychological conditions, "pharmaceutical selves" (BIEHL 2005), ethics and experiences of illness with the broader social world, colonial history, and the ways in which bodies are produced and experienced within post-colonial realities and regimes of coloniality, both in the past and the present (BIEHL & MORAN-THOMAS 2009).

Post- and decolonial approaches have therefore led medical anthropologists to investigate the unequal dynamics between powerful economic, political, and state institutions and more politically marginalized or peripheral realities in Global North contexts, such as the health and well-being of migrant people (SANGARAMOORTHY & CARNEY 2021). Knowledge structures and modes of experience that mirror the violent relations inherent in colonialism or present in modern regimes of coloniality, along with hierarchical gender divisions (JOLLY 2021; MBAYE 2019; DAS 2008) have been further goals of these strands of study on subjectivity. Through careful analysis of historical processes, medical anthropology, critical medical anthropology and other cognate disciplines within the medical humanities have pointed out how forms of global domination and hierarchy are unequivocally connected to forms of colonial hierarchy, gender discrimination, and the subjugation of bodies that trace back to the colonial and imperial past (LUGONES 2007; 2011; MBAYE 2018: 107-143). In the book edited by GOOD, DELVECCHIO, HYDE and PINTO (2008), medical anthropologists provide an exploration of postcolonial subjectivities that not only consider colonial encounters and violence but also emphasize the resistance and contradictions generated by regimes and institutional apparatuses of post-coloniality and contemporary coloniality (GOOD, DELVECCHIO, HYDE & PINTO 2008: 15). Importantly, this focus on social, historical, political, and economic phenomena has not undermined the acknowledgment of coeval processes equally relevant to the formation of subjectivities and related forms of citizenship. For instance, globalization, neoliberal policies, medicalization as well as nationalism (AÇIKSÖZ 2020) in relation to forms of chronicity and disability constitute further factors in the formation of subjectivities. In the edited volume (GOOD, DELVECCHIO, HYDE & PINTO 2008), detailed ethnographic studies provide, in fact, a deeper understanding of how various historical and social processes have influenced selves and subjectivities in various human groups in connection to past colonial regimes they were subjected to (COMAROFF & COMAROFF 2003). These critical perspectives have also described how experiential and material states such as psychological traumas and/or various types of disabilities and debility (LIVINGSTON 2005) have been shaped by processes of colonialism, post-slavery, imperialism, systemic racism, and (neo)coloniality (GINSBURG & RAPP, 2020: S9; GRECH & SOLDATIC 2016). As I will show in the next section, postcolonial subjectivities and individual experiences have been also determined, influenced and governed by global health regimes in Global South contexts (OBRIST & EEUWIJK 2020: 784). In this regard, significant attention has been given to analyses concerning: experiential states within (neo)colonial forms of governmentality, the formation of subjectivities under conditions of legal, juridical, and social marginality, as well as the sedimentation of colonial and postcolonial orders as well as the biomedical production of specific pathologies and categorizations of "normality" (GOOD, DELVECCHIO, HYDE & PINTO 2008: 18–25).

Another research topic in which the entanglements between medical anthropology and post- and decolonial approaches is visible in regard to inquiries about subjectivities concerns the analysis of the connections between mobility, states of social marginality and the difficulties affecting migrant peoples in accessing healthcare systems in Global North countries. For instance, SANGARAMOORTHY (2019) has investigated the interrelation between citizenship and marginality in the case of Mexican migrant women who work in US while experiencing injury, instability and disability. From research like the one by Sangaramoorthy, it clearly emerges the relevance of forms of care put in place by migrant subjects as well as the tremendous impact that racialized dynamics between patients and physicians have of these individuals. Although not directly framed in the article, these issues significantly impact the subjectivities and selves of migrant people, especially these individuals experience difficult access to healthcare systems along with the trauma resulting from forced mobility.

Besides, ethnographic analysis of subjectivities in Global South contexts, the intertwinements between medical anthropology and post- and decolonial perspectives appear visible in the methodological exploration of the anthropologist's positionality in the field. The acknowledgement of the "situated" (HARAWAY 1988) nature of anthropological research and the ways anthropological analyses are conducted and produced (ADAMS, BURKE & WHITMARSH 2014) have become major topics within medical anthropology. Stemming from the critical points raised by SPIVAK (1988), who provocatively asked if the "subalterns" could participate in these debates, as well as internal critiques against the concept of "culture" (GUPTA & FERGUSON 1992), this new line of inquiry has questioned socio-cultural position of anthropologists while producing knowledge about their empirical works.

Decentering global health

While the previous parts of the text delve deeper into the entanglements between post- and decolonial approaches and research in relation to the formation of subjectivities in postcolonial Global South settings, this section intends to explore how post- and decolonial approaches have become instrumental in uncovering the colonial roots of practices inherent to global health interventions and actions as well as their immobilities and disconnectivites. (DILGER & MATTES 2018). Scholars working on this topic have repeatedly outlined that grounded assumptions in global health actions are mainly and primarily centered around ideas of the Global North narratives, epistemologies and etiological systems. Against indigenous and local healing systems, these assumptions have therefore perpetuated power inequalities beyond the traditional North/South divide reinforcing existing power imbalances through extractivist practices as well as the marginalization of populations which are still subjected to colonial logics nowadays. As stated by NDLOVU-GATSHENI (2013), such practices could be described as "parasitic."

Since the 1980s and 1990s, socio-cultural and medical anthropologists (FEIERMAN 1985; VAUGHAN 1991; FEIERMAN & JANZEN 1992; TILLEY 2011) have discussed how science and biomedicine and their related epistemologies and histories have been disseminated across the world during and after the colonial period, imposing specific Eurocentric empirical and conceptual regimes based on social, political and economic disparities. Such inequalities, these scholars argue, have been further amplified by the unequal distribution of funding, hierarchical health policies and agendas as well as humanitarian and biomedical interventions. These debates have therefore remarked the global scale on which medicine has operated so far, questioning its origins and purposes (CRANE 2013). Additionally, science and medicine have been described as intricately woven into the Global North socio-economic and political systems and closely intertwined with colonial and post-colonial forms of sovereignty and "regimes of coloniality" (NDLOVU-GATSHENI 2013). Furthermore, these critical viewpoints have emphasized the inherently colonial nature of medicine not only in the past but also in the present. Hence, NDLOVU-GATSHENI (2013) has poignantly argued that a significant portion of the world's population, particularly in various African countries, continues to live under (neo)colonial regimes which materialize through the presence of international agencies, humanitarian organizations, and transnational unequal connections in the field of global health (BIRUK 2018; DILGER, KANE & LANGWICK 2012; PACKARD 2016; PRINCE & MARSLAND 2014).

The perpetuation of transformed versions of Global North coloniality stems from the multiple and articulated ways this geopolitical "empire" has been deeply influencing and structuring the social, economic, and political processes that facilitated its spread and dominance over centuries

(BURBANK & COOPER 2012). Undergoing processes of adaptation and transformation (GEISSLER & MOLYNEUX 2011), imperial and colonial forms of Global North medicine and science have been disseminated to diverse geographical contexts. Such trend not only has been visible since the independence of many African countries but has been vehemently foregrounded by the recent traumatic events linked to the Ebola outbreak in West Africa, the rise of the Black Lives Matter (BLM) movement, and the identification of economic, social, racial, and gender inequalities during the Covid-19 pandemic (ABIMBOLA & PAI 2020; BÜYÜM, KENNEY, KORIS, MKUMBA & RAVEENDRAN 2020; LAWRENCE & HIRSCH 2020).

Through various ethnographies and essays, scholars in medical anthropology have described these issues, unveiling tensions and contradictions inherent to the global spread of medical and scientific approaches (FASSIN 2020). Enabling the creation and promotion of global health practices on a planetary scale, existing inequalities between Global North and South contexts have outlined how the origin of global health problems lies in the structural socio-political-economic unbalance between various geographical contexts. In this regard, BEAGLEHOLE and BONITA (2010) have shed light on the representations of Global North health epistemologies and medical practices to combat diseases and health issues in various countries of the Global South as universalistic. The presence of "colonial apparatuses" of global health (RICHARDSON 2020) as well as the interactions between post-colonial states, health systems, and international agencies (GEISSLER 2015) have even more cemented the coloniality of such health-related interventions all around the world. Furthermore, the production of data and numerical indices in public and global health practices have further enhanced the unequal fabrication of health identities and data (KINGORI & GERRETS 2019; SANGARAMOORTHY & BENTON 2012).

Scholars at the intersection of medical anthropology and post- and decolonial approaches have therefore raised critical concerns about such universal and universalistic displays of global health structures and practices. Hence, AFFUN-ADEGBULU and ADEGBULU (2020) show that, while the deficiencies of Global South health systems for combatting the spread of diseases and pandemics have been always underlined, the rooting causes behind the onset and diffusion of health-related issues have been overlooked or barely addressed. For instance, structural disparities that afflict vulnerable populations in the Global South have not fully taken into consideration by global health institutions and practitioners. Instead of bridging the gap between Global North and South health contexts, global health infrastructures have thus reinforced power asymmetries and perpetuated forms of social suffering resulting from political and economic inequalities (ABIMBOLA & PAI 2020). To improve this situation, AFFUN-ADEGBULU and ADEGBULU (2020) propose alternative solutions that go beyond the one-size-fits-all approach inherent to Global North-based biomedical and global health interventions. The production and implementation of context-specific strategies that are able to address diverse health challenges faced by different populations and their will could be one solution. Additionally, AFFUN-ADEGBULU and ADEGBULU (2020) emphasize the need to remove all forms of supremacy, oppression, and racism from scientific and biomedical practices in global health and call for decentralizing knowledge platforms, promoting mutual learning, diversifying power structures, and treating health as a fundamental human-rights goal rather than an act of charity.

Many scholars in medical anthropology and other disciplines in the health humanities and social sciences (ADAMS, BURKE & WHITMARSH 2014; ADAMS, BEHAGUE, CADUFF, LÖWY & ORTEGA 2019; MONTENEGRO, BERNALES & GONZALES-AGUERON 2020) thereby stress the importance of contextualizing global health, Global North biomedicine, and science within historical and socio-cultural dynamics. Therefore, they assert that it is vital to understand and take into account the origins and implications of science and biomedicine by considering social forms of privilege, the relevance of political economies, and the will of reinforcing Eurocentric and Global North types of knowledge (ADAMS, BURKE & WHITMARSH 2014; ADAMS, BEHAGUE, CADUFF, LÖWY & ORTEGA 2019; MONTENEGRO, BERNALES & GONZALES-AGUERON 2020). By adopting such a critical approach to global health practices and interventions, global health practitioners and institutions could promote more inclusive and equitable visions of health future. According to ANDERSON (2014), however, this is not enough as biomedicine in Global South contexts has always integrated decolonial and indigenous critiques about the racially biased biomedical practices that exclude large segments of the population under intervention. In these instances, global medicine's malleability has led to the recognition of hybrid care models and alternative health practices, while simultaneously reinforcing epistemological hierarchies that prioritize Global North biomedical knowledge (ANDERSON 2014: 3822).

By summarizing the critical approaches to global health interventions and actions provided by many scholars in both medical anthropology and other cognate disciplines within the spectrum of medical humanities, it emerges that post- and decolonial critical perspectives not only have shed light on the structural inequalities and inequities inherent to both humanitarian and non-humanitarian global health practices but also has exposed how Global North biomedicine and sciences, with their histories and imperial tendencies, engage in various forms of knowledge extraction from many world regions. In order to complicate this picture even more, the coloniality of global health does not only appear outside of the Global North political borders but are also reproduced and perpetuated within them. For example, SANGARAMOORTHY (2014) shows how HIV/AIDS prevention efforts - which take place in both Global North and South contexts alike – consider individuals' ethnicity, gender, nationality, and "race" and their "affinity concepts" (M'CHAREK 2023) as relevant determinants for comprehending the risk to contract and spread diseases. Although these categories could appear neutral, they actually stem from the same inequalities and regimes of coloniality that have materialized through histories of violence, slavery, oppression and colonization.

Decolonial practices and the rediscovery of indigenous knowledge

The article has thus far focused on how post- and decolonial ideas and approaches have sparked meaningful reflections within medical anthropology and other disciplines within the broader group of medical humanities and social sciences.

These reflections encompass two key areas: first, the (neo)colonial character of global health practices, and second, a deeper exploration of post-colonial subjectivities in relation to health, diseases, disability and well-being. Hence, this section develops an analysis of the influences of post- and decolonial perspectives to medical anthropological research in outlining how these approaches have contributed to ethnographic works and anthropological reflections that recognize the inherent value of indigenous healing practices and systems. Rather than evaluating them solely in comparison to "standard" Global North ideas, narratives, practices and infrastructures around health and well-being, medical anthropologists have documented the relevance of alternative indigenous knowledge about the body and human health.

Such new research perspectives stem from criticism about the previous main anthropological focus on social suffering, structural violence and material poverty within Global South healthcare systems (KLEINMAN, DAS & LOCK 1997; DAS, KLEINMAN, RAMPHELE & REYNOLDS 2000). As elicited by MKHWANAZI (2016), certain strands of research in medical anthropology have tended to produce one-dimensional analyses of complex aspects related to medicine, health, and well-being in Africa and other regions. These attention to specific negative characteristics of African lives risk perpetuating a "single story" that solely provides portrayals and images of suffering, disrupted healthcare systems, and socio-economic inequalities. At the same time, this approach also overlooks the multifaceted socio-cultural and political practices through which people in Global South contexts try to get healed, fight against ailments and diseases and endeavor to embody well-being. For instance, LOCK and NICHTER (2002) note that local populations in Global South settings, such as Indonesia, enact forms of resistance against biomedicine because they see it as a type of colonization. Such resistance manifests through support to local healing systems by lay people or state administrations. To enhance anthropological knowledge about these intricate practices, FASSIN (2020) calls for the need for medical anthropologists to consider the structural conditions in which subjects live, along with the social and economic contexts of their experiences, before conducting any analysis of health and healing practices within specific socio-cultural settings.

In a bid to overcome these challenges and venture into new research frontiers beyond the realms of the "coloniality of knowledge" (NDLOVU-GATSHENI 2013), medical anthropologists have thus turned their attention to multiple and decolonial histories and practices concerning notions of health, illness, and disability from and in Global South contexts. For instance, scholars have outlined not only the colonial structures in place through which disabilities are framed but also the ways forms of bodily non-normativity are conceived of and experienced in many Global South settings (FRIEDNER & ZOANNI 2018; GINSBURG & RAPP 2020; GRECH & SOLDATIC 2016).

By analyzing research on local health systems and indigenous practices, OBRIST and EUWIJK (2020) have emphasized the importance of decolonizing global health (as discussed in the previous section) and examining local health practices in light of/contrast to influences exercised by Global North medical and scientific ideas and interventions. In relation to medical anthropology research in Africa, this special attention to local and regional healing practices is not new as it has had a long history within the discipline (JANZEN 2012). Many anthropologists, in particular, have shown interest in the ways in which healing practices intersect not only with ritual, magical, and religious ideas and epistemologies (JANZEN 1978) but also with underlying modes of radical critique against Global North modernity, ideas of development, and ways of life imposed by contemporary neoliberal capitalism (SCHERZ 2018).

This focus on local forms of care and healing has prompted medical anthropologists to question not only practices but also "indigenous" health systems and their ecologies of care and solidarity (DUCLOS & CRIADO 2020). Such systems are in fact seen to possess their own epistemologies and etiologies as well as have a conception of care and illness that transcends the human body to intersect with more-than-human beings and elements inhabiting the environment. This decolonial perspective in medical anthropology has led to examine the reproduction of indigenous knowledge within Global North systems of governance and medical institutions. These configurations reveal the circulation and re-circulation of non-Global North medical knowledge and systems of care as well as processes of indigenous reshuffling/hybridization/creation that differ from the medical and scientific knowledge and practices implemented by Global North enterprises in various world localities. The presence of institutionalized ideas of medical pluralism within healthcare systems based on Global North instructions and epistemologies (MKHAWANAZI 2021) has prompted some medical anthropologists, like LANGWICK (2011), to raise questions about the etiologies and epistemologies on which these "indigenous" systems of care, within Euro-American-codified healthcare systems in Tanzania, are based (LANGWICK 2011).

Developing these research directions, medical anthropologists have started to document indigenous forms of care. These research directions have been born out of postcolonial contexts (MBEMBE 2001) considered as sites for the intermingling, creolization, and intersections between Global North medicine and sciences, and local curative knowledge and etiologies. Importantly, such hybridizations are not confined to exchanges solely between regions in the Global South and North. Historical and contemporary instances demonstrate exchanges of healing practices even between areas within the Global South, such as the long-standing presence of Chinese medicine in East Africa (HSU 2022). Regarding the political aspects tied to indigenous health practices, OBRIST and EUWIJK (2020: 784) refer to NIEZEN'S (2003) early interest in Global South curative practices and the development of global movement of "international indigenism." As underlined above, in fact, the term "indigenous" have been documented to begin circulating among scholars and activists as early as the 1980s. Being conceived of by movements defending the social integrity of communities in the Global South and pursuing the recognition of alternative health practices at the international level, "international indigenism" has been based on sense of identity as well as forms of belonging to people with deep attachments to their lands and "cultures" believed to be "from time immemorial" (NIEZEN 2003: 4).

However, the use of indigenous medical knowledge within systems of coloniality means that care practices are experienced and reshaped through the lens of Global North medicine, science, and the sovereignty wielded by economic and political structures established by countries in the Global North. Studies in medical anthropology (HSU 2009; LAPLANTE 2015) have illustrated how indigenous medicinal herbs and various local healthcare systems (FÚNEZ-FLORES 2022: 10) in Africa and China are reintegrated into the circuit of Global North medicine through agreements between states, local communities, and pharmaceutical industries. Amidst these extractive dynamics, commercialization interests involve all parties but the final revenues from these activities are unevenly distributed, leading to frictions and conflicts among all the actors involved.

To summarize, this section has briefly hinted at the interest by some scholars in medical anthropology in the existence, circulation, production, and enactment of indigenous healing practices along with Global North health interventions and healthcare systems already in place in many Global South localities. Although the anthropological scholarly sources considered here are not exhaustive, I aim to highlight how identity formation around decolonial and alternative notions, epistemologies, and etiologies of health and well-being are a few of the key characteristics of indigenous healing knowledge. Additionally, it is pertinent to explore how Global North healthcare systems, even outside Euro-American political borders, have integrated indigenous practices within formal systems through forms of medical pluralism. This process of integration also involves elements of extraction. Much like during time of colonization and colonial settlements, prevailing healthcare systems have incorporated specific types of knowledge from alternative sources without fully recognizing them.

Conclusion

This review article has attempted to shed light on the mutual influences and connections between post- and decolonial approaches and some of the more recent ethnographic explorations and epistemological developments in medical anthropology. The analysis presented here has focused on the entanglements between post- and decolonial reflections and research within medical anthropology. Among the many lines of interest, the article has shown three strands that emerged prominently.

The first strand concerns the influence exercised by post- and decolonial reflections on self and subjectivities in studies conducted by scholars in medical anthropology and other disciplines within the range of medical humanities. From the texts analyzed, it emerges that the analytical focus on the social, economic, political and cultural dynamics is connected to post- and decolonial analysis of processes of decolonization and contemporary states of coloniality. The second strand of research inaugurated by this intersection is concerned with the neo-colonial character of medical-humanitarian and global health interventions in various areas of the Global South. In this regard, the article has elicited how various scholars have emphasized the hegemony exercised by the scientific and biomedical categories on which Global North medicine is based. In return, I have also pointed out the lack of epistemological exchanges between such global health actions and local Global South healing systems and practices. Finally, the last section has highlighted how medical anthropology has contributed to an analytical look at Global South systems and practices of care and healing by highlighting relationships and frictions between indigenous healing practices and Global North biomedical epistemologies and systems.

Therefore, post- and decolonial theoretical and empirical essays and texts have thus had the merit of exploring the multiple nuances of the colonial history of Global North science and medicine. Additionally, they have also illuminated the ways in which this set of epistemological, empirical, intellectual practices came into unbalanced contact with the knowledge and healing realities of populations in the Global South, during and after the event of colonization and its political and historical end (VAUGHAN 1991; ARNOLD 1993; ANDERSON 2006). While the interconnections between post- and decolonial approaches and medical anthropology have proved fruitful from various perspectives, these studies, however, risk producing a series of idyllic descriptions of the recurring nationalistic teleology that followed the historical process of decolonization. As pointed out by ANDERSON (2014), following CHAKRABARTY (2000), post-colonial and decolonial influences in medical anthropology have inadvertently described both local readjustments and contestations against Global North medicine and science, bringing out subjectivities in the populations of the Global South. At the same time, such perspectives have also had the demerit of describing the repetition of practices inherent in postcolonial (neo)nationalistic systems of thought aimed at cementing political powers within post-colonial states, in so doing, creating essentialized separate realities. Notwithstanding this, studies in medical anthropology have provided and provide valuable case studies to unearth the colonial genealogies of global health and medicine (ANDERSON 2014: 376). Such analyses have in fact brought out and described the multiple and complex forms of resistance enacted by various subjects such as, for instance, people living in Global South settings, and/or persons forcibly experiencing mobility. In nutshell, the entanglements between post- and decolonial approaches and studies in medical anthropology have unveiled epistemological, etiological and imaginative pluriverses expressed by Global South healing practices.

Such epistemological orientations in medical anthropology have made it possible to unmask how systems of thought and "situated knowledge" (HARAWAY 1988) within the Euro-American world have travelled between various sites and have undergone multiple dislocations, transformations and resistances, within unbalanced power dynamics. Such intertwinements have given rise to the proliferation of hybrid forms of healing practices and epistemologies. Hence, post-colonial and decolonial perspectives have had the merit to emphasize the relevance of etiologies and practices of care and healing that have developed in contact with and/or in contrast to epistemologies pertaining to Global North science and medicine. The decentralized perspective and a radical critique of ethnographic practices and forms of writing within medical anthropology has been a further contribution from post- and decolonial perspectives that have tended to diversify analyses and studies within the discipline. As noted earlier, the interconnections between post- and decolonial approaches and the research conducted in medical anthropology have enabled the uncovering of new notions of health, illness and disability (MARSLAND & STAPLES 2021; STAPLES 2020; STAPLES & MEHROTRA 2016).

Besides a positive evaluation about the entanglements between these two strands of research, it is also necessary to highlight the negative sides of these interconnections. First, the most known centers for knowledge production within medical anthropology are still nowadays located within Global North European and US-based universities, institutions and public events. This hinders the development of discussions about the ways through which anthropological reflections about healing, well-being and mental health have been developed in other world contexts such as Latin America (BARUKEL 2014; MENÉNDEZ 2018). Furthermore, the "diffusion" of theories and ethnographic practices in medical anthropology is strongly determined by the use of English as a vehicular language. This issue has prevented the flourishing of decolonial scholarships about health, illness and disability from other localities within the globalized versions of medical anthropology. Furthermore, the "irony" of some of the post- and decolonial approaches and theories by scholars who inhabit powerful, privileged and ambiguous positions, such those imbricated within the Harvard Medical School and its machinery, exacerbate the existing distance between medical anthropology, as a predominant white space, and the decolonial practices (HERRICK & BELL 2022: 1475).

While, throughout the article, I preferred to focus on the fruitful aspects of the entanglements between post- and decolonial approaches and medical anthropology and other disciplines within medical humanities, the negative aspects of these intertwinements exist. Together with a deeper analysis of these aspects, future research and critical interventions on this topic may also try to elicit in which ways theories and ethnographic data in medical anthropology and other disciplines within the group of medical humanities have been used and read by scholars who define themselves as post- and decolonial independently from their disciplines of reference. This could show how data and theories produced within medical anthropology circulate among scholars belonging to other disciplines and the wider public. As a further final limitation of the present fragmented review, I should also mention the fact that the three research areas examined here have seldomly touched upon intersected questions regarding gender, disability, chronicity, emotions and environmental health or one health which are relevant topics raised by post- and decolonial scholars interested in health, healing and the body. Furthermore, relevant topics such as critical studies of forensic anthropology (M'CHAREK 2023) and its emotional consequences (OLARTE-SIERRA 2019) as well as anthropological analysis of science, technologies and society (KLEINMAN & MOORE 2014), whose topics intersect with the general interests of scholars in medical anthropology at large, have been not considered in this text.

Given such limitations, the multiple lines of research inaugurated by the fruitful intersection between medical anthropology and post- and decolonial reflections and their mutual influence remain important. Hence, one can conclude by stating that this is the direction in which to go in order to unveil today's pressing issues such as global warming, gender inequalities, racism and discrimination in health and technologies. In other words, post- and decolonial perspectives and approaches in medical anthropology allow for the unveiling of other modes of care by highlighting structural and racially-based inequalities that afflict many areas of the Global South and marginalized communities in Global North settings. For these reasons, a medical anthropology that is both post- and decolonial contributes to affirming and describing the presence of epistemological, empirical and analytical realities and practices that, despite the totalizing impulses of Global North ideas of modernity, continue to exist and resist.

Acknowledgments

I thank the following persons for their insightful suggestions and useful comments on previous drafts of the article: Janina Kehr, Aminata Cécile Mbaye and all the members of the Health Matters Research Group at the University of Vienna, Department of Social and Cultural Anthropology. Thanks go to the two anonymous reviewers for their careful and detailed comments and reading of earlier drafts of the manuscript and editors of Curare, Ehler Voss and Philipp Goll, for their assistance and support throughout the writing process.

Notes

1 I use the conventional terms "Global South" and "Global North" to delineate macro-geopolitical and geographical areas with their histories, political dynamics and social configurations. However, such geographical and geopolitical scales are no more precise than in the past due to the presence of complex, manifold and multi-centered power global and regional dynamics. Furthermore, as highlighted by DADOS and CONNELL (2012), "North-South terminology, then, like core-periphery, arose from an allegorical application of categories to name patterns of wealth, privilege, and development across broad regions" that do not correspond to the complexity of the present-day world. Therefore, readers should be aware of the profound limitations of such terminology.

2 Special thanks to Janina Kehr for suggesting possible ways to figure out the intricacies and genealogies around the relations between medical anthropology and critical medical anthropology since the late 1980s. Unfortunately, I do not have here enough space to highlight this history.

References

ABADÍA-BARRERO, CÉSAR E. 2022. Medicine: Colonial, postcolonial, or decolonial? In SINGER, MERRILL; ERICKSON, PAMELA I. & ABADÍA-BARRERO, CÉSAR E. (eds) *A Companion to Medical Anthropology*. Hoboken: Wiley Blackwell: 373–387.

ABIMBOLA, SEYE & PAI, MADHUKAR 2020. Will global health survive its decolonisation? *The Lancet* 396, 10263: 1627–1628.

AÇIKÖZ, SALIH C. 2020. Prosthetic debts. Economies of war disability in neoliberal Turkey. *Current Anthropology* 61, S21: S76–S86.

ADAMS, VINCANNE; BEHAGUE, DOMINIQUE; CADUFF, CARLO; LÖWY, ILANA & ORTEGA, FRANCISCO 2019. Re-Imagining global health through social medicine. *Global Public Health* 14, 10: 1383-1400.

---; BURKE, NANCY J. & WHITMARSH, IAN 2014. Slow research: Thoughts for a movement in global health. *Medical Anthropology* 33, 3: 179-197.

AFFUN-ADEGBULU, CLARA & ADEGBULU, OPEMIPOSI 2020. Decolonising global (public) health: From western universalism to global pluriversalities. *BMJ Global Health* 5, 8: e002947.

ALLEN, JAFARI S. & JOBSON, RYAN C. 2016. The decolonizing generation: (Race and) theory in anthropology since the eighties. *Current Anthropology* 57, 2: 129-148.

ANDERSON, WARWICK 2002. Introduction: Postcolonial technoscience. *Social Studies of Science* 32, 5–6: 643–658.

--- 2006. *Colonial Pathologies: American Tropical Medicine, Race, and Hygiene in the Philippines*. Durham: Duke University Press.

---2009. From subjugated knowledge to conjugated subjects: Science and globalisation, or postcolonial studies of science? *Postcolonial Studies* 12, 4: 389-400.

--- 2014. Making global health history: The postcolonial worldliness of biomedicine. *Social History of Medicine* 27, 2: 372–384.
ARIS, YASMEEN 2021. The reluctant native: Or, decolonial ontologies and epistemic disobedience. *HAU: Journal of Ethnographic Theory* 11, 1: 256–263.
ARNOLD, DAVID 1993. *Colonizing the Body: State Medicine and Epidemic Disease in Nineteenth-Century India*. Berkeley: University of California Press.
BAER, HANS A.; SINGER, MERRILL; SUSSER, IDA (eds) 2004. *Medical Anthropology and the World System*. Westport: Praeger.
BARUKEL, AGUSTINA 2014. *Decolonialidad y salud mental. Perspectivas de un diálogo*. XI Congreso Argentino de Antropología Social, Rosario.
BIEHL, JOÃO 2005. *Vita: Life in a Zone of Social Abandonment*. Berkeley: University of California Press.
--- & MORAN-THOMAS, AMY 2009. Symptom: Subjectivities, social ills, technologies. *Annual Review of Anthropology* 38:267–288.
---; GOOD, BYRON J. & KLEINMAN, ARTHUR (eds) 2007. *Subjectivity: Ethnographic Investigations*. Berkley and Los Angeles: University of California Press.
BEAGLEHOLE, ROBERT & BONITA, RUTH 2010. What is global health? *Global Health Action* 3, 1: 5142.
BHABHA, HOMI 1994. *The Location of Culture*. London: Routledge.
BHAMBRA, GURMINDER K. 2014. Postcolonial and decolonial dialogues. *Postcolonial Studies* 17, 2: 115-121.
BIRUK, CRYSTAL 2018. *Cooking Data: Culture and Politics in an African Research World*. Durham: Duke University Press.
BURBANK, JANE & COOPER, FREDERICK 2012. The empire effect. *Public Culture* 24, 2: 239–247.
BÜYÜM, ALI M.; KENNEY, CORDELIA; KORIS, ANDREA; MKUMBA, LAURA & RAVEENDRAN, YADURSHINI 2020. Decolonising global health: If not now, when? *BMJ Global Health* 5, 8: e003394.
CESAIRE, AIME 2000. *Discourse on Colonialism*. New York: Monthly Review Press.
CHAKRABARTY, DIPESH 2000. *Provincializing Europe: Postcolonial Thought and Historical Difference*. Princeton: Princeton University Press.
CHEN, MEL Y.; KAFER, ALISON; KIM, EUNJUNG & MINICH, JULIE A. (eds) 2023. *Crip Genealogies*. Durham: Duke University Press.
COMAROFF, JANE & COMAROFF, JOHN L. 2003. Ethnography on an awkward scale: Postcolonial anthropology and the violence of abstraction, *Ethnography* 4 (2): 147–179.
--- *Theory from the South: Or, how Euro-America is Evolving toward Africa*. New York: Paradigm.
CRANE, JOHANNA T. 2013. *Scrambling for Africa: AIDS, Expertise, and the Rise of American Global Health Science*. Ithaca: Cornell University Press.
DADOS, NOUR & CONNELL, RAEWYN 2012. The Global South. *Contexts* 11, 1: 12–13.
DAS, VEENA 2008. Violence, gender, and subjectivity. *Annual Review of Anthropology* 37:283-99.

---; KLEINMAN, ARTHUR; RAMPHELE, MAMPHELA & REYNOLDS, PAMELA 2000. *Violence and Subjectivity*. Berkeley: University of California Press.
DE CASTRO, VIVEIROS 2013. The relative native. *HAU: Journal of Ethnographic Theory* 3, 3: 473–502.
DERIDDER, MARIE; EYEBIYI, ELIETH P. & NEWMAN, ANNEKE 2021. Le decolonial turn: Quels échos, résonances et chantiers pour l'APAD? *Anthropologie & Développement*, Hors-série: 331–346.
DE SOUSA SANTOS, BOAVENTURA & MENESES, MARIA P. 2019. Conclusion: Toward a post-abyssal world. In DE SOUSA SANTOS BOAVENTURA & MENESES, MARIA P. (eds) *Knowledge Born in the Struggle: Constructing the Epistemologies of the Global South*. New York: Routledge: 241–245.
DEVISCH, RENÉ & NYAMNJOH, FRANCIS (eds) 2011. *The Postcolonial turn: Re-Imagining Anthropology and Africa*. Bameda: Langaa RPCIG.
DIAGNE, SOULEYMANE B. & AMSELLE, JEAN-LOUP 2020. *In Search of Africa: Universalism and Decolonial Thought*. Cambridge: Polity Press.
DILGER, HÄNSJORG; KANE, ABDOULAYE & LANGWICK, STACEY A. (eds) 2012. *Medicine, Mobility, and Power in Global Africa. Transnational Health and Healing*. Bloomington: Indiana University Press.
DILGER, HÄNSJORG & MATTES, DOMINIK 2018. [2017]. Im/mobilities and dis/connectivities in medical globalisation: How global is Global Health? *Global Public Health*, 13, 3: 265–275.
DU BOIS, WILLIAM E.B. 1979. *The World and Africa*. New York: International Publishers.
DUCLOS, VINCENT & CRIADO, TOMÁS S. 2020. Care in Trouble: Ecologies of support from below and beyond. *Medical Anthropology Quarterly* 34, 2: 153–173.
FANON, FRANZ 1963 [1959]. *The Wretched of the Earth*. New York: Grove Press.
--- 1965 [1961]. *A Dying Colonialism*. New York: Grove Press.
---1986[1952]. *Black Skin, White Masks*. London: Pluto Press.
FARMER, PAUL 2005. *Pathologies of Power: Health, Human Rights and the New War of the Poor*. Berkeley and Los Angeles: University of California Press.
FASSIN, DIDIER 2001. Culturalism as ideology. In OBERMEYER, CARLA M. (ed) *Cultural Perspectives on Reproductive Health*. Oxford: Oxford University Press: 300-317,
---2020. Epilogue: In search of global health. Global health and the new world order. In GAUDILLIÉRE, JEAN-PAUL; BEAUDEVAIN, CLAIRE; GRADMANN, CHRISTOPH; LOVELL, ANNE M. & PORDIÉ, LAURENT (eds) *Global Health and the New World Order. Historical and Anthropological Approaches to a Changing Regime of Governance*. Manchester: Manchester University Press: 230–246.
FEIERMAN, STEVEN 1985. Struggles for Control: The social roots of health and healing in modern africa. *African Studies Review* 28, 2/3: 73.
FEIERMAN, STEVEN; JANZEN, JOHN M. (eds) 1992. *The Social Basis of Health and Healing in Africa*. Berkeley: University of California Press.

FLUEHR-LOBBAN, CAROLYN 2000. Antenor Firmin: Haitian pioneer of anthropology. *American Anthropologist* 102, 3: 449–466.

FÚNEZ-FLORES, JAIRO I. 2022. Decolonial and ontological challenges in social and anthropological theory. *Theory, Culture & Society* 39, 6: 21-41.

GAMLIN, JENNIE; GIBBON, SARAH; SESIA, PAOLA M. & BERRIO, LINA 2020. *Critical Medical Anthropology: Perspectives in and from Latin America*. London: UCL Press.

GEISSLER, WENZEL P. & MOLYNEUX, CATHERINE (eds). 2011. *Evidence, Ethos and Experiment: The Anthropology and History of Medical Research in Africa*. New York: Berghahn Books.

GEISSLER, WENZEL P. (ed) 2015. *Para-States and Medical Science: Making African Global Health*. Durham: Duke University Press.

GILROY, PAUL 1993. *The Black Atlantic: Modernity and Double Consciousness*. Harvard: Harvard University Press.

GINSBURG, FAYE & RAPP, RAYNA 2020. Disability/Anthropology: Rethinking the parameters of the human: An introduction to Supplement 21. *Current Anthropology* 61, S21: S4-S15.

GLISSANT, EDOARD 1989. *Caribbean Discourse: Selected Essays*. Charlottesville: University of Virginia Press.

GOOD, BYRON J.; DELVECCHIO GOOD, MARY-JO; HYDE, SANDRA T. & PINTO, SARAH (eds) 2008. *Postcolonial Disorders*. Berkeley: University of California Press.

GRABOYES, MELISSA 2018. *The Experiment Must Continue: Medical Research and Ethics in East Africa, 1940–2014*. Athens: Ohio University Press.

GRECH, SHAUN & SOLDATIC, KAREN (eds) 2016. *Disability in the Global South: The Critical Handbook*. Cham: Springer.

GUPTA, AKHIL & FERGUSON, JAMES 1992. Beyond "Culture": Space, identity, and the politics of difference. *Cultural Anthropology* 7, 1: 6-23.

HARAWAY, DONNA 1988. Situated knowledges: The science question in feminism and the privilege of partial perspective. *Feminist Studies* 14, 3: 575-599.

HARRISON, FAYE V. 2016. Theorizing in ex-centric sites. *Anthropological Theory* 16, 2-3: 160-176.

HERRICK, CLARE & BELL, KIRSTEN 2021. Epidemic confusions: On irony and decolonisation in global health. *Global Public Health* 17, 8: 1467–1478.

HSU, ELISABETH 2009. Chinese propriety medicines: An "alternative modernity?" The case of the anti-malarial substance artemisinin in East Africa. *Medical Anthropology* 28, 2: 111-140.

--- 2022. *Chinese Medicine in East Africa: An Intimacy with Strangers*. New-York, Oxford: Berghahn Books.

--- & POTTER, CAROLINE 2012. Medical anthropology in Europe: Shaping the field. *Anthropology and Medicine* 19, 1: 1-6.

ILLICH, IVAN 1974. Medical nemesis. *The Lancet* 303, 7863: 918-921.

JANZEN, JOHN M. 1978. *The Quest for Therapy in Lower-Zaire*. Berkeley: University of California Press.

JANZEN, JOHN M. 2012. Afri-global medicine: New perspectives on epidemics, drugs, wars, migrations, and healing rituals. In DILGER, HÄNSJORG, KANE, ABDOULAYE, LANGWICK, STACEY A. (eds). *Medicine, Mobility, and Power in Global Africa. Transnational Health and Healing*. Bloomington: Indiana University Press: 115-137.

JOBSON RYAN C. 2020. The case for letting anthropology burn: Sociocultural anthropology in 2019. *American Anthropologist* 122, 2: 259–271.

JOLLY, JALLICIA 2021. At the crossroads: Caribbean women and (black) feminist ethnography in the time of HIV/AIDS. *Feminist Anthropology* 2, 2: 224–241.

KEHR, JANINA 2018. Colonial hauntings: Migrant care in a French hospital. *Medical Anthropology* 37, 8: 659–673.

KING, CHARLES 2020. *The Reinvention of Humanity. How a Circle of Renegade Anthropologists Remade Race, Sex and Gender*. London and New York: Penguin.

KINGORI, PATRICIA & GERRETS, RÉNE 2019. The masking and making of fieldworkers and data in postcolonial Global Health research contexts. *Critical Public Health* 29, 4: 494–507.

KLEINMAN, ARTHUR; DAS, VEENA & LOCK, MARGARET M. 1997. *Social Suffering*. Berkley and Los Angeles: University of California Press.

KLEINMAN, DANIEL L. & MOORE, KELLY 2014. *Routledge Handbook of Science, Technology, and Society*. London, New York: Routledge.

LANGWICK, STACEY 2011. *Bodies, Politics, and African Healing: The Matter of Maladies in Tanzania*. Bloomington: Indiana University Press.

LAPLANTE, JULIE 2015. *Healing Roots: Anthropology in Life and Medicine*. New York: Berghahn Books.

LAWRENCE, DAVID & HIRSCH LIOBA S. 2020. Decolonising global health: Transnational research partnerships under the spotlight. *International Health* 12, 6: 518–523.

LIVINGSTON, JULIE 2005. *Debility and the Moral Imagination in Botswana*. Bloomington: Indiana University Press.

LOCK, MARGARET & NICHTER, MARK (eds) 2002. *New Horizons in Medical Anthropology: Essays in Honour of Charles Leslie. Theory and Practice in Medical Anthropology and International Health*. New York: Routledge.

--- & NGUYEN, VINH-KIM 2010. *An Anthropology of Biomedicine*. Chichester: Wiley-Blackwell.

LUGONES, MARÍA 2007. Heterosexualism and the colonial/modern gender system. *Hypatia* 22, 1: 186–209.

---2011. Toward a decolonial feminism. *Hypatia* 25, 4: 742–759.

MAHMUD, LILITH 2021. Feminism in the house of anthropology. *Annual Review of Anthropology* 50, 1: 345–361.

MARSLAND, REBECCA & STAPLES, JAMES 2021. Diversifying medical anthropology. *Medical Anthropology* 40, 1: 1–2.

MARZAGORA, SARA 2016. The humanism of reconstruction: African intellectuals, decolonial critical theory and the opposition to the 'posts' (postmodernism, poststructuralism, postcolonialism). *Journal of African Cultural Studies* 28, 2: 161–178.

MBAYE, AMINATA C. 2018. *Les Discours Sur l'Homosexualité au Sénégal*. München: AVM. Edition.

MBAYE, AMINATA C. 2019. Queer political subjectivities in Senegal: gaining a voice within new religious land-

scapes of belonging. *Critical African Studies* 10, 3: 301–314.
Mbembe, Achille 2001. *On the Postcolony*. Berkeley: University of California Press.
Mberu, Blessing U.; Haregu, Tilahun N.; Kyobutungi, Catherine & Ezeh, Alex C. 2016. Health and health-related indicators in slum, rural, and urban communities: A comparative analysis. *Global Health Action* 9, 1: 33163.
M'charek, Amade 2023. Curious about race: Generous methods and modes of knowing in practice. *Social Studies of Science* 53, 6: 826-849.
Menéndez, Eduardo L. 2018. Antropología médica en América Latina 1990-2015: Una revisión estrictamente provisional. *Salud Colectiva* 4, 3: 461–481.
Mignolo, Walter D. 2021. *The Politics of Decolonial Investigations*. Durham: Duke University Press.
––– & Walsh, Catherine E. 2018. *On Decoloniality: Concepts, Analytics, Praxis*. Durham: Duke University Press.
Mkhwanazi, Nolwazi 2016. Medical Anthropology in Africa: The Trouble with a Single Story. *Medical Anthropology* 35, 2: 193-202.
––– 2021. Postcolonial medicine in African contexts. In Lüddeckens, Dorothea; Hetmanczyk, Philipp; Klassen, Pamela & E., Stein, Justin B. (eds) *The Routledge Handbook of Religion, Medicine, and Health*. London and New York: Routledge: 363-375
Montenegro, Christian; Bernales, Margarita & Gonzales-Agueron, Marcela 2020. Teaching global health from the south: Challenges and proposals. *Critical Public Health* 30, 2: 127–129.
Mudimbe, Valenti-Yves 1988. *The Invention of Africa: Gnosis, Philosophy, and the Order of Knowledge*. Bloomington: Indiana University Press.
Ndlovu-Gatsheni, Sabelo S. 2013 *Empire, Global Coloniality and African Subjectivity*. London, New York, Shanghai: Berghahn Books.
Niezen, Ronald 2003. *The Origins of Indigenism: Human Rights and the Politics of Identity*. Berkeley: University of California Press.
Obrist, Brigit & Van Eeuwijik, Peter 2020. Medical anthropology in, of, for and with Africa: Three hotspots. *Medical Anthropology* 39, 8: 782–793.
Olarte-Sierra, María Fernanda 2019. Of flesh and bone: emotional and affective ethnography of forensic anthropology practices amidst an armed conflict. *Tapuya: Latin American Science, Technology and Society* 2, 1: 77–93.
Packard, Randall 2016. *A History of Global Health: Interventions into the Lives of Other Peoples*. Baltimore: Johns Hopkins Press.
Prince, Ruth, Marsland, Rebecca (eds) 2014. *Making and Unmaking Public Health in Africa: Ethnographic and Historical Perspectives*. Athens: Ohio University Press.
Quijano, Aníbal 2000. Coloniality of power and Eurocentrism in Latin America. *International Sociology* 15, 2: 215–232.
–––2007. Coloniality and modernity/rationality. *Cultural Studies* 21, 2: 168–178.
Richardson, Eugene T. 2020. *Epidemic illusions: On the Coloniality of Global Health*. Cambridge: MIT Press.
Robinson, Cedric 2021 [1983]. *Black Marxism: The Making of the Black Radical Tradition*. London: Penguin Classics.
Said, Edward W. 2003 [1978]. *Orientalism: Western conceptions of the Orient*. London: Penguin.
Sangaramoorthy, Thurka 2014. *Treating AIDS. Politics of Difference, Paradox of Prevention*. New Brunswick: Rutgers University Press.
––– 2018. "Putting band-Aids on things that need stitches": Immigration and the landscape of care in rural America. *American Anthropologist* 120, 3: 487–499.
––– 2019. Liminal living: Everyday injury, disability, and instability among migrant Mexican women in Maryland's seafood industry. *Medical Anthropology Quarterly* 33, 4: 557–578.
––– & Benton, Adia 2012. Enumeration, identity, and health. *Medical Anthropology* 31, 4: 287–291.
––– & Carney, Megan 2021. Immigration, mental health and psychosocial well-being. *Medical Anthropology* 40, 7: 591–597.
Savransky, Martin 2017. A decolonial imagination: Sociology, anthropology and politics of reality. *Sociology* 51, 1: 11–26.
Scherz, China 2018. Stuck in the clinic: Vernacular healing and medical anthropology in contemporary sub-Saharan Africa. *Medical Anthropology Quarterly* 32, 4: 539–555.
Scheper-Hughes, Nancy & Lock, Margaret M. 1987. The mindful body: A Prolegomenon to future work in medical anthropology. *Medical Anthropology Quarterly* 1, 1: 6–41.
Singer, Merrill 2004. Critical medical anthropology. In Ember, Carol J. & Ember, Melvin (eds) *Encyclopedia of Medical Anthropology: Health and Illness in the World's Cultures*. New York: Kluwer Academic/Plenum Publishers: 23–30.
Spivak, Gayatri 1988. Can the subaltern speak? In Nelson, Cary & Grossberg, Lawrence (ed) *Marxism and the Interpretation of Culture*. Chicago: University of Illinois Press, Chicago: 271-313
Staples, James 2020. Decolonising disability studies? Developing South Asia-specific approaches to understanding disability. In Mehrotra, Nilika (ed). *Disability Studies in India*. Singapore: Springer Singapore: 25-41
Staples, James & Mehrotra, Nilika 2016. Disability studies: Developments in anthropology. In Grech, Shaun & Soldatic, Karen (eds). *Disability in the Global South: The Critical Handbook*. Cham: Springer International Publishing: 35-49,
Tilley, Helen 2011. *Africa as a Living Laboratory. Empire, Development, and the Problem of Scientific Knowledge, 1870-1950*. Chicago: University of Chicago Press.
Trouillot, Michel-Ralph 1991. Anthropology and the savage slot: The poetics and politics of otherness: In Fox, Richard G. (ed). *Recapturing Anthropology: Working in the Present*. Santa Fe: School of American Research Press: 17–44,
Vaughan, Megan 1991. *Curing their Ills: Colonial Power and African Illness*. Stanford: Stanford University Press.

VAN WOLPUTTE, STEVEN. 2004. Hang on to your self: Of bodies, embodiment, and selves". *Annual Review of Anthropology* 2004. 33:251–69

VERGÈ, FRANÇOISE 2021. *Decolonial Feminism*. London: Pluto Press.

WHITMARSH, IAN 2009. Hyperdiagnostics: Postcolonial Utopics of Race-Based Biomedicine. *Medical Anthropology* 28, 3: 285–315.

WILLIAMS, ERICA L. 2022. Centering black women: Critique of mainstream anthropology form the margins at HBCU. *Cultural Anthropology* 37, 3: 404–411.

This article has been subjected to a double blind peer review process prior to publication.

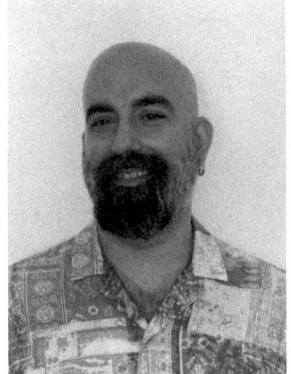

Giorgio Brocco, is a lecturer and postdoctoral fellow at the University of Vienna, Department of Social and Cultural Anthropology, where he is associated with the research group "Health Matters." Based on his doctoral research, Giorgio is currently working on his first monograph, tentatively titled "Trajectories of Albinism: Subjectivities, Experiences, and Narratives in Tanzania," in which he documents the life experiences of people with albinism in Tanzania. Giorgio's new research project explores the various ways humans conceive, interact with, and imagine toxicity and the afterlives of artificial molecules in the French overseas departments of Martinique. Over the years, Giorgio's research has been published in peer-reviewed journals, book chapters, and blog posts. Furthermore, he is also the editor of the recent Berghahn Books Series "Disability and Chronicity Through the Ethnographic Lens."

University of Vienna
Department of Social and Cultural Anthropology
Universitätsstraße 7
1010 Wien
e-mail: giorgio.brocco@univie.ac.at

Healthcare Workers' Experiences during the COVID-19 Pandemic in Argentina
A Syndemic Approach to Hospitals

ANAHI SY

Abstract The SARS-CoV-2 pandemic put into evidence the need to think in syndemic terms, as all health issues co-exists with environmental, social, economic and political factors that exacerbate any epidemic. In this work we propose the concept of "syndemic" to analyze what happened in public hospitals of Argentina, from a socio-epidemiological perspective. In methodological terms, semi-structured interviews with workers were conducted in two phases: initially, at the onset of the pandemic in Argentina, using WhatsApp, and subsequently, as the pandemic progressed, through virtual meeting platforms. The content analysis of the narratives makes it possible to identify how health workers, in many situations, are the architects of problem-solving strategies that emerge during the pandemic: managing shortages (of supplies, for example) and providing care – even at risk to their own health. We also identified deliberative spaces of "dialogue-work" among workers (meetings, crisis committees, union activities), recognized as environments of support, care and/or self-care during the pandemic. In these spaces some challenges facing the health sector must be seen syndemically. We conclude by analyzing the potential of applying the concept of syndemic to public health problems and policies in hospital institutions from a socio-epidemiological perspective, highlighting the transformative process of workers to attend to emergency situations. These dimensions are crucial in developing health policies in synch with other processes of socio-epidemiological change, which occur both within hospitals and within the population that uses public health services.

Keywords hospital – syndemic – COVID-19 pandemic – healthcare workers – socio-epidemiology

Introduction

The declaration of the coronavirus pandemic has highlighted that any approach aiming to understand and address health-disease processes at the population level, recognize environmental risks, and promote more balanced and sustainable ecosystems must necessarily begin with considering the interactions of humans with other living things and the shared environment they inhabit (WALSH et al. 2020; ROCK et al. 2009).

CHABROL & KEHR (2020) propose that COVID-19 emerged at a time when, in Southern European countries such as France and Spain, important social movements in defense of public health were under way; the pandemic interrupted mass-mobilization while also fueling continued reflection on the gradual degradation of working conditions and quality of care in public hospitals due to under-staffing and under-financing. In Argentina, a similar process was unfolding, evidenced from previous years, for example, by the downgrading of the Ministry of Health to a department, resulting in a reduction in personnel and funding, with the consequent degradation in working conditions and salaries (SY et al. 2021).

In Latin American countries, COVID-19 pandemic overlaps with endemic diseases (tuberculosis, Chagas, dengue, hepatitis, and HIV, among others, called "neglected diseases"), seasonal diseases (such as the flu and other respiratory diseases) and diseases that have acquired an epidemic or pandemic status (obesity, diabetes, and hypertension, among others). The situation is potentiated not just fear of contagion, but also actual experiences of stigmatization, racism, gender inequalities, inequalities in the access to information, exposure to different types of violence, the availability of social protection policies and programs as well as access to health care, among others (FRONTEIRA et al. 2021).

Ethnographic studies evidence that hospitals are not closed, total institutions but are continuations and condensations of society at large. Van der GEEST and FINKLER (2004) contrast new hospital ethnography with earlier functionalist models. They state that life in the hospital should not be regarded in contrast with life outside the hospital. STREET and CLEMAN (2012) highlight the hospital is not an island and cite recent articles have emphasized the permeability of the hospital: the movement of patients, staff, and visitors in and out of the institution and the social relationships, inequalities, and cultural values that they carry with them (e.g., MOONEY & REINARZ 2009; QUIRK; LELLIOTT & SEALE 2006). Moreover, it is argued that those social and cultural continuities are not merely external impingements on biomedicine. Biomedical practices and diagnostic styles are themselves adapted to the social and cultural conditions of the country in which a hospital is located (e.g., FINKLER 2004; GIBSON 2004; see also BERG & MOL 1998). While the COVID-19 pandemic has rendered the image of hospitals as solutions for health problems even more powerful and unquestioned, it has also shown the fragility, overwhelmedness and chronic strain of these institutions, aggravated by decades of outsourcing and austerity policies that have left many of them drained of personnel, maintenance and means.

In Latin America, and specifically in Argentina, ethnographic studies (CROJETOVIC 2010; GARCÍA et al. 2017; SY et al., 2021; MOGLIA & SY 2022 and 2023) illustrate the permeable character of hospital practices in contexts of scarce resources and extraordinary demand. These studies highlight how the subjectivity, creativity, and agency of workers shape processes of care and attention, as well as communication and interpersonal relationships.

Our hypothesis is that in the hospital space, during the pandemic, there is a synergistic interaction between pre-existing precarious working conditions and emergent problems, such as physical and mental exhaustion, promoting the development of new forms of working and new capacities that are unpredictable in the context of uncertainty.

In this sense, we revisit the concept of syndemic, introduced by the anthropologist Merrill Singer in 1990 to talk about the HIV/AIDS epidemic. He proposed understanding the synergistic interaction of health problems that coexist with environmental, social, economic and political factors that exacerbate any epidemic (SINGER 1996).

This biocultural synthesis involves: 1) the intertwinement with the most important health problems at the local level; 2) the way in which individuals and their community understand health-disease; 3) the intervening social, political and economic dimensions, as well as the environmental conditions that can contribute to health or to the development of disease. This dialectical proposal drives the concept of syndemic (SINGER 1996 and 2003).

More recently SINGER and colleagues (2003) have broadened this concept to analyze its application to public health programs and policies. This entails a syndemic orientation to the prevention of as well as to the health problems associated with an epidemic, considering these connections when developing health policies in tune with other processes of social change so as to generate the conditions necessary for collective health. The concept of syndemic challenges the way disease has traditionally been conceptualized and defined, as a differentiated, discrete and disjunctive entity that exists (in theory) separate from other diseases and the social groups and contexts in which they are found (SINGER & CLAIR 2003).

Such an expansion of the concept posits the existence of "community health" for both social scientists and those who develop policies. In this sense the concept operates as a theory that would make it possible to predict how to intervene effectively to mitigate risks to public health (TSAI et al. 2017).

This syndemic model shares fundamental premises with the field of public health and with collective health in particular. Such premises have been described in detail – with greater emphasis in one dimension or another – from the schools of thought of Latin American Social Medicine (LAURELL 1986), critical epidemiology (BREILH 1995 and 1997), also Collective Health; ethnoepidemiology (ALMEIDA FILHO 1992, 1993, 2000 and 2020) and socio-epidemiology or sociocultural epidemiology (MENÉNDEZ 1990, 1992, 2008 and 2009;

HARO 2010; HERSCH-MARTÍNEZ & HARO 2007; HERSCH-MARTÍNEZ 2013; SY 2017).

In very general terms, what can be highlighted in any of these schools of thought is the need to consider any health problem (whether or not it is epidemic) in the socio-cultural, political and economic context in which it occurs, understanding that the problem at the same time emerges from these conditions, which in turn also impact the persistence, chronicity or the possibility of caring for health effectively. Disease is not conceived of as an individual but rather as a collective, social, or community problem (the terminology varies by author).

In seeking to replace the term pandemic for that of syndemic, emphasis is placed on that broader view; these concepts and perspectives acquire new value in light of the present pandemic.

Analyzing the present situation as a syndemic – much in the same way as analyzing it from a socio-epidemiological perspective – means thinking beyond the SARS-CoV-2 virus, incorporating an analysis of the global problem of social inequalities and living conditions, that is, how the population lives, falls ill and dies, in addition to considering the synergy resulting from the interaction between COVID-19 and other epidemic or endemic diseases.

This pandemic has irreversibly deteriorated the health of many sectors of the population, even those who have not contracted COVID-19; the increase in unemployment and poverty, the mental health crises and emergencies or the worsening of previously existing chronic diseases are some examples, among others.

Recent research developed in Latin America also makes use of the concept of syndemic; ALMEIDA-FILHO highlights a proliferation of concepts such as syndemic, infodemic, pandemic, to propose the need to develop a "pandemiology" (2021: 18). MASTRANGELO et al. (2022) signal that in Argentina, COVID-19 emerged in a syndemic manner with infectious and chronic diseases as well as those associated with poverty (dengue, tuberculosis and measles). They suggest that this multi-morbidity is simultaneous, consecutive, and preexisting in the marginalized neighborhoods with a high index of unmet basic needs in which the authors' research takes place. In this sense, the April 2022 editorial of *Cadernos de Saúde Pública* criticizes the thesis that this is a "democratic disease," highlighting that all epidemics are at the same time biological, social and historical phenomena that express themselves unequally in the population, seen in the inequities in the risk of infection, illness or death, as well as the possibility of accessing care. In this context, as it is now known, the COVID-19 morbidity and mortality burden falls principally upon the poorest, revealing and deepening the enormous social inequalities in health already existing in Brazil (WERNECK 2022) and also in other countries. WERNECK (2022) therefore calls for the incorporation of the concepts of syndemic and intersectionality in epidemiological studies, citing the work of HORTA et al. (2022), who, in the same issue of the journal, demonstrate the lack of access to health care during the first months of the pandemic in the most disadvantaged groups of the population, which makes it possible to foresee the impact in chronic diseases the care of which was postponed. In Argentina, the work of REMORINI et al. (2021) makes reference to the local expressions of the syndemic; they posit it in relation to the impact on and implementation of responses in the everyday work of health services, from the perspective of applied anthropology. Unlike these works, our study proposes that the syndemic does not "act upon" or "express itself in" but rather is a constitutive part of what occurs in hospitals and among its workers. Here we propose to explore from a socio-epidemiological perspective the syndemic of the COVID-19 in health institutions, particularly public hospitals.

In this sense, we propose the syndemic involves health institutions, where the uncertainty, new work protocols, and physical and mental exhaustion of the workers interact synergistically with the prior working conditions (work precarity, supply shortages, among others), requiring the development of new forms of working and new capacities, necessary in contexts of uncertainty. Simultaneously, this situation has demanded new strategies of government, in which the epidemiological data is insufficient to understand and address the problem. The circulation of people can be measured, permitting an understanding of the increase or decrease in the number of new cases and deaths, but it has been seen that there is no measure that works to intervene in human behavior. Although it is true that the circulation of a virus can be limited with vaccinations, this pandemic involves much more than a virus; it has involved living conditions, the way in which people live and die – having irreversibly deteriorated the health of many population groups – and it has challenged the forms of work and the work capacities of the health sector as well as demanded of the State in general new government strategies [SY *et al.* 2021].

Although the virus does not seem will stop circulating, the challenge of intervening in this new socio-epidemiological reality that the pandemic has produced will remain.

Our proposal is to discuss a little-examined and little-visualized dimension of the syndemic that unfolds within the health institutions. We base our work in the narratives of health workers in hospitals of the southern area of the metropolitan region of Buenos Aires, where the majority of hospitals in the metropolitan area are located, as well as where indicators related to health, overcrowding, poverty and violence are most concerning.

Theoretical-methodological framework

Although it is possible to think that "globalization" has tended to homogenize health problems and populations, and indeed the COVID-19 epidemic has acquired worldwide dimensions in epidemiological terms, the way in which the disease affects populations is not homogenous; the social and cultural inequalities that characterize Latin American countries represent a limit to statistical standardization or generalization. As is proposed with the concept of syndemic, an epidemic health problem does not have its origin in the risk behaviors of people and social collectives in a way isolated from their living conditions, their access to health care and their ability to meet basic needs such as food, work or housing, among others. This category also allows us to reflect upon the differences and inequalities that preexist the COVID-19 pandemic and their differential impact by gender, age, ethnicity or social class, among other dimensions.

Latin America is characterized by its diversity and its ethnic, racial, economic and environmental inequalities, among others, which coexist and overlap in ways that can be more or less contradictory. In these contexts the pandemic also presents consequences that cannot be described, much less addressed, exclusively from a modern epidemiology point of view.

The socio-epidemiological approach developed in this work has its precedents in Latin American authors such as MENÉNDEZ (2008 & 2009), SY (2017 & 2018) and SY *et al.* (2021), seeking to overcome the biological and positivist biomedical bias that characterizes a large part of modern epidemiological research in order to examine this pandemic not explicitly intending to do so "in syndemic terms" per se. Doing so entails an openness to ethnographic-type research to examine unexplored issues and model new scientific objects in the field of collective health, recognizing the socio-historical character of the discipline of epidemiology itself. It also requires the construction of models of interpretation of health-disease processes[1] in modern societies capable of integrating both perspectives through the application of methodological strategies that competently combine quantitative and qualitative approaches in a single ethno-epidemiological strategy. One of the central premises is that health-disease phenomena are social processes and, understood as such, are also historical, complex, fragmented, conflictive, dependent, ambiguous and uncertain (ALMEIDA FILHO 1992; 2000). Whith "Socio-epidemiology" or "socio/ethno-epidemiology" we highlight the need to integrate the methods, techniques and theory of medical anthropology, ethnography and epidemiology (HERSCH MARTÍNEZ & HARO 2007; MENÉNDEZ 2008, 2009; ÁLVAREZ 2008; HARO 2010; HERSCH MARTINEZ 2013). This perspective does not just seek to change the statistical representation of a phenomenon but rather to obtain a conceptual development that makes it possible to understand the historical and social base of the unequal distribution of health in human populations. Thus, socio-epidemiology is a discipline whose ultimate purpose is to transform concrete health realities. From the perspective of Latin American socio-epidemiology, the subject is considered not only the unit of description and analysis, or as is traditionally considered, "the object of study," but also is included as a transformative agent that produces and not just reproduces the social structure and meanings (MENÉNDEZ 2009).

These perspectives are closely related to North American Critical Medical Anthropology (they share a Marxist legacy). A recent criticism of the concept of syndemic, published in *Social Science and Medicine*, signals the absence of references to intersectionality (SANGARAMOORTHY & BENTON 2021). The response posits that syndemic theory stems from Critical Medical Anthropology (BULLED & SINGER Y OSTRACH 2022). In 1995, Singer had already clearly stated that from this perspective: 1) health is profoundly political; 2) the mission of the theory is emancipatory and aims not just to understand but also to change the patterns of oppression and exploitation that occur with respect to health; 3) a commitment to change is established as a fundamental aspect of the discipline (SINGER 1995). These assertions are very familiar in the field of collective health as a whole, and in the field of sociocultural epidemiology in particular.

It is from this theoretical-methodological approach that we propose situating this study in hospitals so as to analyze the syndemic reality they experience in the context of the coronavirus pandemic.

The area of study is the southern region of the Metropolitan Area (MA) of the province of Buenos Aires. According to the 2010 census, the population of the province of Buenos Aires is 15,625,084 inhabitants, 9,916,715 of which correspond to the MA (INDEC 2012). The southern region of the MA has the highest population density, with 3,747,486 inhabitants. According to INDEC data (2021), in the second semester of 2020, 40.9% of homes in the *partidos* [jurisdictions unique to the province of Buenos Aires, similar to counties] of Greater Buenos Aires were at poverty level and 4.5% were considered to be indigent[2]. This region concentrates the largest number of Zonal and Interzonal General Hospitals in the province, a total of 20.[3]

The sample of people interviewed was made up of general hospital workers (of zonal or interzonal hospitals) from the southern area of the MA. The selection criteria for interviewees was: a) that their workplace (at least one, in the event of more than one job) be one of the aforementioned general hospitals; b) that they worked at the institution (whether prior to or at the time of the interview) during the period of the coronavirus pandemic. These sampling criteria ensure achieving the greatest possible diversity of workers, not just professionals but also technical and administrative staff.

In this sense, in a first exploratory stage, carried out between May and August 2020, contact with the workers was established via WhatsApp in order for them to narrate their experiences. A message was sent through institutional networks inviting workers to participate in the research, offering information about the study objectives and the ethical precautions that would be taken. When a worker responded with interest in participating, we provided them with greater detail through a WhatsApp audio message or a personal call. These first contacts also referred us to others who might be interested in participating (reaching a total of 41 workers; 34 female and 7 male). In the second stage of the study, occurring between May and November 2021, a total of 38 semi-structured interviews were carried out (24 female and 14 male), mostly via Zoom, GoogleMeet or Jitsi, although some were in-person. Staff of different areas such as cleaning, administration, medical care, mental health, social work, nursing, biochemistry and security were interviewed in order to reveal the views and experiences of different social actors involved in the hospital during the pandemic, as is proposed by socio-epidemiology.

The processing of the whatsApp audio and the interviews recorded included a full transcription of the audio and content analysis of the narratives. Initially, a comprehensive and thorough reading of the transcribed text was carried out, oriented at obtaining an overall view of the full set of narratives obtained and the elaboration of categories and theoretical concepts, as well as an explanation of the preliminary presumptions orienting the analysis. Next, certain descriptions and inferences were elaborated and definitive emergent categories were constructed in articulation with the data and theoretical categories.

This project was carried out in the framework of the research grant "PISAC-COVID-19: Argentine Society in the Postpandemic" (2020) of the Agencia Nacional de Promoción de la Investigación, el Desarrollo Tecnológico y la Innovación, Argentina.

It is also connected to an international network of research teams examining the experiences of health workers during the COVID-19 pandemic in 22 countries. This network is coordinated by the Rapid Research Evaluation and Appraisal Lab (RREAL) at the University College of London in the United Kingdom.

The data was obtained in accordance with the ethical precautions established by the Argentine Ministry of Health in the document "Guía para Investigaciones con Seres Humanos" (Res. MSAL 1480/2011). The overall project encompassing this study was approved by the Research Ethics Committee of the Juan H. Jara National Institute of Epidemiology (Record N°059/2016, FOLIO 107. Comittee of Human Research Minutes N°2, 09/02/2016, Code SY 01/2020).

Results

> "We went to work because it was our job and we'd chosen it before the pandemic, but nobody wanted to be a hero, ok? We all had to do it because it was our job."

The people interviewed organized their narratives according to their lived experiences, shared among those who work in hospitals and health centers but not always coinciding with the "official" narratives, such as the organization of data into epidemiological weeks or according to stages (from 1 to 5, in which different activities were allowed). During this time of epidemiological emergency, in which we were in contact with different hospital workers from the Greater Buenos Aires area, we could identify experiences that situate those who work in the health field in a unique framework of space and time. We organize our results based on this temporality narrated to us by those at the center of this work.

Not seeing the forest for the virus

The start of 2020 attracted our attention towards a virus moving in an unpredictable way, giving rise to the idea of it "escaping from a laboratory" in China, although finally its zoonotic origin was established (REYES et al. 2021).

On January 12, 2020, Chinese scientists made public the genome of the new coronavirus, the cause of a new human disease: COVID-19 (WHO 2020b).

Rapidly we found ourselves living in a reality that felt part science fiction movie and part apocalyptic catastrophe. There was a proliferation of images from China that at the time seemed farfetched – people with plastic bottles covering their whole faces or with surgical suits fumigating streets or involved in violent confrontations in incomprehensible situations.

On March 2, 2020, the first case of coronavirus was confirmed in Argentina and on March 7 the first death was reported in Latin America. On March 11 the World Health Organization (WHO) granted pandemic status to the expansion of SARS-CoV-2, highlighting the speed of the virus's spread and the passivity of the governments worldwide (OMS 2020). At the same time it was highlighted that COVID was not just a crisis in the area of public health but affecting society as a whole, and governments were urged to take measures oriented at the prevention of infection and minimize the virus's impact. On March 12, 2020, the Argentine government signed the Decreto de Necesidad y Urgencia (Declaration of Emergency) that established a health emergency, enabling the Ministry of Health to adopt the necessary public health measures to avoid propagation of the virus. As a corollary, on March 19, 2020, Preventative and Obligatory Social Isolation was declared. Only those known as "essential workers" had permission to circulate. In general, health workers were considered "essential," although not all of them; there were primary health care centers closed at the start of the pandemic and hospital services that were "put on pause," workers without protocols to follow, with uncertainty about the obligation of going to work (or not) and in what way, to do what, how to reach patients and users that needed them urgently, for psych treatments or for dental emergencies or for medication for a chronic illness.

> "This issue that during the pandemic there aren't other illnesss, no? Because there are people who need continuity in their treatment, these situations of risk that haven't been easy in mental health."

The quotation emphasize the fact that lot of people does not receive care for chronic or emergent health problems except for COVID-19. In this context "new" care strategies were developed, certain territory-based practices appeared, in the home of the users themselves or via telephone.

Another important issue was the shrinking of the staff in the health system in general, because people went on leave or because they were part of the population defined as "at risk."

In the institutions, rotating work shifts were established so as to reduce the exposure of the whole staff at the same time. These shifts meant more hours in the day but fewer overall days, thereby guaranteeing coverage and, in the event that isolation was necessary, a smaller group of people who would be required to isolate.

A critical example at the start of the pandemic was availability the personal protective equipment (PPE), in addition to the discussions about its utility as a type of protection from or prevention of infection, and about who should use it and when. This situation stirred old rivalries among professionals: At the beginning, the infectious diseases specialists fought everyone to not use a mask, they wanted to work in the emergency room without a mask themserlves. There was a big crisis between the staff and the infectious diseases specialists, everyone brought their own mask. They say: "At first everything was very tense".

In some cases, during this first period, access to equipment occurred through donations or the direct purchase of the workers themselves.

We have to get through the winter

These issues highlighted at the start of the pandemic were accented and others were added in the winter, during what was known as the "first wave." Regarding this situation, one worker explains:

> "We had to buy our clothes, we had to deal with the bad pay. The work isn't worse than before the pandemic, the risk is greater than before, and people are worse to the health staff, they're more violent, more toxic".

Although the shortages of supplies as well as the situations of violence towards the staff or the low salaries are problems that pre-exist the pandemic, they became more visible and magnified especially when there was a sharp increase in the number of cases, intensifying unease and discomfort.

While violence was recognized as pre-existing, it reemerged in this context, especially visible to those in charge of hospital security. A health care worker ironically says:

> "In March of this year, a person came in, I was covering the emergency room. And a guy came in who wanted to be seen right away, but I explained that the protocol was that he had to go through triage to get his temperature taken (…) And the man spit green mucus in my face. And when I told my boss what had happened he said 'well, it's part of the job'. The supervisor higher up told me 'ok, but let it go, it's over now'."

These narratives reveal how violent situations are naturalized within the institutions and those who suffer them are revictimized. In this case the security staff, in the context of the pandemic, were doubly exposed: to violence but also to infection as the result of interactions of this type with those in need of hospital care.

In this context there were also those who took leave or quit for health or personal reasons, leaving their job in the hospital: With the increase in demand, scarcity was once again magnified:

> "In nursing human resources have been historically scarce. These are problems from even before I started working at the hospital (…) this goes beyond the pandemic".

Another preexisting issue that worsened during the pandemic is the lack of space and cleanliness in the hospitals:

> "In the middle of a COVID outbreak in our service (residency) we had to fight for them to clean our bathroom, they hadn't come to clean the area where we sleep for three months".

New demands also appeared: "the emergency room became an intensive care unit and we aren't intensivists." Old rivalries reemerged, connected to institutionalized inequalities among doctors and nurses, linked to professional and gender hierarchies that preexist the pandemic: It's disproportionate, you know, it's always been like that and it'll continue to be like that, it's like machismo, ok? There's a huge difference between men and women, here there's a huge difference between doctors and nurses. Here we're still in the stone ages, they think we're errand boys, "bring the bedpan," "change the diaper." This got worse in the pandemic [...] the nursing profession grew a lot during the pandemic [...] but there's no recognition of that.

Low salaries and multiple jobs are also a pre-pandemic epidemic:

> "And don't get me started on what salaries we make, it's so little, we doctors earn a little more but this nurse who is vital, who is ... nothing would work without her (...) has to have two jobs, so they come, that is, they work 12 hours a day and get here totally exhausted".

A health care worker ironically says

> "Don't congratulate me so much, just pay me what I'm worth; I'm just saying, just a minor little detail [ironic tone]".

The adjustment variable in these situations in the body itself, the health of the workers. In the case of women, many are also heads of households depending entirely on their salary and domestic labor for the reproduction of the domestic life in their homes:

> "You start rethinking a bunch of things, I've always had two jobs, and that's when I started rethinking things and saying 'Is all of this worth it?' At the end of the day, if something happens to me, my kids will be left all alone."

The simultaneity of problems at an institutional level, reflected in the narratives, reaches the subjective, individual dimension:

> "After a long shift, when it was a hard shift, you come back to your house and feel empty, you feel like you gave it your all and you've earned your rest, but you also feel like you don't have anything, like your life doesn't belong to you, you feel like you came home to your house and suddenly your life is nothing...you were 32 hours at the hospital and you get home at 5 in the afternoon and you don't have the energy to do anything, it's so hard, and of course there's the contact with death, the contact with people dying."

Workers situate their hope in the immediate future. "It's winter now, we have to get through the winter [...] we hope that the spring comes soon". The major expectation was around the vaccination to change the situation.

The second wave

During the second wave these problems worsened and magnified, the lack of roms and workers fatigue and exhaustion were increased; "I had to sedate four patients on the same night because there was no room in critical care".

Workers, and especially the area of social work, recognize problems have to do more with the precarization of the lives of people, they stopped seeing and stopped accompanying "even if it's not something COVID related, or it is but in a more complicated way".

As is evident in the quote, workers recognize that COVID acts syndemically on populations, even when they don't give it that name, they recognize the worsening of the clinical state of chronic diseases and the deterioration of living conditions as a determinant of health-disease.

There is unease expressed in the narratives resulting from the unique circumstances in synergistic interaction with pre-existing issues. This synergy among epidemics at the population level also manifests itself at the hospital level, among its workers: they spoke of episodes of COVID-19 infection, hypertension, rashes, headaches, panic attacks, extreme anxiety, fear, stiffness, and worsening of the state of chronic diseases, as well as "sadness, deep sadness" throughout this period.

In search of the next horizon

In the same way that problems that magnify and worsen during the pandemic can be identified, there are also relational dimensions that intervene synergistically in supporting health workers. In this sense, the place of the "team" in moments of anxiety or despair is valued; the team is the space in which "paralysis" is prevented and a response to the "fear" and "paranoia" emerging in these circumstances is given, especially in solitary moments.

> "The pandemic put on the table some issues that I understand are like a certainty in our work logic, that is, we couldn't have gone through this pandemic without all the teamwork we'd been carrying out beforehand [...] it somehow puts into evidence that you have to plan things, you have to

work in teams, [...] nothing new, right? But I think it really imposed itself strongly".

Unions, crisis committees and team meetings were spaces of support for workers during the crisis, with them stating "we couldn't have tolerated it any other way." Although we asked about spaces of emotional or psychological support formally offered during the pandemic, the institutional proposals did not go beyond the institution's own area of psychology, that is, seeing one's own colleagues, with the intimidating situation that this generated. There were also individual responses to start therapy or pharmacological treatment, with personalized therapeutic accompaniment.

A horizon of hope with the vaccines can be detected. Hospitals have now become spaces in which the workers feel "safer than outside." There's a certain stability and predictability of PPE, protocols and protection measures.

Although workers seek a future horizon in which "a return to normalcy" is possible, the transition to the post-pandemic requires certain considerations in the sense that there is no returning to a previous state but rather a continuity toward a new socio-epidemiological reality. From this place it is necessary to consider and re-consider the reality of those who today provide care with respect to who they were two years ago. A return to a previous state is implausible, no one comes back unchanged from situations like those experienced in the pandemic; even continuing like nothing had happened would be disruptive, because the circumstances have changed.

The workers discern consequences of the syndemic in the future, in particular in the socio-epidemiological profiles of those who seek care in the public health sector. The secondary effects of sequelae of COVID will have to be cared for, as well as the health situations that were postponed during the pandemic:

"A lot of surgeries are being reprogrammed and that's wrong. It's wrong at the level of the patient's health, but at the level of the health system there's no alternative: I don't have beds in the care units, I can't make them up, so I can't operate."

There are cases of scheduled operations and other situations more connected to chronic diseases, the treatments of which were interrupted or discontinued, with a corresponding worsening of the clinical picture.

These issues present a novel scenario in public health, a new socio-epidemiological reality with some conclusions that require consideration:

"The lessons aren't for each health service, they're for the health system [...]. It doesn't work, you have the public system, the social security system and the private system, with zero coordination, zero. So the public system ends up absorbing everything that the private and social security systems can't or don't want to absorb in the pandemic [...]. The country's health system needs to be reformed because like this it works badly, no, it works terribly. And there's no awareness in the population that it's not working."

This narrative expresses the need to establish deep transformations. Talk to "zero coordination" refers to the fragmentation of the health system in Argentina composed by public, social security and private parts. Although it is true, as FRANCO and MERHY (2017) explain, the work processes in health materialize in the actors – individual and collective – that produce them, we should not lose sight of the local scenarios in which those processes take place. The pandemic generated a new situation at the macro level that had unique expressions in hospitals, contributing to the visibilization of certain problems and highlighting some social actors while invisibilizing others. In this sense, our work did not limit itself to exclusively interviewing workers that directly treated COVID cases, but rather, in accordance with our theoretical framework, posits the necessity of dialoging with all hospital workers situated in their unique work scenarios. This allows us to see that the distribution and concentration of processes affecting health are not the same for all the personnel, with differences produced in relation to, for example, gender, hierarchy and labor inequalities existing within the institutions.

Discussion and final considerations

From the syndemics framework, it becomes clear that during the pandemic, hospitals faced a convergence of existing issues such as endemic and epidemic diseases and social demands with newly emerging or situational problems and challenges, all arising from the necessity to respond to the health emergency. The pandemic established new, centralized forms of organization, norms and management decisions that came into tension with the limits of autonomy of workers to produce health, with impacts that could have been reflected in their work with users and in their relationship with colleagues or other hospital workers. Those interviewed narrated that their everyday work was carried out in a context of scarcity of PPE, human resources and infrastructure, which demands constant readjustment and adaptation between the ideal and the possible.

These transformations show that their everyday work also affects the health of hospital workers. An often invisibilized or naturalized dimension in the narratives of these workers is that beyond the exposure to COVID infection, a number of new situations of violence, tension and stress appear in hospitals; a closeness to death is developed in a way that, according to the interviewees' narratives, they had never experienced before.

In this sense, granting descriptive and analytic priority to the different experiences and perspectives of those who work in the health field though their own narratives allows for a comprehension of certain dimensions that contribute to fragilizing and violating the health of the workers themselves, connected not only to the unexpected events of the pandemic that we are analyzing (as it is unfolding), but also to pre-existing problems that become magnified during the epidemiological emergency: working multiple jobs, low salaries and the inadequate infrastructure of the hospital are recurring topics. These dimensions highlight the syndemic character that the pandemic acquires within health institutions, in this case hospitals.

A recent work of Eduardo Menéndez (2020) posits that the fundamental space in which COVID-19 is combatted has been and continues to be that of self-care, which constitutes one of the structures that micro-groups generate in order to live and survive. Menéndez highlights that this reality remains hidden in politics and medicine, invisibilizing where the true power of containment of the pandemic lies. In our work, while our focus is on a very particular part of the population – health workers – we also could posit that an enormous power of containment, care and self-care lies in the health teams. Health care workers, in a number of situations, are architects of problem-solving strategies that emerge in the situation of the pandemic: managing scarcity (of PPE, for example) and offering care even at risk to one's own health. This is expressed in certain meanings and subjectivities shared among these workers within each institution: first, prioritize the care of the patient's health, and then one's own health or wellbeing. In relation to this dimension, different spaces of dialogue among workers (work meetings, crisis committees, union activity) are recognized as spaces of support for getting through this period of the pandemic and are valued as spaces of care or self-care.

In these deliberative dialogue-work spaces, some challenges facing the health sector (connected especially to the syndemic character of the pandemic) can also be seen, especially postponement in the care of chronic diseases, in ambulatory care, in surgical interventions and in neglected endemic health problems. The Pan-American Health Organization (2020) posits that services for the prevention and treatment of noncommunicable diseases (NCDs) have been gravely affected since the start of the COVID-19 pandemic in the region of the Americas. According to a survey carried out by the Pan-American Health Organization/World Health Organization (PAHO/WHO), since the start of the pandemic, routine health services were reorganized or suspended and many ceased to provide attention to people in treatment for diseases like cancer, cardiovascular disease and diabetes. Similarly, many health workers who usually provide this care were redirected to other areas for COVID care. Ambulatory health care services were partially or totally suspended in many countries, like Argentina. These interruptions have affected the care of people with NCDs, diabetes, hypertension, oral care and rehabilitation (PAHO 2020).

At present, health workers identify difficulties associated with this situation and, from our socio-epidemiological perspective, must appeal to their experience and knowledge of the territory to implement strategies that allow them to solve the problems that can be discerned in the present and that become important challenges for the near future.

In this way, the consideration of the syndemic within the health institutions themselves shows the complexity of dimensions that remain hidden or invisibilized from a macro perspective or from a conventional perspective of epidemiology of health systems and services. Examining the unique character of the worker and their work and of the teams in each institution contributes to the development of public health measures and interventions within these institutions that favor the health of their workers and of the general population, attentive to the needs felt by those who carry out their work there.

In this sense, we propose an innovative approach to syndemic by applying this concept to healthcare workers in the hospitals in which old and new problems interact synergistically. It is crucial to consider dimensions that are intrinsically connected, taking as a starting point those collective dialogue-work spaces among workers as a fundamental cohesive force for promoting any change or social transformation that materializes within the institution.

Notes

1 From Latin American theorizations health-disease process is defined as a multidimensional phenomenon that involves not only biological and clinical aspects but also social, cultural, economic, and political factors. It emphasizes how these dimensions interact and determine the health and disease of populations, highlighting social inequities and structural conditions that influence health outcomes.

2 Defined as the condition in which a person or household lacks the economic resources to cover essential basic needs for daily subsistence.

3 https://www.gba.gob.ar/saludprovincia/regiones_sanitarias

References

ALMEIDA FILHO, NAOMAR 1992. Por una etnoepidemiología. Esbozo de un nuevo paradigma epidemiológico. *Cuadernos Médico Sociales* 61: 43–47.

--- 1993. La práctica teórica de la epidemiología social en América Latina. *Salud y Cambio* 10, 3: 25–31.

--- 2000. La ciencia tímida. Ensayos de deconstrucción de la Epidemiología. Buenos Aires: Lugar Editorial:11–56.

--- 2020. Etnoepidemiología y salud mental: perspectivas desde América Latina. *Salud Colectiva*, 16:e2786. DOI: 10.18294/sc.2020.2786.

--- 2021. Sindemia, infodemia, pandemia de COVID-19: Hacia una pandemiología de enfermedades emergentes. Salud Colectiva, 17:e3748 doi: 10.18294/sc.2021.3748.

BERG, MARC & ANNEMARIE, MOL 1998. *Differences in medicine: Unraveling practices, techniques, and bodies.* Durham, NC: Duke University Press: 1–12.

BREILH, JAIME 1995. Epidemiology's Role in the Creation of a Humane World: Convergences and Divergences Among the Schools. *Social Science & Medicine* 41, 7: 911–914. http://hdl.handle.net/10644/3286.

--- 1997. A epidemiologia na humanização da vida: convergências e desencontros das correntes. In Barata, R.b.; Barreto, M.l.; Filho, N. Almeida & Veras ,R.p. (eds) *Equidade e saúde: contribuições da epidemiologia.* Rio de Janeiro: Fiocruz/Abrasco: 23–37.

CHABROL, FANNY & KEHR, JANINA 2020. The Hospital Multiple: Introduction. *Somatosphere.* https://somatosphere.com/2020/hospital-multiple-introduction.html/ [10.7.2024]

CROJETHOVIC, MARÍA 2010. El efecto de la informalidad en la dinámica organizacional. El análisis de los hospitales públicos de la Provincia de Buenos Aires. *VI Jornadas de Sociología de la UNLP*. Universidad Nacional de La Plata. Facultad de Humanidades y Ciencias de la Educación. Departamento de Sociología, La Plata. https://www.aacademica.org/000-027/338 [10.7.2024].

FARMER, PAUL 1996. On suffering and structural violence: A View from below. *Daedalus* 125, 1: 261–283. https://www.jstor.org/stable/20027362

FRONTEIRA, INÊS; SIDAT, MOHSIN; MAGALHÃES, JOÃO PAULO; CUPERTINO DE BARROS, FERNANDO PASSOS ; DELGADO, ANTÓNIO PEDRO; CORREIA, TIAGO, DANIEL-RIBEIRO, CLÁUDIO TADEU & FERRINHO, PAULO 2021. The SARS-CoV-2 pandemic: A syndemic perspective. *One health* 12, 100228. https://doi.org/10.1016/j.onehlt.2021.100228

FINKLER, KAJA 2004. Biomedicine globalized and localized: Western medical practices in an outpatient clinic of a Mexican hospital. *Social Science & Medicine* 59: 2037–2051.

GUADALUPE, GARCÍA MARIA; LAURA, MARIA (Recoder) & SUSANA MARGULIES 2017. Space, time and power in hospital health care: contributions based on the ethnography of an obstetric center. *Salud Colect* 13: 391–409.

GIBSON, DIANA 2004. The gaps in the gaze in South African hospitals. *Social Science & Medicine*, 59: 2013–2024.

HARO, JESÚS ARMANDO (ed) 2010. *Epidemiología Sociocultural. Un diálogo en torno a su sentido, métodos y alcances.* Buenos Aires: Lugar Editorial: 10–32.

HERSCH-MARTÍNEZ, PAUL 2013. Epidemiología sociocultural: una perspectiva necesaria. *Salud Publica Mex.* 55: 512–518. http://www.scielosp.org/pdf/spm/v55n5/v55n5a9.pdf [10.7.2024].

INSTITUTO NACIONAL DE ESTADÍSTICAS Y CENSOS 2012. *Censo Nacional de Población, Hogares y Viviendas 2010. Censo del Bicentenario.* Buenos Aires, Argentina: INDEC. https://www.indec.gob.ar/ftp/cuadros/poblacion/censo2010_tomo2.pdf [10.7.2024].

--- 2021. Incidencia de la pobreza y la indigencia en 31 aglomerados urbanos. Segundo semestre de

2020. *Condiciones de vida* 5, 4. Buenos Aires, Argentina: INDEC. https://www.indec.gob.ar/uploads/informesdeprensa/eph_pobreza_02_2082FA92E916.pdf [10.7.2024].

Laurel, Asa Cristina 1986. El estudio social del proceso salud-enfermedad en América Latina. *Cuadernos Médicos Sociales* 37: 3-18.

Menendez, Eduardo Luis 1990. *Antropología médica en México. Hacia la construcción de una epidemiología sociocultural. Antropología médica Orientaciones, desigualdades y transacciones.* Distrito Federal, México: CIESAS: 24-49.

--- 1992. Salud pública: sector estatal, ciencia aplicada o ideología de lo posible. La crisis de la salud pública: reflexiones para el debate Washington DC: OPS. Publicación Científica N° 540: 103–122.

--- 2008. Epidemiología sociocultural: propuestas y posibilidades. Región y Sociedad, 20(2): 5–50. http://www.redalyc.org/articulo.oa?id=10209802 [10.7.2024].

--- 2009. *De Sujetos, saberes y estructuras. Introducción al enfoque relacional en el estudio de la Salud Colectiva.* Buenos Aires, Argentina: Lugar Editorial:11–63.

--- 2020. Consecuencias, visibilizaciones y negaciones de una pandemia: los procesos de autoatención. *Salud Colectiva* 16:e3149. doi: 10.18294/sc.2020.3149 [10.7.2024].

Moglia, Brenda & Sy, Anahi 2022. A metaethnographic approach to rationality and emotionality in the health care processes in hospitals in Latin América. *Saude e Sociedade* 31, 2: 1–14. DOI: 10.1590/S0104-12902022210140es.

--- & Sy, Anahi 2023. Chronic disease care during the covid-19 pandemic. An analysis of the narratives of public hospital workers in the Buenos Aires suburbs (Argentina). *Enero-Abril* 41, 1: 1–11 DOI: https://doi.org/10.17533/udea.rfnsp.e349651.

Mooney Graham & Jonathan Reinarz (eds) 2009. *Permeable walls: Historical perspectives on hospital and asylum visiting.* Amsterdam, Netherlands: Rodopi.

OMS-OPS 2020. La COVID-19 afectó el funcionamiento de los servicios de salud para enfermedades no transmisibles en las Américas. https://www.paho.org/es/noticias/17-6-2020-covid-19-afecto-funcionamiento-servicios-salud-para-enfermedades-no [10.7.2024].

Quirk, Alan, Lelliott, Paul & Seale, Clive 2006. The permeable institution: an ethnographic study of three acute psychiatric wards in London. *Social science & medicine* (1982) 63, 8: 2105–2117. DOI: https://doi.org/10.1016/j.socscimed.2006.05.021

Remorini, Carolina; Teves, Laura; Pasarin, Lorena & Castro, Mora 2021. Expresiones locales de la sindemia COVID-19: estrategias de los trabajadores de salud en Argentina. *Cuadernos Médicos Sociales* 61, 3: 19–35. https://cms.colegiomedico.cl/https-cms-colegiomedico-cl-wp-content-uploads-2021-11-suplementoantropologia2021-pdf/ [10.7.2024].

Reyes, Lenisse, Lilibeth Ortiz, Maxwell Abedi, Yenifel Luciano, Wilma Ramos, Pablo J. de JS. Reyes 2021. Misinformation on COVID-19 origin and its relationship with perception and knowledge about social distancing: A cross-sectional study. *PLOS ONE* 16(3): e0248160. DOI: https://DOI.org/10.1371/journal.pone.0248160.

Rock, Melanie, Bonnie Buntain, Jennifer Hatfield, Benedikt Hallgrímsson 2009. Hallgrímsson, Animal-human connections, "one health," and the syndemic approach to prevention. *Social Science & Medicine* 68: 991–995. DOI: https://doi.org/10.1016/j.socscimed.2008.12.047

Sangaramoorthy, Turka & Adia Benton (2021). Intersectionality and syndemics: a commentary. *Social Science & Medicine* 68: 1-3 113783. DOI: https://doi.org/10.1016/j.socscimed.2021.113783.

Singer, Merrill 1990. Reinventing medical anthropology: toward a critical realignment. Social Science & Medicine, 30, 2: 179-187. DOI: 10.1016/0277-9536(90)90078-7.

--- 1995. Beyond the Ivory Tower: critical praxis in medical anthropology. *Medical Anthropology Quarterly*, 9(1): 80–106. DOI: https://doi.org/10.1525/maq.1995.9.1.02a00060.

--- 1996. A Dose of Drugs, a Touch of Violence, a Case of AIDS: Conceptualizing the SAVA Syndemic. *Free Inquiry in Creative Sociology* 24, 2: 99-110. Recuperado de: https://ojs.library.okstate.edu/osu/index.php/FICS/article/view/1346.

Singer, Merrill & Clair Scott 2003. Syndemics and public health: reconceptualizing disease in bio-social context. *Medical Anthropology Quarterly* 17(4): 423-41. DOI: 10.1525/maq.2003.17.4.423.

Street, Alice & Coleman, Simon 2012. Introduction: Real and Imagined Spaces. *Space and Culture* 15(1): 4-17. DOI: https://doi.org/10.1177/1206331211421852.

Sy, Anahi 2017. Socio/Ethno-epidemiologies: proposals and possibilities from the Latin American production. *Health Sociology Review* 26(3): 293–307. DOI: https://doi.org/10.1080/14461242.2017.1368402

--- 2018. Mujeres, Migrantes Y "Locas". Trayectorias De Internación Psiquiátrica Entre 1895 Y 1940 En Argentina. *Trayectorias Humanas Trascontinentales* 3: 5–19. DOI: https://doi.org/10.25965/trahs.754.

---, Moglia, Brenda & Derossi, Paula 2021. Todo se transformó completamente: experiencias de atención a la pandemia de COVID-19 en el ámbito de la salud pública. Rev. Salud Pública, 26(2): 60–72. https://revistas.unc.edu.ar/index.php/RSD/article/view/33077 [10.7.2024]

---Moglia, Brenda; Derossi, Paula& Aragunde, Gisele 2021. La urgencia bajo la lupa: una revisión de la producción científica sobre servicios de emergencia en hospitales desde la etnografía. Cad. *Saúde Pública* 37, 1: e00026120 DOI: 10.1590/0102-311X00026120

C Tsai, Alexander; Mendenhall, Emily; A Trostle, James & Kawachi, Ichiro 2017. Co-occurring epidemics, syndemics, and population health. *The Lancet* 389(10072): 978–982. DOI: 10.1016/S0140-6736(17)30403-8.

Van Der Geest, Sjaak & Finkler, Kaja 2004. Hospital ethnography: introduction. *Soc Sci Med* 59, 10:1995–2001. DOI: 10.1016/j.socscimed.2004.03.004

Walsh, Michael G.; Sawleshwarkar, Shailendra; Hossain, Shah & Mor, Siobhan M. 2020. Whence the next pandemic? The intersecting global geography of the animal-human interface, poor health systems and air transit centrality reveals conduits for high-impact spillover. *One Health* 11 (100177). DOI: 10.1016/j.onehlt.2020.100177.

World Health Organization 2020a. La OMS caracteriza a COVID-19 como una pandemia. https://www.paho.org/es/noticias/11-3-2020-oms-caracteriza-covid-19-como-pandemia [10.7.2024].

--- 2020b. Listings of WHO's response to COVID-19. https://www.who.int/news/item/29-06-2020-covid-timeline [10.7.2024].

Zinsstag, Jakob; Schelling, Esther; Wyss, Kaspar & Mahamat, Bechir 2006. Potential of cooperation between human and animal health to strengthen health systems. *The Lancet* 366(9503): 2142–5. DOI: 10.1016/S0140-6736(05)67731-8.

This article has been subjected to a double blind peer review process prior to publication.

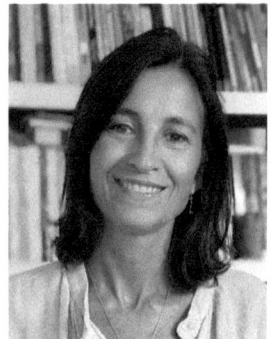

Anahi Sy, Dr., is a Social Anthropology and health researcher. Bachelor's degree in Anthropology and a Ph.D. in Natural Sciences from the National University of La Plata (Buenos Aires, Argentina). Fellow Researcher at the Institute of Justice and Human Rights from National Council for Scientific and Technical Research (CONICET, Argentina). Professor at the Department of Community Health. National University of Lanús (UNLa). Her work focuses on health care alternatives and indigenous peoples, socio/ethno-epidemiology and mental health in psychiatric institutions and general hospitals, from an ethnographic perspective. She has worked as a consultant in UNICEF Argentina projects, in the Ministry of Health and Social Development of Argentina. Additionally, she is a member of the coordinating committee of the Argentine Network of Anthropology and Health (RedASA) and serve on the Research Ethics Committee at the University of Gran Rosario (UGR), Argentina.

e-mail: anahisy@gmail.com

FORUM
FORUM

Alternative Religiosität und „natürliche" Geburt
Religionswissenschaftliche Bemerkungen zu Robbie Davis-Floyd

JILL MARXER & JOHANNES ENDLER

2022 widmete sich die zweite Ausgabe der *Curare* dem Schwerpunktthema *Lebensanfänge und -enden. Ethnographische Erkundungen und methodologische Reflexionen*. Der vorliegende Aufsatz greift das Thema Lebensanfang und Geburt abermals auf und widmet sich zu diesem Zweck den Schriften der US-amerikanischen Anthropologin und Aktivistin ROBBIE DAVIS-FLOYD (geb. 1951). Die Herausgeberinnen des genannten *Curare*-Schwerpunktes bezeichnen DAVIS-FLOYDS *Birth as an American Rite of Passage* (1992) als Klassiker (REHSMANN & SIEGL 2022: 8). Sie selbst sagt über sich:

> For three generations of practitioners, activists, and policymakers in the fields of childbirth, obstetrics, midwifery, and maternity care, I have served as the international public face of anthropology. [...] My anthropological work has heavily influenced the language and supported the direction of the movements for the humanization of birth in the US, Europe, and particularly Latin America (DAVIS-FLOYD 2021).

Die Feststellung, ihre anthropologische Arbeit habe die Sprache aktivistischer Bewegungen – deren Angehörige DAVIS-FLOYDS Forschungsgegenstand darstellen – stark beeinflusst, ist bemerkenswert. Anders als in den Beiträgen in „Lebensanfänge" finden sich bei DAVIS-FLOYD kaum methodologische Reflexionen über die eigene Positionalität und die Interferenzen zwischen Ethnologie und Feld. Ihre erklärte Absicht ist es, bestimmte Vorstellungen, wie eine Geburt idealerweise begleitet werden sollte und welche Erfahrungen die Gebärende dabei machen könne, zu popularisieren. Sie stellt damit ein Orientierungswissen zur Verfügung, das von Befürworter*innen einer „natürlichen" oder „ganzheitlichen" Geburt angeeignet werden kann und Geburtsnarrative im Feld prägt, die ihrerseits zur Basis von Forschungsdaten werden können.

Ziel unseres religionswissenschaftlich angelegten Beitrages ist es, Davis-Floyds Vorstellungen und Empfehlungen zur Geburt – die idealerweise eine spirituelle Erfahrung für die Gebärende und ihre Helferinnen sei – herauszuarbeiten und als Ausdruck der alternativreligiösen Kultur ihrer Zeit zu analysieren.

Holistische Geburtsbegleitung

DAVIS-FLOYD ist Vertreterin einer *engaged anthropology*[1] wie sie in den 1970er und 80er Jahren gerade in Bezug auf Forschungen über Geburt üblich war. Beispielhaft sei die IV. Internationale Fachtagung der Arbeitsgemeinschaft Ethnomedizin (AGEM) genannt, die 1978 unter dem Titel *Die Geburt aus ethnomedizinischer Sicht* stattfand. Im Vorwort zum gleichnamigen und die Konferenz vertiefenden *Curare*-Sonderband (1983) beklagte KIRCHHOFF die sterile Atmosphäre moderner Kreißsäle. Technische Fortschritte hätten zwar zu einer Senkung der Mütter- und Kindersterblichkeit beigetragen, dennoch gebe es eine intensive Bewegung gegen die „familienfeindliche" Geburtshilfe. Die Schulmedizin mit ihrer berechtigten Forderung nach Sicherheit für Mutter und Kind dürfe sich auch der Forderung nach Sinnerfahrung nicht verschließen (KIRCHHOFF 1983: 6). Die AGEM nahm damit im Gefolge der nordamerikanischen *Anthropology of Birth*,[2] zu der auch DAVIS-FLOYD zählt, Impulse aus den Gesundheits- und Frauenbewegungen auf und verfolgte eine gesellschaftspolitische Agenda. Mit ethnomedizinischen[3] Forschungen in außereuropäischen Kulturen und der kritischen Analyse der modernen Geburtshilfe wollte man dazu beitragen, in den Industriegesellschaften eine „menschlichere"[4] Geburtsbegleitung zu etablieren, die die Bedürfnisse werdender Mütter in den Mittelpunkt stellt und ihre Erfahrungen ernst nimmt. In Geburten, die von Hebammen begleitet werden und außerhalb des ärztlichen Zugriffs auf „natürliche" Weise ablaufen, erblickte man dabei ein emanzipatorisches Aufbegehren gegen patriarchale Strukturen.

Davis-Floyd stellt Medikalisierung und Patriarchat nun eine „natürliche" Spiritualität gegenüber. „Spirituality is everywhere in birth, if only we have eyes to see it" schreibt sie im Vorwort des Sammelbandes *Sacred Inception. Reclaiming the Spirituality of Birth in the Modern World* (Delaporte & Martin 2018: xxiii) und deutet damit an, es gebe eine kontextunabhängige spirituelle Dimension der Geburt, die für jede Frau offenbar wird, sofern keine Hindernisse im Weg stehen. Um diese Dimension zu erfahren, müssen sich Gebärende und Geburtshelferinnen laut Davis-Floyd am „holistischen" Paradigma orientieren. Dieses sei eines von drei Haltungen, welche die Geburtspraktiken im Westen und zunehmend auf der ganzen Welt bestimmen:

> The *technocratic model* stresses mind-body separation and sees the body as a machine; the *humanistic model* emphasizes mind-body connection and defines the body as an organism; the *holistic model* insists on the oneness of body, mind, and spirit and defines the body as an energy field in constant interaction with other energy fields (Davis-Floyd 2001: 5).

Es handelt sich hier nicht nur um ein analytisches Modell, um empirische Daten zu ordnen, sondern um eine normative Gegenüberstellung. Das technokratische Modell spiegele die westlichen Werte der Profitmaximierung und der patriarchalen Institutionen wider. Das Krankenhaus sei am Modell der Fabrik orientiert, in dem die defekte Maschine – die Frau – repariert werden muss, um ein ansprechendes Produkt – das Baby – herzustellen (vgl. Davis-Floyd 2001: 5).

Das Anliegen des humanistischen Modells hingegen sei die Reformation des medizinischen Systems von innen: „Humanists wish simply to humanize technomedicine – that is, to make it relational, partnership-oriented, individually responsive, and compassionate" (Davis-Floyd 2001: 10). Sie praktizierten selbst keine komplementär- oder alternativ-medizinischen Heilverfahren[5], seien aber grundsätzlich aufgeschlossen dafür. „Most will not undergo the radical shift in values that permits them to go beyond compassion to employ the healing power of that mysterious thing called energy in overcoming disease" (Davis-Floyd 2001: 15).

Dieser radikale Schritt, so Davis-Floyd, wird erst im holistischen Modell vollzogen, bei dem man Logik und rigide Klassifikationen überschreite und Kreativität und Intuition auf überraschende Weise zum Vorschein kämen. Als Beispiele für holistische Positionen nennt sie einen Klassiker der neopaganen Wicca-Bewegung (Starhawk 1979) und das *Farm Midwifery Center*, eines der ersten außerklinischen Geburtshilfezentren der USA, das durch Ina May Gaskins Klassiker *Spiritual Midwifery* (1974) bekannt wurde.[6] Holistisch Praktizierende gehen davon aus, dass das menschliche Wohlbefinden vom Fließen einer Energie, aus der alle Menschen bestehen, abhänge und arbeiten mit einem breiten Spektrum von Methoden wie Akupunktur, Homöopathie, Reiki oder Magnetfeldtherapie.[7] Auch wenn eine Hebamme das Fenster öffne, Musik einschalte, mit der Gebärenden tanze oder sie mit ihrem Partner eine Zeit lang alleine lasse, könne man von energetischen Interventionen sprechen (vgl. Davis-Floyd 2001: 17).

Ein holistischer Ansatz käme nach Davis-Floyd nicht nur den gebärenden Frauen zugute, sondern transformiere auch die Ärztinnen und Hebammen, die den „Paradigmenwechsel" von der technokratischen Medizin zur ganzheitlichen Heilkunst vollzogen haben. „The quest to recover healing in medicine reflects a virtual hunger for a spiritual dimension of life; it indicates a willingness to honor a transcendent, transpersonal aspect of existence" (Dossey 1998: x), ist im Vorwort zu Davis-Floyds *From Doctor to Healer* zu lesen. Holistische Ärztinnen und Hebammen treten in diesem Sinn als spirituelle Expertinnen auf, die gebärenden Frauen einen Raum eröffnen können, in dem die Geburt als Ereignis mit spiritueller Bedeutung erfahren werden kann. Mehr noch gelte dies für sogenannte Doulas (gr. Δούλη: Dienerin), nicht-medizinische Geburtshelferinnen, die Frauen ganzheitlich und spirituell begleiten (vgl. Davis-Floyd 2015). Der Begriff Doula, der eine alte Tradition suggeriert, wurde tatsächlich erst in den 1970er Jahren durch die Anthropologin und Still-Aktivistin Dana Raphael popularisiert (vgl. Raphael 1976) und ist ein Beispiel dafür, wie einem

Konzept eine „invented tradition" (Hobsbawm & Ranger 1992) beigefügt und damit Legitimität zugesprochen werden kann. Mit der Religionssoziologin Danièle Hervieu-Léger gesprochen, fungiert die vermeintlich jahrtausendealte Tradierung des Doulawissens als eine „chain of memory" (Hervieu-Léger 2000). Tradition von Erinnerungsketten als transgenerationales Wissen validiert und legitimiert also eine Glaubensvorstellung.

Religionswissenschaftliche Einordnung

Die Rede von Ganzheitlichkeit und der energetischen Verbundenheit allen Seins ist aus religionswissenschaftlicher Perspektive ein Merkmal von alternativer Spiritualität (vgl. STOLZ 2005: 122), wie sie in der anglo-amerikanischen New Age Bewegung der 1970er und 1980er Jahren populär wurde (vgl. BOCHINGER 1994: 137; HAMMER 2001; HANEGRAAFF 1996; HEDGES & BECKFORD 2000; POSSAMAI 2005; SUTCLIFFE 2002.). Der Begriff Spiritualität wird heute überwiegend als alternative, individualisierte und nicht-institutionalisierte Religiosität verstanden, die in vielen Gegenden der Welt Schnittmengen mit alternativen Heilverfahren und der Wellnesskultur aufweist.

Sich selbst beschreibt DAVIS-FLOYD als eine Person, die nach langer Suche ihre eigene Form der Spiritualität entdeckt hat, was ebenfalls typisch für den alternativ-religiösen Diskurs ist. Nach der presbyterianisch geprägten Kindheit sei sie als junge Studentin mit mexikanischem Schamanismus und einer New Age-Heilungsgruppe in Kontakt gekommen und von einer Forscherin zur glühenden Adeptin dieser Gruppe geworden. Schließlich habe sie sich auch von dieser äußeren Autorität abgewandt und übe seitdem nur mehr Praktiken aus, die in Übereinstimmung mit einem reflektierten, selbst gewählten Glaubenssystem stehen (vgl. DAVIS-FLOYD & LAUGHLIN 2016). In ähnlicher Weise reklamieren die Frauen in PAMELA KLASSENs religionswissenschaftlicher Studie über amerikanische Hausgeburten eine positiv konnotierte Spiritualität für sich, die sie als „a more personal, immediate, and authentic sacrality" (KLASSEN 2001a: 65) verstehen und von eher negativ bewerteter Religion abgrenzen.[8]

Dieses Verständnis des Begriffes „Spiritualität" kann innerhalb der sogenannten „alternativen Religiosität" verortet werden. Aus Sicht des Feldes ist Spiritualität dabei eine Perspektive auf das gesamte Leben und weniger eine spezifische Praxis oder Lehre (vgl. LÜDDECKENS & WALTHERT 2010: 43). HUBERT KNOBLAUCH beschreibt „Spiritualität" als eine soziale Form der Religion, die in Distanz zu großen religiösen Organisationsformen steht und auf direkte, unmittelbare, persönliche Erfahrung anstelle von „Glaube aus zweiter Hand" abstellt (vgl. KNOBLAUCH 2006: 92). Die zunehmende emische Verwendung des Spiritualitätsbegriff nimmt KNOBLAUCH zum Anlass, diesen auch in der Religionswissenschaft als analytischen Begriff zu nutzen: „[D]er Begriff spielt im Vokabular der religiösen Akteure eine große Rolle. Deswegen scheint es auch sinnvoll, diesen, wie man sagen könnte: Akteursbegriff als Ausgangspunkt für weitere Konzeptionalisierungen zu nehmen, die wissenschaftlich anschlussfähig sind" (KNOBLAUCH 2005: 125).[9]

Es lässt sich jedoch auch die Ablehnung einer metasprachlichen Verwendung von Spiritualität feststellen, da „die Übernahme objektsprachlicher Begriffe in die fachsprachliche Terminologie einer Fremdbestimmung unseres Forschungsgegenstandes" (ZEUGIN 2020: 24) gleichkomme und nicht mehr zwischen emischer und etischer Perspektive differenziert werden könne. LÜDDECKENS zufolge lässt sich die genannte Normativität der Unterscheidung von spirituell und religiös vermeiden, indem man „Religion" als „umbrella term" verwendet (vgl. LÜDDECKENS 2018: 171f.).[10] In der religionswissenschaftlichen Fachsprache findet sich darum auch der Begriff der (alternativen) Religiosität anstelle von Spiritualität. Dadurch bietet sich die Möglichkeit der Beschreibung jener Phänomene, die im Feld als *spirituell* und aus religionswissenschaftlicher Sicht als *Religion* bezeichnet werden können (vgl. MEZGER 2018: 27).[11] Alternative Religiosität fasst Ausprägungen von Religion, die auf das Individuum bezogen sind und eine Alternative zur traditionellen Religion und zum religiösen Mainstream bieten.[12]

In Europa und Nordamerika beträgt der Anteil derer, die angeben, sich über einen längeren Zeitraum hinweg intensiv mit alternativ-religiösen Praktiken beschäftigt zu haben, etwa 4–8% der erwachsenen Bevölkerung. Ein Viertel bis ein Drittel nehmen zumindest ab und zu derartige Angebote in Anspruch. Dabei fällt auf, dass es sich bei über zwei Drittel der Personen, die alternativ-religiöse Aktivitäten anbieten oder in Anspruch nehmen, um Frauen handelt.[13] EEVA SOINTU und LINDA WOODHEAD (2008) zufolge sind entsprechende Praktiken für Frauen deshalb so attraktiv, weil im Kontext alternativer Religiosität „traditionelle" Praktiken und Diskurse von Weiblichkeit zugleich legitimiert und unterlaufen werden, wobei die Autorinnen vor allem die angloamerikanische Mittelklasse im Blick haben. So erfahren etwa „weiblich" konnotierte Tätigkeiten im Zusammenhang mit Beziehungsarbeit und körperlich-emotionaler Pflege eine hohe Wertschätzung in alternativ-religiösen Milieus. Subversives Potential sehen SOINTU und WOODHEAD hingegen in der in alternativ-religiösen Kreisen oft wiederholten Botschaft, man müsse erst für sich selbst sorgen, bevor man anderen helfen könne. Dazu gehöre, körperliche und emotionale Wünsche nicht zu unterdrücken und sich auch Genuss zu erlauben, ohne dabei ein „schlechtes Gewissen" zu haben. Wo Autor*innen, die dem Milieu eher ablehnend gegenüberstehen, Narzissmus und einen Mangel an sozialem und politischem Engagement orten,[14] sehen SOINTU und WOODHEAD ein spezifisch weibliches Aufbegehren gegen traditionelle Rollenmuster, in denen Frauen stets das Wohl anderer im Blick haben sollen.

DAVIS-FLOYD hebt einerseits die „typisch weibliche" heilsame Beziehung zwischen Geburtshelferin und Gebärender hervor und versteht die Geburt andererseits als transformativ-ekstatische Erfahrung, die zu persönlichem Wachstum der Frau führt – ein Topos, der im Sinne von SOINTU und WOODHEAD seine Attraktivität durch die Opposition zu traditionellen Weiblichkeitsdiskursen (der anglo-amerikanischen Mittelklasse) gewinnt. In der alternativen Religiosität liegen für beide Aspekte passende Deutungshorizonte bereit und es überrascht daher nicht, dass sich DAVIS-FLOYDS Verständnis von Spiritualität gerade in diesem Kontext entfaltet. KLASSEN kommt in ihrer Studie über zuhause gebärende Frauen zu einem ähnlichen Schluss: „Since religious traditions, contemporary clergy, and medical professionals, generally speaking, have not been concerned with the transformative possibilities of birth for a woman, women have turned elsewhere to find ways to make religious sense of childbirth" (KLASSEN 2001a: 83).

Spirituelle Geburtserfahrungen

Die „holistische" Geburt wird von DAVIS-FLOYD als spirituelle Erfahrung *par excellence* gerahmt. Durch die Freisetzung von Oxytocin – ein biologischer Vorgang – komme es zu veränderten Bewusstseinszuständen und „the feelings of sacredness and spirituality that often wash over us during sex with a person we truly love and during labor, birth, and what is called the Golden Hour after birth" (DAVIS-FLOYD 2018: xxiii). Im Folgenden sollen Berichte über diese Erfahrungen, die DAVIS-FLOYD behandelt, näher untersucht werden.

DAVIS-FLOYD schreibt über ihre traumatische erste Geburt und die Entscheidung, sich durch eine radikale Änderung ihrer Lebensweise, die sie als einseitig intellektuell und damit nicht „ganzheitlich" erkannt habe, auf ihre zweite Geburt besser vorzubereiten. Diesmal findet die Geburt nicht im Krankenhaus, sondern zu Hause statt und wird von einer Doula, ihrem Ehemann, zwei Hebammen, einem Masseur, einem weiteren Freund und einem Fotografen begleitet. Sie beschreibt im Zusammenhang mit dieser Hausgeburt ein Ritual, in dem Kerzenlicht, gemeinsames Singen, Massagen, eine große Geburtswanne und ein frisch bezogenes Bett eine Rolle spielen. Zeitweise kommt eine Sauerstoffmaske zur Anwendung, da DAVIS-FLOYD biomedizinische Unterstützung nicht generell ablehnt, sondern nur deren Anwendung mit einer „technokratischen" Geisteshaltung. Nachdem sie aufhört, gegen den Schmerz anzukämpfen, beobachtet sie eine Veränderung:

> I felt that I, body and soul, *became the pain*, and once there was no more separation between me and the pain, there was no more pain! I lay there on the bed, utterly relaxed, breathing softly, in total peace, floating somewhere above my body. I could hear the midwives whispering „Good, that's really good." [...] That magical, highly spiritual, altered state of consciousness is what midwives call „laborland", and if you are in it, those around you should protect you from any interruption that might snap you out of it (DAVIS-FLOYD 2018: xv).

Die Erfahrung der völligen Hingabe ist für DAVIS-FLOYD eine bedeutende Lehre fürs Leben, die durch das Gebären gewonnen werden kann. Als der Schmerz mit aller Macht zurückkommt, ist in ihr bereits eine bislang ungeahnte Entschlossenheit gereift, mit der sie schließlich ihr Kind zur Welt bringt. In ganz ähnlicher Weise schreibt auch die Pflegewissenschaftlerin WENDY BUDIN:

> The challenge of giving birth today is to develop confidence and trust in one's inner wisdom and allow nature to do its thing. When this is accomplished, a woman's body is often permeated and nourished by spiritual energy and guidance. She emerges from her labor bed with a renewed sense of her body's strength and power and with an enhanced spirituality (BUDIN 2001: 38).

Die hier beschriebene Spiritualität der Geburt hat etwas mit dem Zusammenspiel von Selbstermächtigung und Hingabe zu tun. Die Gebärende trifft zunächst eine bewusste Entscheidung für ein bestimmtes „Geburtssystem" und demonstriert damit ihre Unabhängigkeit von herrschenden (medizinischen) Konventionen. Sie ist in dieser Entscheidung nicht allein, sondern wird von einer Gemeinschaft von Helfer*innen begleitet. Auf dem Höhepunkt der Anstrengungen und Schmerzen kommt es schließlich zu einer Verschiebung: Die Frau tritt als handelndes Subjekt zurück und kommt in einen Zustand, in dem ihr etwas geschieht, in dem sie einen Prozess durchläuft, der außerhalb ihrer Verfügungsmacht liegt. Diese Selbstermächtigung speise sich außerdem aus weiblichem, inkorporiertem Wissen: Das Geburtswissen sei im Körper der Gebärenden angelegt und die Frau damit inhärent spirituell.

Dieser Zustand geht für DAVIS-FLOYD mit einer Veränderung des Bewusstseins, einem „altered state of consciousness", einher. Körperliche Empfindungen werden mit Bezug auf eine spirituelle Energie beschrieben, die leiblich wahrnehmbar sei. Auch für die Frauen in KLASSENS Studie ist die Geburt ein intensives Erlebnis, welches die Gebärende mit ihren innersten Gefühlen konfrontiere (vgl. KLASSEN 2001a: 68). Damit einher gehe die Hingabe zur Geburt als Naturkraft, die Zugang zu übernatürlichen Kräften ermögliche (vgl. KLASSEN 2001b: 801). Diese Erfahrung ist mit der Hingabe an die Natur und den eigenen Körper als Teil derselben verbunden und nicht etwa in einem traditionell monotheistischen Sinn mit der Hingabe an und der Vereinigung mit Gott. Aus religionswissenschaftlicher Perspektive kann die von KLASSEN beschriebene Deutung als alternativ-religiös gefasst werden: Geburt wird in der Schnittmenge von Weiblichkeit, Holismus und Natur kontextualisiert und die eigene Erfahrung und Empfindung essentialisiert.[15] Mit STOLZ gesprochen, kann Geburt aus dieser Perspektive als spirituelle Selbstverwirklichung verstanden werden und zwar „in holistischer, synkretistischer und naturverbundener Art und Weise" (STOLZ 2005: 123).

Das Verweilen in „laborland", das spirituelle Zentrum in DAVIS-FLOYDS Erzählung, dauert nicht lange an und ist auch kein Selbstzweck. Vielmehr gehe es darum, durch dieses Moment der Hingabe und des Loslassens das Vertrauen in die eigene Kraft zu stärken und den Prozess der Geburt gut zu Ende zu bringen. Das Bewusstsein der eigenen Stärke, die in der spirituell verstandenen Verbindung zur Natur wurzelt, soll auch nach der Geburt beibehalten und in den weiteren Lebensvollzug integriert werden. Für DAVIS-FLOYD gibt es strukturelle Gründe, warum viele Frauen diese Erfahrungen nicht machen können – ein Grund sei das technokratische System, dem sie ausgeliefert seien. Zudem betont sie aber die eigene Verantwortung am Beispiel ihrer eigenen Geschichte:

> I had spent my whole adult life as an academic, an intellectual disconnected from my body and living mostly in my head. How could I then expect to suddenly become connected with my body in the way I needed to in order to have the natural birth I had wanted, yet had done no internal work to prepare for? (DAVIS-FLOYD 2018: x)

Um – überspitzt formuliert – eine perfekte Geburt zu erleben und sie zu einem einschneidenden spirituellen Erlebnis zu machen, bedarf es viel Vorbereitung. Noch expliziter formuliert etwa die Sozialanthropologin SHEILA KITZINGER, ebenfalls eine zentrale Figur der frühen *Anthropology of Birth*, diesen Appell in ihrem Ratgeber *Wie soll mein Kind geboren werden* (KITZINGER 1986). Den Soziologinnen ROSE und SCHMIED-KNITTEL zufolge enthält diese Konstruktion einerseits die Verheißung, die bevorstehende Krise mit eigener Kraft meistern zu können. Andererseits lädt sie den Individuen ein enormes Maß an Verantwortung auf, da sie es sind, die über die Güte des Geburtsverlaufs entscheiden. Die Entbindung werde narzisstisch aufgeladen und als biografische Klimax mit orgiastischen Anklängen stilisiert (vgl. ROSE/SCHMIED-KNITTEL 2011: 87–89; PELLENGAHR 2001: 269). Es gehe nicht mehr nur darum, ein Kind zu gebären, sondern ein „Geburtserlebnis" zu erfahren, was mit Erfolgsdruck und Versagensängsten für werdende Mütter einhergehe. Diese Form der Geburtskultur könne als Ausdruck einer individualistischen „Erlebnisgesellschaft" (SCHULZE 2000) verstanden werden.

Eine spirituelle Geburtserfahrung ist bei DAVIS-FLOYD allerdings nicht isoliert von den Menschen zu denken, die die Gebärende umgeben und mit ihrer vertrauensvollen Anwesenheit einen Raum öffnen, in dem sie sich fallen lassen kann.[16] Auch für die Frauen in KLASSENS Studie ist die Geburt keine rein individualistische Angelegenheit:

> [I]n addition to this experiential, therapeutic character, the religion provoked by home birth is also seen as saturated with a kind of power that is not only personal and self-rewarding, but transformative of society and relationships. Thus it is an inner-directed religion often accompanied by a strong political voice and a deep sense of ‚mission' to let other women know of choices in childbirth (KLASSEN 2001a: 68).

Zu ähnlichen Schlüssen kommt auch die Religionswissenschaftlerin ANN DUNCAN in ihrer Arbeit über das *Sacred Living Movement* (2017). Dieses Netzwerk bietet Retreats, Publikationen und eine Online-Community an, in denen Schwangerschaft und Geburt als spirituell bedeutsame Übergangsrituale gerahmt werden. Schwangere berichten von der einzigartigen Gemeinschaft, die bei den Retreats unter den Teilnehmenden entstehe. Spiritualität der Geburt bezieht sich dabei nicht nur auf ein besonderes „Geburtserlebnis", sondern auf die gemeinschaftlich erlebte Zeit der Schwangerschaft, in der Schwangere die Verbindung zu ihren „Schwestern" und den Frauen, die diese Erfahrung vor ihnen durchlebt haben, rituell begleitet werden. Das Zelebrieren der Schwangerschaft[17] kann als weiblich begangenes Übergangsritual verstanden werden und vereint Vorstellungen von Natürlichkeit, Holismus, Weiblichkeit und Spiritualität.

Fazit

ROBBIE DAVIS-FLOYD beschreibt die Geburt ihrer ersten Tochter als traumatisches Erlebnis, das zu einem Wendepunkt in ihrem Leben werden sollte. Die Suche nach Antworten auf die Frage, warum ihre Geburt in dieser Weise verlaufen war, führte zu einer regen Publikationstätigkeit, tatkräftigem Engagement im Gesundheitsbereich und einem grundlegenden Wandel ihrer persönlichen Lebensführung.[18] Die „Früchte" dieser Entwicklung hätten sich bei der Geburt ihres Sohnes gezeigt, die sie als kathartische spirituelle Erfahrung beschreibt. DAVIS-FLOYD positioniert sich damit als Rollenvorbild, bei dem die Geburt der Kinder zu einer inneren spirituellen Neugeburt führten.

In vorliegendem Beitrag wurde DAVIS-FLOYDS Verständnis von Spiritualität herausgearbeitet und kontextualisiert. Dabei zeigte sich erstens die wechselseitige Durchdringung von Anthropologie und sozialen Strömungen zur Förderung natürlicher Geburt, auf die etwa auch MARGARET MACDONALD (2007: 55) hinweist. Zweitens wurde deutlich, dass DAVIS-FLOYDS Spiritualität der Geburt Züge einer spezifisch spätmodernen Religiosität aufweist, die vornehmlich weiblich konnotiert ist und mit den Merkmalen Ganzheitlichkeit, Natürlichkeit und Erfahrungsbezogenheit beschrieben werden kann.

Diese Ergebnisse weisen auf einen Punkt hin, der für Studien im Bereich Geburt und Spiritualität bedenkenswert ist: Davis-Floyd und ihre Befragten partizipieren an einem alternativ-religiösen Schwangerschaftsdiskurs. Geburtserzählungen, die als zentrale Analysequellen herangezogen werden, schöpfen dabei aus einem geteilten Orientierungswissen, welches die Erzählenden stets aufs Neue aktualisieren und modifizieren. Dieses Orientierungswissen ist seinerseits nicht zuletzt durch anthropologische Publikationen mitgestaltet, wodurch sich ein partiell selbstreferenzielles System ergibt. Damit ist selbstverständlich nicht gesagt, dass Geburtserzählungen keine „verlässlichen" Daten darstellen oder gar den Erfahrungen Gebärender generell zu misstrauen ist. „Rather, we might approach birth stories as narrative constructions that are always produced within particular contexts", wie Molly Fitzpatrick (2019: 5) ausführt. Weitere Geburtsforschungen könnten sich stärker reflektierend mit diesen Narrationen, die am Schnittpunkt zwischen „direkter" Erfahrung und kulturell verfügbarem diskursivem Wissen angesiedelt sind, auseinandersetzen, wobei ethnologische und religionswissenschaftliche Reflexionszugänge eine fruchtbare Verbindung eingehen können.

Anmerkungen

1 Zu Geschichte und potenziellen Dilemmata der engaged anthropology in den USA vgl. Low & Engle Merry 2010.
2 Einen Überblick über die Geschichte der Anthropology of Birth als eigenständigen Forschungsansatz geben Davis-Floyd 1992; Davis-Floyd & Sargent 1997; Ginsburg & Rapp 1991, 1995; Inhorn & Birenbaum-Carmeli 2008; Lock 1993. Sargent & Gulbas 2011 situieren ethnologische Forschungen zur Geburt im weiter gefassten Feld der Anthropology of Reproduction.
3 Zu Diskussionen der Begriffe Ethnomedizin, Medizinethnologie oder Medizinanthropologie, die sich alle in deutschen Texten über Anthropology of Birth finden, siehe beispielsweise Lux 2003, Greifeld 2003 und Brown & Hatfield Timajchy 1997.
4 Vgl. die Beiträge in Schiefenhövel & Gottschlak-Batschkus 1995.
5 Davis-Floyd spricht von „alternative therapies", heute verwendet man den Begriff CAM (complementary and alternative medicine) und verweist damit auf „ a diverse array of treatment modalities and diagnostic techniques that are not presently considered part of conventional/mainstream medicine and emphasize a holistic approach towards health care" (Ernst 2008: 2).
6 Ina May Gaskin ist Hebamme und Vorreiterin der „natürlichen Geburt", deren Werk noch heute rezipiert wird.
7 Während diese Praktiken Ende des 20. Jahrhunderts deutlich als „alternativ" markiert waren, erfahren sie heute zunehmende Akzeptanz und werden zum Teil auch in biomedizinischen Kontexten ergänzend angewendet. Vgl. z.B. Gunther Brown 2013 und Ruggie 2004 oder für die Akzeptanz asiatischer Körperpraktiken Karstein & Benthaus 2018.
8 Zu dieser Gegenüberstellung vgl. Fuller 2001, Hood 2003 und Sinclair, Pereira & Raffin 2006. Zur Geschichte des Begriffs „Spiritualität" vgl. Bochinger 1994.
9 Im angelsächsischen Raum sind religionswissenschaftliche und religionssoziologische Befürworter*innen der metasprachlichen Verwendung u.a. Sutcliffe & Bowman 2000, Heelas 2007 und Heelas & Woodhead 2005 oder Woodhead 2010: 37: „the term ‚spirituality' can be defined in a way that helps us identify and make sense of observable patterns in practices and discourses in the contemporary religious landscape". In diesem Diskurs der Spiritualitätsrezeption finden sich weniger Assoziationen zum christlichen Kontext, sondern eher zu einem buddhistischen und Semantiken des New Age (vgl. Sutcliffe & Bowman 2000, Knoblauch 2009 und 2005: 128 oder Bochinger 1994).
10 Lüddeckens lehnt sich hier an Hanegraaf an „who also uses religion as an umbrella term, but differentiates between ‚a religion' (institutionalized) and ‚a spirituality' (individual), both of them being ‚religion'." (Lüddeckens 2018: 172). Religion ist nach Hanegraaf „any symbolic system which influences human action by providing possibilities for ritually maintaining contact between the everyday world and a more general metaempirical framework of meaning" (2000: 295).
11 Auch Religion ist in der religionswissenschaftlichen Verwendung ein Produkt des Diskurses und besteht nicht a priori (vgl. dazu Stausberg 2012).
12 Die Zunahme alternativer Formen von Religiosität heisst keine singuläre Entscheidung, mehrheitlich bewegt sich die Person gleichermassen in alternativen und traditionellen Religionsformen: „Diese Grenze zwischen ‚alternativ' und ‚traditionell' verläuft aber nicht zwischen den Individuen, sondern ein und dieselbe Person kann sich beider Arten von Glaubenskonzepten und -praktiken bedienen" (Mezger 2018: 33). Vgl. Bochinger, Engelbrecht, & Gebhardt 2009.
13 Vgl. Höllinger & Tripold 2012: 121 und 128–129 in Übereinstimmung mit Heelas & Woodhead 2005 und Houtman & Aupers 2008.
14 Vgl. grundlegend Lasch 1980 und Bellah, Madsen, Sullivan, Swidler & Tipton 1985.
15 Zu Natur vgl. Stolz & Schneuwly Purdie 2014: 71f.; Boddy 1989 und Albanese 1991. Zu Holismus vgl. Stolz & Schneuwly Purdie 2014: 71f.; Höllinger & Tripold 2012, 26; Knoblauch 2009: 126–127; Heelas & Woodhead 2005. Zu eigener Erfahrung vgl. Knoblauch 2009: 130; Höllinger & Tripold 2012: 26.
16 Für eine Ausarbeitung dieses relationalen Ansatzes vgl. Wojtkowiak & Crowther 2018: 18–19.
17 Für die Ritualisierung von Schwangerschaft und Geburt vgl. Wojtkowiak 2020.
18 Vgl. http://www.davis-floyd.com/autobiography/.

Literatur

Albanese, Catherine L. 1991. *Nature Religion in America. From the Algonkian Indians to the New Age.* Chicago: University Of Chicago Press.
Bellah, Robert N.; Madsen, Richard; Sullivan, William M.; Swidler, Ann & Tipton, Steven M. 1985. *Habits of the Heart. Individualism and Commitment in American Life.* Berkeley: University of California Press.
Bochinger, Christoph 1994. *„New Age" und moderne Religion.* Gütersloh: Kaiser Gütersloher Verlagshaus.
---, Christoph, Engelbrecht Martin & Gebhardt, Winfried (Hg) 2009. *Die unsichtbare Religion in der sichtbaren Religion – Formen spiritueller Orientierung in der religiösen Gegenwartskultur.* Stuttgart: Verlag W. Kohlhammer.
Boddy, Janice 1989. *Wombs and alien spirits. Women, men, and the Zar cult in northern Sudan.* Madison: University of Wisconsin Press.
Brown, Peter & Hatfield Timajchy, Kendra 1997. Art. „medical systems". In Barfield, Thomas (Hg). *Dictionary of Anthropology*, Malden: Blackwell Publishers: 318-320.
Budin, Wendy C. 2001. Birth and Death: Opportunities for Self-Transcendence. *Journal of Perinatal Education* 10,2: 38-42.
Crowther, Susan & Hall, Jenny (Hg) 2018. *Spirituality and Childbirth Meaning and Care at the Start of Life.* London und New York: Routledge: 13-29.
Davis-Floyd, Robbie 2021. How to Make Medical Anthropology Useful to Healthcare Practitioners, Activists,

and Policy-Makers: Lessons Learned. *Somatosphere. Science, Medicine and Anthropology*. http://somatosphere.net/2021/medical-anthropology-practice-policy-activism.html/ [14.9.2023].

--- 2018. Foreword. In DELAPORTE, MARIANNE & MARTIN, MORAG (Hg.). *Sacred Inception. Reclaiming the Spirituality of Birth in the Modern World*. London: The Rowman & Littlefield Publishing Group: vii-xxvii.

--- 2015. Foreword. In CASTAÑEDA, ANGELA N. & JOHNSON SEARCY, JULIE (Hg.) *Doulas and Intimate Labour. Boundaries, Bodies, and Birth*. Demeter Press: xiii-xxx.

--- 2001. The technocratic, humanistic, and holistic paradigms of childbirth. *International Journal of Gynecology & Obstetrics* 75: 5–23.

--- 1992. *Birth as an American Rite of Passage*. Berkeley: University of California Press.

--- & LAUGHLIN, ROBERT 2016. *The Power of Ritual*. Brisbane: Daily Grail Press.

--- & SARGENT, CAROLYN 1997. Introduction. The Anthropology of Birth. In DAVIS-FLOYD, ROBBIE/SARGENT, CAROLYN (Hg) *Childbirth and authoritative knowledge. Cross-Cultural Perspectives*. Berkeley: University of California Press. 1–51.

DOSSEY, LARRY 1998. Forword. In DAVIS-FLOYD, ROBBIE & ST. JOHN, GLORIA (Hg) *From Doctor to Healer. The transformative Journey*. New Brunswick: Rutgers University Press: ix–xi.

DUNCAN, ANN 2017. Sacred Pregnancy in the Age of the „Nones". *Journal of the American Academy of Religion* 85,4: 1089–1115.

ERNST, EDZARD 2008. *Oxford Handbook of Complementary Medicine*. Oxford: Oxford University Press.

FITZPATRICK, MOLLY 2019. Birth story interviews. On the assumptions hidden in our research methods. *Medical Anthropology Theory*. https://doi.org/10.5167/uzh-185188.

FULLER, ROBERT C. 2001. *Spiritual, but not Religious. Understanding Unchurched America*. Oxford: Oxford University Press.

GASKIN, INA MAY 1974. *Spiritual Midwifery*. Sommertown: Book Publishing Company.

GINSBURG, FAYE D. & RAPP, RAYNA 1995. *Conceiving the New World Order. The Global Politics of Reproduction*, Berkeley: University of California Press.

--- 1991. The Politics of Reproduction. *Annual Review of Anthropology* 20: 311–343.

GREIFELD, KATHARINA (Hg) 2003. *Medizinethnologie. Eine Einführung*. Reimer: Berlin.

GUNTHER BROWN, CANDY 2013. *The Healing Gods. Complementary and Alternative Medicine in Christian America*. Oxford: Oxford University Press.

HANEGRAAFF, WOUTER 2000. New Age Religion and Secularization. *Numen* 47,3: 288–312.

--- 1996. *New Age Religion and Western Culture. Esotericism in the Mirror of Secular Thought*. Leiden, New York & Köln: Brill.

HAMMER, OLAV 2001. *Claiming Knowledge. Strategies of Epistemology from Theosophy to the New Age*. Leiden, Boston, & Köln: Brill.

HEDGES, ELLIE & BECKFORD, JAMES 2000. Holism, Healing and the New Age. In SUTCLIFFE, STEVEN & BOWMAN, MARION (Hg). *Beyond New Age. Exploring Alternative Spirituality*. Edinburgh: Edinburgh University Press: 169–187.

HEELAS, PAUL 2007. The Holistic Milieu and Spirituality. Reflections on Voas and Bruce. In KIERAN FLANAGAN & JUPP, PETER C. (Hg). *A Sociology of Spirituality*. Aldershot: Ashgate: 63–80.

--- & WOODHEAD, LINDA 2005. *The Spiritual Revolution. Why Religion is Giving Way to Spirituality*. Malden, Oxford & Carlton: Blackwell Publishing.

HERVIEU-LÉGER, DANIÈLE 2000. *Religion as a Chain of Memory*. Cambridge, Malden: Polity Press.

HOBSBAWM, ERIC & RANGER, TERENCE 1992. *The Invention of Tradition*. Cambridge: Cambridge University Press.

HOOD, RALPH W. 2003. The Relationship between Religion and Spirituality. In GREIL, ARTHUR L. GREIL & BROMLEY, DAVID G. (eds). Defining Religion. Investigating the Boundaries Between the Sacred and Secular. Amsterdam, London: JAI (Religion and the Social Order 10): 241–265.

HÖLLINGER, FRANZ & TRIPOLD, THOMAS 2012. *Ganzheitliches Leben. Das holistische Milieu zwischen neuer Spiritualität und postmoderner Wellness-Kultur*. Bielefeld: Transcript.

HOUTMAN, DICK & AUPERS, STEF 2008. The Spiritual Revolution and the New Age Gender Puzzle: the Sacralisation of the Self in Late Modernity (1980-2000). In AUNE, KRISTIN, SHARMA, SONYA & VINCETT, GISELLE (Hg). *Women and Religion in the West. Challenging Secularization*. London & New York: Routledge: 99–118.

INHORN, MARCIA & BIRENBAUM-CARMELI, DAPHNA 2008. Assisted Reproductive Technologies and Culture Change. *Annual Review of Anthropology* 37: 177–196.

KARSTEIN, UTA & BENTHAUS, APEL FRIEDERIKE 2012. Asien als Alternative oder Kompensation? Spirituelle Körperpraktiken und ihr transformatives Potential (nicht nur) für das religiöse Feld. In GUGUTZER, ROBERT & BÖTTCHER MORITZ (Hg) *Körper, Sport und Religion. Zur Soziologie religiöser Verkörperungen*. Wiesbaden: Springer VS: 311–339.

KIRCHHOFF, HEINZ 1983. Vorwort. In SCHIEFENHÖVEL, WULF / SICH, DOROTHEA (Hrsg) *Die Geburt aus ethnomedizinischer Sicht. Beiträge und Nachträge zur IV. Internationalen Fachtagung der Arbeitsgemeinschaft Ethnomedizin über traditionelle Geburtshilfe und Gynäkologie in Göttingen 8.–10.12.1978*. Wiesbaden: Vieweg+Teubner: 5–6.

KITZINGER, SHEILA 1986. *Wie soll mein Kind geboren werden*. München: Kösel.

KLASSEN, PAMELA 2001a. *Blessed Events. Religion and Home Birth in America*. Princeton: Princeton University Press.

--- 2001b. Sacred Maternities and Postbiomedical Bodies: Religion and Nature in Contemporary Home Birth.

Signs: Journal of Women in Culture and Society 26,3: 775–809.
KNOBLAUCH, HUBERT 2009. *Populäre Religion. Auf dem Weg in eine spirituelle Gesellschaft*. Frankfurt am Main, New York: Campus Verlag.
––– 2006. Soziologie der Spiritualität. In BAIER, KARL (Hg) *Handbuch Spiritualität. Zugänge, Traditionen, interreligiöse Prozesse*. Darmstadt: WBG: 91-111.
KNOBLAUCH, HUBERT 2005. Einleitung: Soziologie der Spiritualität. *Zeitschrift für Religionswissenschaft* 13,2: 123–131.
LASCH, CHRISTOPHER 1980. *Das Zeitalter des Narzissmus*. München: Steinhausen.
LOCK, MARGARET 1993. Cultivating the Body: Anthropology and Epistemologies of Bodily Practice and Knowledge. *Annual Review of Anthropology* 22: 133–155.
LOW, SETHA M. & ENGLE MERRY, SALLY 2010. Engaged Anthropology: Diversity and Dilemmas: An Introduction to Supplement 2. *Current Anthropology* 51: 203–226.
LÜDDECKENS, DOROTHEA 2018. Complementary and Alternative Medicine (CAM) as a Toolkit for Secular Health-Care. The De-differentiation of Religion and Medicine. In LÜDDECKENS, DOROTHEA & SCHRIMPF, MONIKA (Hg) *Medicine, Religion, Spirituality: Global Perspectives on Traditional, Complementary, and Alternative Healing*. Bielefeld: Transcript: 167–199.
––– & WALTHERT, RAFAEL 2010. Das Ende der Gemeinschaft? Neue religiöse Bewegungen im Wandel. In LÜDDECKENS, DOROTHEA & WALTHERT, RAFAEL (Hg) *Fluide Religion. Neue religiöse Bewegungen im Wandel. Theoretische und empirische Systematisierungen*. Bielefeld: Transcript: 19–53.
LUX, THOMAS 2003. *Kulturelle Dimensionen der Medizin. Ethnomedizin – Medizinethnologie Medical Anthropology*. Reimer: Berlin.
MACDONALD, MARGARET 2007. *At Work in the Field of Birth: Midwifery Narratives of Nature, Tradition, and Home*. Nashville, TN: Vanderbilt University Press.
MEZGER, MIRJAM 2018. *Religion, Spiritualität, Medizin*. Bielefeld: Transcript.
PELLENGAHR, ASTRID 2001. Von der „programmierten" zur „natürlichen" Geburt. Zur kulturellen Konstruktiion von Geburtsvorstellungen und deren Wandel in der Gegenwart. In BREDNICK, ROLF; SCHEIDER, ANETTE & WERNER, UTE (Hg) *Natur-Kultur. Volkskundliche Perspektiven auf Mensch und Umwelt*. Münster: Waxmann. 269–280.
POSSAMAI, ADAM 2005. *In search of New Age Spiritualities*. Aldershot u.a: Ashgate.
RAPHAEL, DANA 1976. *The Tender Gift: Breastfeeding*. New York: Schocken Books.
REHSMANN, JULIA & SIEGL, VERONIKA 2022. Lebensanfänge und -enden. Ethnographische Erkundungen und methodologische Reflexionen: Introduction to the Special Issue. *Curare. Zeitschrift für Medizinethnologie* 45,2: 7–16.
ROSE, LOTTE & SCHMIED-KNITTEL, INA 2011. Magie und Technik: Moderne Geburt zwischen biographischem Event und kritischem Ereignis. In VILLA, PAULA-IRENE; MOEBIUS, STEPHAN & THIESSEN, BARBARA (Hg) *Soziologie der Geburt. Diskurse, Praktiken und Perspektiven*. Frankfurt am Main: Campus-Verlag.
RUGGIE, MARY 2004. *Marginal to Mainstream. Alternative Medicine in America*. Cambridge: Cambridge University Press.
SARGENT, CAROLYN & GULBAS, LAUREN 2011. Situating Birth in the Anthropology of Reproduction. In *A Companion to Medical Anthropology*. Hoboken: John Wiley: 289–303.
SCHIEFENHÖVEL, WULF; SICH, DOROTHEA & GOTTSCHLAK-BATSCHKUS, CHRISTINE E. 1995. (Hrsg) *Gebären – Ethnomedizinische Perspektiven und neue Wege*. Berlin: VWB – Verlag für Wissenschaft und Bildung.
SCHULZE, GERHARD 2000. *Die Erlebnisgesellschaft. Kultursoziologie der Gegenwart*. Frankfurt am Main: Campus.
SINCLAIR, SHANE; PEREIRA, JOSE & RAFFIN, SHELLEY 2006. A Thematic Review of the Spirituality Literature within Palliative Care. *Journal of Palliative Medicine* 9,2: 464–479.
SOINTU, EEVA & WOODHEAD, LINDA 2008. Spirituality, Gender, and Expressive Selfhood. *Journal for the Scientific Study of Religion* 47,2: 259–276.
STARHAWK 1979. *The Spiral Dance. A Rebirth of the Ancient Religion of the Great Goddess*. New York: Harper & Row.
STAUSBERG, MICHAEL 2012. *Religion. Begriff, Definitionen, Theorien. Religionswissenschaft*. Berlin: Walter de Gruyter.
STOLZ, JÖRG 2005. Der Erfolg der Spiritualität. Gesellschaftsentwicklung und Transzendenzerfahrung am Beispiel der Schweiz. In LEUTWYLER, SAMUEL & NÄGELI, MARKUS (Hg) *Spiritualität und Wissenschaft*. Zürich: vdf Hochschulverlag: 121–132.
STOLZ, JÖRG & SCHNEUWLY PURDIE, MALLORY 2014. Vier Gestalten des (Un-)Glaubens. In STOLZ, JÖRG; KÖNEMANN, JUDITH; SCHNEUWLY PURDIE, MALLORY; ENGLBERGER, THOMAS & KRÜGGELER, MICHAEL (Hrsg) *Religion und Spiritualität in der Ich-Gesellschaft. Vier Gestalten des (Un-) Glaubens*. Zürich: Edition NZN bei TVZ: 65–78.
SUTCLIFFE, STEVEN 2002. *Children of the New Age. A History of Spiritual Practices*. London, New York: Routledge.
––– & BOWMAN, MARION 2000. Introduction. In SUTCLIFFE, STEVEN & BOWMAN, MARION (Hg) *Beyond New Age. Exploring Alternative Spirituality*. Edinburgh: Edinburgh University Press: 1–13.
WOJTKOWIAK, JOANNA 2020. Ritualizing Pregnancy and Childbirth in Secular Societies: Exploring Embodied Spirituality at the Start of Life. *Religions* 11,9: 458.
WOODHEAD, LINDA 2010. Real religion and fuzzy spirituality? Taking sides in the sociology of religion. In HOUTMAN, DICK & AUPERS STEFF (Hg) *Religions of Modernity. Relocating the Sacred to the Self and the Digital*. Leiden, Boston: Brill: 31–48.
ZEUGIN, BARBARA 2020. *Selbstermächtigung am Lebensende. Eine religionswissenschaftliche Untersuchung alternativer Sterbebegleitung in der Schweiz*. Göttingen: Vandenhoeck & Ruprecht.

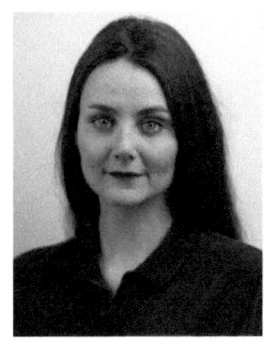

Jill Marxer, Dr., ist Religionswissenschaftlerin und derzeit Postdoktorandin und Koordinatorin der Sigi Feigel Gastprofessur für Jüdische Studien der Universität Zürich sowie wissenschaftliche Mitarbeiterin am Religionswissenschaftlichen Seminar der Universität Zürich. In ihrem ethnografischen Dissertationsprojekt erforschte sie Doulas in der deutschsprachigen Schweiz. Aktuell fokussiert sie sich auf Realisierungen und Konnotationen von Eruv und der Konzeption von Ort(en) und Raum in verschiedenen zeitgenössischen jüdischen Gemeinschaften. Ihre Forschungsschwerpunkte beinhalten Geburt und Lebensanfang, Religion und Medizin, Alternative Religiosität und zeitgenössisches Judentum.

Universität Zürich
Religionswissenschaftliches Seminar
Kantonsschulstrasse 1, CH-8001 Zürich
e-mail: jill.marxer@rws.uzh.ch

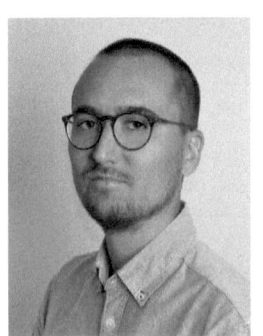

Johannes Endler, Dr., promovierte über Diskurse zu Zeugung, Schwangerschaft und Geburt in alternativ-religiöser Ratgeberliteratur seit dem neunzehnten Jahrhundert und ist Sozialarbeiter im Bereich der Sozialpsychiatrie. Von 2019 bis 2023 war er Stipendiat der Österreichischen Akademie der Wissenschaften am Institut für Religionswissenschaft der Universität Wien. Seine Forschungsinteressen umfassen die Beziehung zwischen religiösen, medizinischen, psychologischen und lebensweltlichen Wissensfeldern in Spiritismus, Okkultismus, Lebensreform, New Age und dem zeitgenössischen holistischen Milieu.

e-mail: endlerjohannes@gmail.com

Radical Applied Clinical Anthropology

JASON W. WILSON & ROBERTA D. BAER

The structure of biomedicine and healthcare delivery is not designed to be patient-centered and will require a radical redesign that drastically shifts the clinical gaze. The shift in gaze will require an implementation of a new applied clinical medical anthropology to identify, describe and resolve the current entanglements that make care delivery so complicated. Those entanglements must be pulled apart and laid bare by utilizing direct observations of patients, providers and healthcare experiences to create new assemblages. A focus on ethnographically informed models is the pathway to shifting the clinical gaze.

MICHEL FOUCAULT (1973) first described the clinical gaze, linking the origin of the concept to the implementation of anatomy-based physician education that led to insider knowledge and asymmetric power relationships between healthcare delivery and healthcare recipient. Anatomy-based education furthered pathophysiological understanding of organic disease concepts, broadening the distance between disease and illness. Others have attempted to find cultural remnants of folk medicine as well as ways to better unite disease/illness concepts, perhaps returning us to some imagined "before", pre-gaze state (KLEINMAN, EISENBERG & GOOD 1978). However, the complexity of modern healthcare systems in the United States are strongly rooted and engrained in a broader capitalism, highly structured, and almost autonomous given the millions of companies, medical supplies, billers, buildings, providers, and patients that reify the system on a daily basis. If there is a cultural context, a cultural system, then it is this neoliberal structure reproducing validity of specific disease definitions and care pathways based on reimbursement strategies that define medical deservingness (RATNA 2020) – who is seen in care pathways and who is not, who has legitimate disease and who goes unnoticed (HOLMES, CASTAÑEDA, GEERAERT, CASTAÑEDA, PROBST, ZELDES AND WILLEN 2020; SHER 1983). The clinical gaze is a lens magnifying this complex network that defines healthcare. This gaze sees what the lens is designed to visualize, not necessarily what diseases patients have or where patients suffer and need clinical pathways of care. The gaze is able to see patients deemed by the healthcare delivery structure as deserving while staying blind to the non-deserving. How can we shift this gaze to be patient-centered?

Applied clinical anthropology is not a new concept but the idea lay dormant for 3 decades (CHRISMAN & MARETZKI 1982; KLEINMAN, CHRISMAN & MARETZKI 1982). NOEL CHRISMAN introduced the idea that anthropologists could navigate the space between disease and illness directly to increase patient compliance (CHRISMAN & MARETZKI 1982). These clinical anthropologists could liaison biomedical care plans to treat disease with patient culture and folk beliefs that made up their illness, largely following the disease/illness paradigm and ethnomedicine concepts being explored at the time (KLEINMAN, EISENBERG & GOOD 1978). That space in between disease and illness or between biomedical culture and local culture/ethnomedicine, it was thought, might be responsible for care plan non-compliance and perpetuation of disease. The assumption that patients chose not to participate in medical care secondary to different belief systems may partially explain small aspects of the variation in compliance but was grossly overstated, leaving out marginalization of asymmetrical power structural determinants of care and care access (SCHEPER-HUGHES 1990; FARMER 2006).

Much of medical anthropology turned to broader, and necessary, critique of the healthcare system, working mostly to identify how power asymmetries, racism, colonialism and gender inequity results in an uneven distribution of healthcare outcomes (SCHEPER-HUGHES 1990). These are necessary critiques but move too far away from the direct patient experience to actually improve human lives.

While anthropology has moved away from static definitions of culture (DE CASTRO 2011), hospital patient experience departments perpetuate "cultural competencies" (AHA 2013) assuming that the reason why the patient does not take her medicine or doesn't always arrive at her appointments is because she is a member of a non-dominant religion, views time differently based on origin stories in her family heritage, doesn't wear jeans to clinic and prefers to not shake hands and to have her husband in the room. These attributes of 'culture' are used to explain, or even justify, observed inequities in care and creation of disparate care delivery (AHA 2013). These explanations and justifications ignore racism, undocumented-status, inability to access health insurance when unemployed, lack of transportation to clinic, family work schedules, domestic violence, misogyny both in her own neighborhood and home, and teetering food insecurity during a pandemic.

We suggest that a radical reconsideration and implementation of an applied clinical anthropology can transform healthcare delivery by directly engaging in the patient-physician interaction and the acute medical encounter. The key to this applied approach is integration of the anthropologist as an actual member of the healthcare team with stated role to consider culture and structural vulnerabilities across current care pathways that contribute to unmet healthcare needs of patients and differential healthcare outcomes. Reimagined applied clinical anthropologists see patients, work with staff and the broader community outside of the hospital or clinic, improve patient centered care models that expand deservingness, link disease and illness, and improve healthcare outcomes. This clinical anthropologist uses these ethnographic observations to inform new pathways, to consider broader assemblages, and to unentangle webs of unaligned incentives across the modern biomedical care delivery space. Clinical operations and direct patient contact are key elements of our new approach that integrates

the broad category of forces that explain health inequities outside of pharmaceuticals and surgeries (social determinants of health) includes issues such as food insecurity, education, sex and gender, geographic residence, homelessness, co-occurring mental illness or substance use (WILLIAMS & SAHEL 2022).

How can social determinant approaches before integrated directly into clinical practice? A neoliberal healthcare system distributes patient care, and patient outcomes, through a hodgepodge conglomeration of drug, device, and procedure delivery, all emphasized through un-aligned incentives (RATNA 2020).

Multiple forms of exploitive, or unchecked, capitalism have been described previously. While capitalism itself may just relate to private business trade and industry operating to produce profit, neoliberalism describes an extreme form of the concept, reducing most government regulations to create supposed free market attributes that allow private entities to further maximize revenues with few barriers. Neoliberalism may have an underlying assumption that creation of profit for the sake of profit creation leads to human progress and should not be inhibited. We are most interested in a related concept of salvage capitalism. Essentially salvage capitalism is the identification of potential profit, potential revenue generation out of human activities that may be taking place for other reasons or in absence of a formalized market. A human illness relates to a narrative during a healthcare encounter. In the United States, that narrative is ultimately packaged into a revenue generating unit called an ICD-10 code (e.g. "Acute Chest Pain" R07.9).

Salvage capitalism (TSING 2009) threads together ways of elevating visibility to some patient populations at the expense of others who go unseen or remain undeserving of care. ICD-10 codes, third party payors, and compliance guideline organizations salvage these revenues creating the illumination of clear pathways in modern healthcare strung along precarious patches of disease and illness. Broadly, this coalition of capitalist forces produce incentives that reify improved care for some patients over others. Over time, reproduction and reification along un-aligned incentives form stochastically entangled care paths that are difficult for patients and providers to navigate but easier for payers and compliance organizations to recognize.

A new clinical anthropology places emphasis on the emergence of pathways of possibility that create newly visible and deserving patient populations such as those with Sickle Cell Disease (SCD), Opioid Use Disorder (OUD), and Hepatitis C Virus (HCV). Pathway development utilizes co-located treatment models that recognize both syndemic and co-occurring diagnoses when present. This anthropology takes into account the broader structure of healthcare delivery as well as the challenges and incentives facing patients, providers and payors. Specifically, our clinical anthropology has been implemented in two broad ways: 1) patient experience, patient shadowing and medical education and (2) creation of care pathways that bring visibility to unseen and vulnerable populations.

Patient experience, shadowing education

An applied clinical anthropology can extend disease-illness gap concepts that may diminish the patient experience of care. Kleinman and colleagues recognized that explanatory models of disease were based on organic precepts and goals of correcting an underlying pathophysiology informed by biomedical and natural science education, while an illness paradigm of many patients focused on symptoms and was likely made up of both ethnomedicine and folk concepts of sickness (KLEINNMAN, EISENBERG & GOOD 1978). Perhaps, by narrowing the gap between explanatory models (disease and illness), patients may have a better experience with the healthcare system.

A modern version of this approach is more complicated, owing to the structural layers that have been added to American healthcare over the past 40 years (healthcare teams, third party payors, attempts to control spending, increased administrative/administrator influence, multiple parties involved in a patient encounter including not just physicians and nurses but also physician assistants and other advanced practice providers and ancillary staff). Patient centered care is now part of the decade old Triple Aim model (a broad set of concepts aimed at improving health, quality, and the patient experience) (IHI, n.d.). How can anthropologists utilize ethnographic methods to inform and apply interventions in medical education, care delivery and continued process improvement that fill the gaps between current state and the vision of Triple Aim implementation.

Hospital Care Assurance Programs (HCAP) and Press-Ganey surveys (Press 2006) are used to track the patient experience across time and across institutions and providers by measuring patient satisfaction (part of the Triple Aim). Percentile differences across institutions result in Centers for Medicare and Medicaid Services (CMS) financial penalties or rewards. More recently, similar data has been tied to individual physicians, affecting their specific Medicare reimbursement rates. While much effort is put into improving facility scores, very little change in those scores becomes persistently hardwired. Most hospitals now have C-suite level Chief Patient Experience Officers and large budgets to employ staff to script and coach providers on potential ways to improve their own satisfaction scores (greet patient, introduce yourself, sit down, wrap up main points with a summary, ask if there are questions).

Our initial attempts to radicalize clinical anthropology were built on this foundation almost 10 years ago when a physician (JW) joined with a medical anthropologist (RB) to invest in a long game strategy aimed at transforming the care experience through medical education and patient shadowing (WILSON, BAER & VILLALONA 2019; WILSON & BAER 2022). In ongoing work, we began teaching an undergraduate course to highly talented students that expressed a desire to attend medical school. Our goal was to reposition patient experience to a front and center process instead of an afterthought in mid-career. To do this, we taught KLEINMAN, EISENBERG & GOOD (1978), HAHN (1996), and other models of culture differences between lay people, biomedical providers and the healthcare system. While we introduced important elements of structural competency evaluation and the impact of structural violence in the clinic, the focus was on gaps in explanatory models and communication issues that explain differences in how a patient and provider view the same encounter very differently. The cornerstone of this model was patient shadowing. Patient shadowing represents the early implementation of ethnographically informed care. Essentially, we re-labeled participant observation as "patient shadowing" to match the nomenclature of premedical students and an academic hospital and then sent our students to sit with multiple patients for the entire patient encounter (WILSON & BAER 2019). Students always remark that they are nervous going into the experience but come out finding this to be the most valuable experience in their education as each student exits the experience with a firsthand knowledge of how care gaps arise, able to witness the culture of medicine, the culture of patients, and the culture created during the physician-patient encounter.

Observations, semi-structured interviews, and quotes from patient shadowing experiences and waiting room observations were thematically coded leading to an ethnographically informed patient-leaflet, laying out what people should expect during a hospital emergency department encounter (WILSON & BAER 2022). Later, we were invited to do a similar seminar for internal medicine resident physicians. After patient shadowing, the medical residents requested that the hospital stop the routine practice of early morning (4am) daily patient blood draws. The practice of 4am blood draws is physician-centered in an attempt to have lab results ready for morning rounds which often begin around 7am. The medical residents noted that daily results rarely impacted clinical outcomes across most patients and the practice of early morning interruption in sleep was not patient centered. We also began to offer patient shadowing and patient centered ethnographic experiences to current medical students during their first year "Doctoring" course and earlier work with premedical students continues through longitudinal cohort surveys as our prior students progress through their medical training and initiate professional life. Will these early experiences shift the clinical gaze over time, integrating patient centered care into the DNA of new physicians?

Healthcare delivery pathways

We cannot just train future healthcare workers to better consider the patient experience while seeing patients. A restructuring of healthcare must occur. Models of sick/not sick, deserving/not deserving must fade away for patients to decide what and where disease and illness are treated as a guiding design of healthcare delivery. Participatory action by those involved in direct patient care and healthcare system design is needed, along with changes to medical education. The goal here is not to improve patient compliance with biomedical care plans but, instead, to reconsider with patients what care plans should be developed and hardwired into healthcare.

The patient encounter that happens over and over again each day in every clinic, hospital and virtual visit, is the level of cultural production and the space where new ways of being for patients, physicians, medical staff and the healthcare system at large are seen or not seen, affirmed or ignored, produced, assembled or disassembled. Here is where we envision situating the applied clinical anthropologist as an active member of the healthcare team, positioned in the liminal spaces where the production of healthcare occurs. The reproduction and performance of these encounters is an ontological transcendence in which disease is made real or not real while patients are made to belong or dismissed, drastically altering healthcare outcomes and mortality.

In this space, the anthropologist can identify and conceptualize the production of culture taking place in patient-physician encounters, the way that healthcare delivery is designed, structured and delivered and the ways in which patients experience that care. How do those encounters embrace potentialities that can either go unrecognized, affirmed, or enhanced to create new patient care pathways? Creation of patient care pathways represent new ontologies in a world of salvage capitalism (TSING 2017). This salvage capitalism is represented by predetermined diagnosis related groups (DRG), reimbursable current procedural terms (CPTs), and international classification of disease (ICD). DRGs, CPTs, ICDs make or break reality of medical disease and patient belonging in the current biomedical model driven by reimbursable visits and the examination and auditing of outside compliance organizations constantly abstracting specific codes. These three letter codes are the reality of practice. A radical anthropology reimagines the design of a healthcare system based on the diseases that patients have and the illnesses they experience, not a response to the designated reimbursable codes. Imagine an emergency medicine physician training curriculum based on the frequency of each complaint for which patients seek care (substance use, mental illness) instead of those that are socially acceptable and deemed deserving of care, both highly reimbursable and monitored for process improvement (heart attack, stroke, sepsis).

But to make visible those diseases, there are complex steps to map out entangled webs of disease-illness, structural vulnerabilities, and use of other codes that hide reality (e.g., abdominal pain for patients with depression, or repeat visits to emergency departments for benign conditions masking food insecurity, mental illness and homelessness or other disease hidden in expression of entangled symptoms). The radical applied clinical anthropologist works in the medical space producing an ethnographically informed care (HENDERSON 2022, WILSON & BAER 2022). While psychological models dominate current care approaches (e.g., trauma informed care) and do add value, that value is based in the approach to the individual patient or an understanding of how individual patients experience disease (BROWN, ASHWORTH, BASS, RITTENBERG, LEVY-CARRICK, GROSSMAN, LEWIS-O'CONNOR & STOKLOSA 2022). Ethnographically informed care does not stand as a mutually exclusive approach to trauma informed care but is useful for broader attempt to reimagine healthcare delivery through collective observations of patient-physician encounters, interviews with patients, interviews with providers and deep knowledge of contextual circumstances driving the presence or absence of established care pathways (WILSON & BAER 2022; HENDERSON 2022). We utilize this approach in our clinical work at an emergency department to develop new ways of improving the patient experience, educating medical students and residents, and treating patients with sickle cell disease, opioid use disorder, HIV and hepatitis, diabetes, firearm violence and, most formally, opioid use disorder. Examples of that work are briefly discussed below.

Ethnographically informed care

Can a critical, clinically applied anthropologist find new ways of working that can bring together the golden triad of patient-centered value, healthcare provider value, and healthcare system value in a way that does not compete to find meaning and purpose in the clinical landscape but instead makes the meaning and purpose of their work obvious to other clinical stake holders, integrating fully into the clinical team. Our applied clinical anthropology is a praxis where research may take place or be generated as a way to demonstrate model success but not as primary end in itself. The goal at the outset for our applied clinical anthropology is to build a new healthcare system, visualizing unseen gaps, assembling and aligning people and systems, and unentangling complicated mixes of training, payer and compliance inertia that guides regular clinical practice for physicians. We envision a radical anthropology in the clinical space with the applied clinical anthropologist moving between roles as interlocutor with multiple groups that must be engaged to reconsider health: physicians, staff, patients, administrators. Think of the disease-illness gap described by KLEINMAN, EISENBERG & GOOD (1978) in the 1970s but made more complex by considering the broader structure of third-party payors, compliance bodies, and collected stories of lived experiences of not just patients but also physicians and others working within the current system.

What does it mean to create ethnographically informed pathways that unentangle and reassemble current clinical realities? Our work to improve care of patients in the emergency department with sickle cell disease, opioid use disorder (OUD), and Hepatitis C Virus (HCV) are all representative of our approach to ethnographically informed assemblage formation (Wilson and Baer 2022). Theoretically, the work of philosophers Delanda, Deleuze and Guatarri, as well as the anthropology of Tsing and Nading, specifically inform our work in their attempts to define and describe assemblages (Delanda 2006; Deleuze Guatarri 1987; Tsing 2017) and complex entanglements (Nading 2019). Methodologically, we extend the descriptive concept of syndemics (two biological disease states linked by same social phenomenon) (Singer, Bulled, Ostrach, and Mendenhall 2017) to an applied treatment approach of co-locating care for co-occurring disorders (HCV and OUD).

To be critical, clinical and applied, the anthropologist can parlay healthcare observations to first unentangle existing structures (Nading 2019) while searching for the precipice of newly forming assemblages. Those assemblages can be formally built out into new and tangible patient care pathways. Extending Tsing's concepts of salvage capitalism (TSING 2017) in the critique of medical coding to generate charges and revenue that create precarious patches (spots where reimbursement leads to semi-permanent care pathways) across a capitalism landscape, new connections can arise to bring those patches together in ways that were not there just a moment ago – providing visibility to patient populations that were unrecognized in the current entanglement. In the past, our ED would follow the CDC guidelines (BRANSON, HANDSFIELD, LAMPE, JANSSEN, TAYLOR, LYSS, CLARK, and the CENTERS FOR DISEASE CONTROL AND PREVENTION 2006) for HCV testing and miss new diagnoses of HCV in patients that inject drugs. While we now see these patients and offer them treatment, most clinical spaces continue to follow the existing algorithm or do not screen for HCV at all, perpetuating spread and missing opportunity for cure. A decade ago, people who use drugs were offered no medical treatment or specific community linkage while now, physicians in our ED initiate lifesaving therapy (buprenorphine) and participate in 'warm hand-off' processes that ensure patients are not lost after ED discharge. Much of this work involves finding connections between those patches of patient-centered care to broader healthcare system and provider incentives or motivations to hardwire new routes of improved outcomes.

Consider first a patient with a myocardial infarction, stroke, or sepsis. In the current healthcare system, provider education, prehospital/EMS, primary care/prevention, pharmaceuticals, compliance organizations (e.g., goals set in the United States by the National Quality Foundation), payment structures (Center for Medicare and Medicaid Services) and reimbursement to individual providers and facilities all align to drive care with less variation from encounter and a common set of expectations among providers and healthcare systems across the United States. These are formalized pathways of care, highly entangled assemblages with patient, provider, administrator incentives aligned. Alignment in healthcare is not a common feature in the United States secondary to different payment sources and associated quality goals for providers and facilities and providers and staff (e.g., nursing). Acute coronary syndrome/coronary artery disease alignment leads to assemblage stability across preventive care, prehospital care, primary care, the emergency department, and the cardiology teams. Patients with a ST-Elevation Myocardial Infarction (STEMI) receive high quality, low variability care across hospitals in the United States.

Patients with Sickle Cell Disease, on the other hand, often receive care below best practice recommendations that is highly heterogenous. In 2016, we recognized our emergency department was delivering highly variable care to patients with SCD Veno-occlusive Crisis (VOC). SCD VOC is a painful condition where sickled cells impede regular blood and microinfarcts in soft tissues and bones occur. As patients with SCD live longer secondary to advances in medical management, they undergo more episodes of these painful conditions and, often, develop a physiological opioid dependence from treatment. The distribution of SCD worldwide is based on evolutionary processes that promote selection of the sickle cell trait which is protective from malaria across geographically affected areas near the equator, including parts of Africa.

In the United States, SCD is structurally distributed with high prevalence in the South secondary to historical enslavement of African people (CDC 2020). Institutional racism and implicit bias of healthcare providers in the south have contributed to uneven care delivery to mostly black patients with SCD VOC. Students conducted participant observation and semi-structured interviews with SCD VOC patients in our hospital, seeking to create a more just, equitable, and evidence-based system of care (Wilson and Baer 2022). Through these ethnographically informed approaches, our hospital has now hardwired utilization of patient-controlled analgesia (PCA) and emphasizes early pain medication delivery after ED arrival. PCA utilization and early drug delivery are WHO/NHLBI best practices (YAWN, BUCHANAN, AFENYI-ANNAN, BALLAS, HASSELL, JAMES & JORDAN 2014) that have resulted in improved patient experiences and decreased hospital admissions by over 10% (OSORNO & WILSON 2018). The long length of stay (LOS) associated with SCD VOC admissions and the "poor payor mix" (a term representing the connection between SCD VOC patients and the likelihood of lower reimbursing Medicaid state/federal insurance), has aligned neoliberal healthcare goals (reduce length of stay on this poorly paying DRG in order to lose less money) and patient care goals, while also removing the opportunity for repeated microaggressions of provider-patient judgement encounters where deservingness of treatment could be decided at the moment of care delivery.

Assemblage formation

A prior graduate student produced an ethnographically informed medication for opioid use disorder (MOUD) pathway that represented roots of new assemblage formation (HENDERSON 2022). 10 years ago, patients that presented to our ED with OUD were given no treatment and few resources. Their mortality at 1 year was higher than that of a person presenting with heart disease (WEINER, BAKER, BERNSON & SCHUUR 2020). HENDERSON, WILSON & MCCOY (2021) constructed the ED BRIDGE to provide buprenorphine to patients with OUD along with a warm hand-off to a community provider (HENDERSON, WILSON & MCCOY 2021). This process required physician engagement and new, two-way relationships with community partners.

The assemblage has more fully begun to form as other work on infectious disease is more clearly linked to OUD pathways. In 2016, JW initiated HIV and HCV non-targeted screening in the ED based on CDC guidelines (2006). Patients with newly diagnosed HCV were difficult to link to care, even though new direct acting antivirals (DAAs) that offered HCV cure in 95% of patients within 12 weeks were available beginning in 2015 (FELD, JACOBSON, HÉZODE, ASSELAH, RUANE, GRUENER, ABERGEL 2015). The traditional demographic of HCV patients shifted from age-cohort ("baby boomers" born between 1945–1965), well-funded (Medicare) people to a non-age-cohort ("millennials" born after 1980) with active or recent drug use and less likelihood of having any third-party insurance or having lower reimbursing state/federal funding (e.g., Medicaid). People who inject drugs (PWID) are also less likely to engage in HCV treatment given the lack of obvious systemic symptoms in the early disease course. Left untreated, those with HCV can develop liver failure or liver cancer. In addition, HCV is highly infectious via injection drug use secondary to the ability of viral particles to remain active on drug paraphernalia.

HCV and OUD are a syndemic created secondary to the biology of HCV (virulent and highly infectious during injection), opioid use disorder (often progresses to injection drug use as physiological dependence develops) and social determinants, social policy and structural causes of drug use. A combination of lower wages, lower education obtainment, less positive outlook for future life happiness, pharmaceutical marketing, federal laws restricting safe injection sites and oral medication supply (both opioids and treatments for opioids) have all combined to place us in a opioid current epidemic that began in the mid 2000s with prescription drug misuse, escalated to injection heroin use and is now best defined by fentanyl. Co-occurring mental health disorders (documented in 80% of our participants) is also an important component of this syndemic.

The classic syndemic description by Singer connected HIV, drug use and domestic violence (Singer, Bulled, Ostrach, and Mendenhall 2017). Other anthropologists have extended syndemic descriptions to diabetes and obesity (MENDENHALL, KOHORT, NORRIS, NDETEI & PRABHAKARAN 2017). The expansion of syndemic models into public health has led to the expansion of the descriptive technique to consider the linkage between social determinants and multiple other acute and chronic disease states and biological conditions. Our clinically applied anthropology extends syndemics from a descriptive model to treatment model, using a syndemic methodology to consider emerging assemblages (OUD programs, HCV linkage and treatment programs) and to design care pathways that manage co-occurring disease. We first implemented the MOUD program in our ED and found that 78% of patients we started on buprenorphine and linked to care also had HCV. Previous to this pathway, our linkage to care rates for HCV were under 30% and only 3% of patients were started on DAA. By co-locating downstream OUD and HCV care (prescription of buprenorphine and DAAs at same site), we established the largest HCV management program for patients in OUD recovery with an over 40% DAA treatment initiation. Our syndemic treatment pathway led to management of OUD and cure of HCV in patients that otherwise would have had no care, a 5% one-year mortality and continued spread of HCV in the community.

Finally, we expanded our newly forming complex assemblage by expanding the territory and scope of our pathway after recognizing that some patients in the ED with HCV were not yet ready to stop using injection drugs in order to start OUD treatment. Those patients attend a syringe exchange program where they undergo onsite testing for HCV. If positive, patients are able to receive DAA treatment at the exchange in a one-of-a-kind program that has the highest rates of HCV treatment in patients still using drugs (an important action to stop the transmission of HCV).

The time is right to reconsider applied clinical anthropologists as direct agents within the healthcare delivery space. This disruption challenges patient experience departments, healthcare providers and social workers to reconsider understanding of social determinants and the role the healthcare system can play in overcoming these burdens to delivery high quality patient-centered care. Those perceived social determinants are neither static burdens to overcome or arbitrarily objective items to be separated from the lived experience of disease. Just as prior concepts of applied clinical anthropology were given up in favor of a critical focus that first examines structural violence and power within relationships between people and institutions, abandonment of cultural competency concepts to are moved past, instead, focusing on ontological emergences within replicated healthcare encounters.

This does not mean that culture does not explain any differences in how patients consume healthcare, how healthcare is accessed or why there are broad disparities across human groups in healthcare outcomes even within local regional space. We are also not suggesting that simply studying structural realities, economic differences, or static demographics will lead to resolution of new disparity formation or solve inequity. Our model of an applied clinical anthropology shifts the lens to the ongoing reproduction and formation of those disparities, suggesting that this is the liminal and hard to see space that the anthropologist must find and magnify as the interesting place for study, healthcare contribution, and improved patient care. Chenhall and Senior (2017) have argued to abandon the static social determinant of disease concept in favor of the dynamic assemblage theory which focuses on disease emergence.

While we do advocate for assemblage theory as the guiding theory to examining, unentangling, and creating new patient care pathways, we actually do not advocate full abandonment of the Social Determinants of Health (SDOH) since this is a language medicine speaks dating back to Virchow who posited that medicine is really social science. Instead, we suggest clinical anthropologists adopt the SDH framework in discussion with medical colleagues but utilize the ontological approach of assemblage formation as a guiding strategy to implement SDOH solutions into healthcare delivery approaches. Traditional anthropological methods relying on participant observation and collection of qualitative data through semi-structured interviews is able to capture lived experiences of patients, providers, and other healthcare stakeholders. Utilizing those insights allows for design of novel care pathways and positions the anthropologist directly into the clinical space. This ethnographically informed care is a radical new clinically applied medical anthropology that can transform the patient experience by shifting the clinical gaze through a shared formative approach to care.

References

American Hospital Association (AHA) 2013. "Becoming a Culturally Competent Health Care Organization." June 2013. https://www.aha.org/ahahret-guides/2013-06-18-becoming-culturally-competent-health-care-organization [08.02.2024].

Branson, Bernard M.; Handsfield, H. Hunter; Margaret A., Lampe; Janssen, Robert S.; Taylor, Robert S.; Lyss, Sheryl B.; Clark, Jill E. & Centers for Disease Control and Prevention (CDC) 2006. Revised Recommendations for HIV Testing of Adults, Adolescents, and Pregnant Women in Health-Care Settings. *MMWR. Recommendations and Reports: Morbidity and Mortality Weekly Report. Recommendations and Reports / Centers for Disease Control* 55 (RR-14): 1–17; quiz CE1–4.

Taylor, Brown; Ashworth, Henry; Bass, Michelle; Rittenberg, Eve; Levy-Carrick, Nomi; Grossman, Samara; Lewis-O'Connor, Annie & Stoklosa, Hanni 2022. Trauma-Informed Care Interventions in Emergency Medicine: A Systematic Review. *The Western Journal of Emergency Medicine* 23 (3): 334–344.

Castro, Eduardo Viveiros de 2011. Zeno and the Art of Anthropology. *Common Knowledge* 17 (1): 128–145.

Centers for Disease Control (CDC) 2020. Data & Statistics on Sickle Cell Disease. Cdc.gov. December 2020. https://www.cdc.gov/ncbddd/sicklecell/data.html [08.02.2024].

Chenhall, Richard D. & Senior, Kate 2018. Living the Social Determinants of Health: Assemblages in a Remote

Aboriginal Community. *Medical Anthropology Quarterly* 32 (2): 177–195.

CHRISMAN, NOEL J. & W. MARETZKI, THOMAS (eds) 1982. *Clinically Applied Anthropology: Anthropologists in Health Science Settings*. 1982nd ed. Dordrecht, Netherlands: Kluwer Academic.

DELANDA, MANUEL 2006. *A New Philosophy of Society: Assemblage Theory and Social Complexity*. London & New York, NY: Continuum International Publishing Group.

DELEUZE, GILLES & GUATTARI, FELIX 1987. *A Thousand Plateaus: Capitalism and Schizophrenia*. 2nd ed. Minneapolis, MN: University of Minnesota Press.

FARMER, PAUL E.; NIZEYE, BRUCE; STULAC, SARA & KESHAVJEE, SALMAAN 2006. Structural Violence and Clinical Medicine." *PLoS Medicine* 3 (10): e449.

FELD, JORDAN J.; JACOBSON, IRA M.; HÉZODE, CHRISTOPHE; ASSELAH, TARIK; RUANE, PETER J.; GRUENER, NORBERT; ABERGEL, ARMAND 2015. Sofosbuvir and Velpatasvir for HCV Genotype 1, 2, 4, 5, and 6 Infection. *The New England Journal of Medicine* 373 (27): 2599–2607.

FOUCAULT, MICHAEL 1973. *The Birth of the Clinic: An Archaeology of Medical Perception*. New York: Pantheon Book.

Hahn, Robert A. 1996. *Sickness and Healing: An Anthropological Perspective*. New Haven, CT: Yale University Press.

HENDERSON, HEATHER; WILSON, JASON W. & MC COY, BERNICE 2021. Applied Medical Anthropology and Structurally Informed Emergency Care in the Evolving Context of COVID-19. *Human Organization* 80 (4): 263–271.

HENDERSON, HEATHER D. 2022. *Applied Anthropology of Addiction in Clinical Spaces: Co-Developing and Assessing a Novel Opioid Treatment Pathway*. Dissertation University of South Florida.

HOLMES, SETH M.; GEERAERT, JEREMY; CASTAÑEDA; CASTANEDA, HEIDE; PROBST, URSULA; ZELDES, NINA; WILLEN, SARAH S. 2021. Deservingness: Migration and Health in Social Context. *BMJ Global Health* 6 (Suppl 1). https://doi.org/10.1136/bmjgh-2021-005107 [08.02.2024].

INSTITUTE FOR HEALTHCARE IMPROVEMENT (IHI) 2021. The IHI Triple Aim. Iihi.org. Accessed June 18, 2021. http://www.ihi.org/Engage/Initiatives/TripleAim/Pages/default.aspx [08.02.2024].

KLEINMAN, ARTHUR; EISENBERG, LEON & GOOD, BYRON 1978. Culture, Illness, and Care: Clinical Lessons from Anthropologic and Cross-Cultural Research. *Annals of Internal Medicine* 88 (2): 251–258.

KLEINMAN, ARTHUR; CHRISMAN, NOEL J.; MARETZKI, THOMAS W. (eds) 1982. *Clinically Applied Anthropology: Anthropologists in Health Science Settings*. 2nd ed. Dordrecht, Netherlands: Springer.

LANGE, KLAUS W. 2021. Rudolf Virchow, Poverty and Global Health: From 'politics as Medicine on a Grand Scale' to 'health in All Policies.' *Global Health Journal* 5 (3): 149–54.

MENDENHALL, EMILY; KOHRT, BRANDON A.; NORRIS, SHANE A.; NDETEI, DAVID & RABHAKARAN, DORAIRAJ 2017. Non-Communicable Disease Syndemics: Poverty, Depression, and Diabetes among Low-Income Populations. *The Lancet* 389 (10072): 951–963.

NADING, ALEX M 2019. *Mosquito Trails: Ecology, Health, and the Politics of Entanglement*. Berkeley, Cal.: University of California Press.

OSORNO-CRUZ, C. & WILSON, JW. Understanding the Sickle-Cell Patient Experience nad New Approaches to Pain Management. Presentation as part of Anthropology and Special Patient Populations in the Emergency Department (TH-160). Society for Applied Anthropology (sfAA), Philadelphia Pennsylvania. Presented by Carlos Osorno-Cruz, April 5, 2018.

PRESS, IRWIN 2006. *Patient Satisfaction: Understanding and Managing the Experience of Care*. 2nd ed. Health Administration Press.

RATNA, HARAN N. 2020. Medical Neoliberalism and the Decline in U.S. Healthcare Quality. *Journal of Hospital Management and Health Policy* 4 (March): 7–7.

SCHEPER-HUGHES, NANCY 1990. Three Propositions for a Critically Applied Medical Anthropology. *Social Science & Medicine* 30 (2): 189–197.

SHER, GEORGE. 1983. Health Care and the 'Deserving Poor.' *The Hastings Center Report* 13 (1): 9–12.

SINGER, MERRILL; BULLED, NICOLA; OSTRACH, BAYLA & MENDENHALL, EMILY 2017. Syndemics and the Biosocial Conception of Health. *The Lancet* 389 (10072): 941–950.

TSING, ANNA 2009. Supply Chains and the Human Condition. *Rethinking Marxism* 21 (2): 148–176.

TSING, ANNA LOWENHAUPT 2017. *The Mushroom at the End of the World: On the Possibility of Life in Capitalist Ruins*. Princeton, NJ: Princeton University Press.

WEINER, SCOTT G.; OLESYA BAKER, DANA BERNSON, AND JEREMIAH D. SCHUUR. 2020. One-Year Mortality of Patients after Emergency Department Treatment for Nonfatal Opioid Overdose. *Annals of Emergency Medicine* 75 (1): 13–17.

WILLIAMS, ANDREW M., AND JOSÉ-ALAIN SAHEL. 2022. Addressing Social Determinants of Vision Health. *Ophthalmology and Therapy*, June. https://doi.org/10.1007/s40123-022-00531-w.

WILSON, JASON W.; BAER, ROBERTA D. & VILLALONA, SEIICHI 2019. Patient Shadowing: A Useful Research Method, Teaching Tool, and Approach to Student Professional Development for Premedical Undergraduates. *Academic Medicine: Journal of the Association of American Medical Colleges* 94 (11): 1722–1727.

WILSON, JASON W. & BAER, ROBERTA D. 2022. *Clinical Anthropology 2.0: Improving Medical Education and Patient Experience*. Lanham, Maryland: Rowman & Littlefield.

YAWN, BARBARA P.; BUCHANAN, GEORGE R.; AFENYI-ANNAN, ARABA N.; BALLAS, SAMIR K.; HASSELL, KATHRYN L.; JAMES, ANDRA H. & LANETTA JORDAN 2014. Management of Sickle Cell Disease: Summary of the 2014 Evidence-Based Report by Expert Panel Members. *JAMA: The Journal of the American Medical Association* 312 (10): 1033.

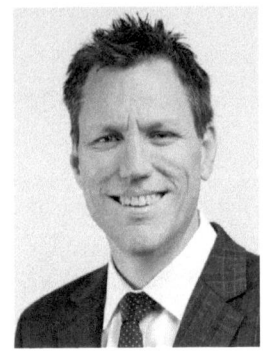

Jason W. Wilson, MD, PhD, is an emergency medicine physician and medical anthropologist. He is the Chairman of Emergency Medicine at the University of South Florida and the Chief of Emergency Medicine at Tampa General Hospital. Dr. Wilson's interests are in the integration of social scientists directly into the clinical space to improve patient care pathways. Dr. Wilson utilizes an ethnographically informed care approach to healthcare design. He has positioned other faculty medical anthropologists in his Department to train students, residents and attending physicians in this approach and to carry out their own clinically applied work. Overall, this approach has allowed the group to tackle social medicine with a unique perspective.

University of South Florida
 Department of Emergency Medicine
Morsani College of Medicine,
e-mail: jwilson2@usf.edu

http://tampaerdoc.com
@tampaERdoc

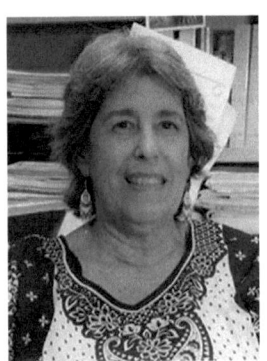

Roberta D. Baer, PhD, is Professor Emerita in the Department of Anthropology, University of South Florida, Tampa, FL., USA. As an applied medical anthropologist, her current interests include Applied Clinical Anthropology, specifically issues related to physician training, firearms injuries, and outreach to underserved communities. She has collaborated with JWW for the last 8 years on projects in hospital settings, as well as in the community.

University of South Florida
Department of Anthropology
4202 E. Fowler Ave.—SOC 107
Tampa, FL. 33620-8100
e-mail: baer@usf.edu

BERICHTE
REPORTS

Krisen, Körper, Kompetenzen. Methoden und Potentiale medizinanthropologischen Forschens

Bericht zur 35. Jahrestagung der Arbeitsgemeinschaft Ethnologie und Medizin (AGEM) in Kooperation mit dem 20. Arbeitstreffen der Kommission Medizinanthropologie der Deutschen Gesellschaft für Empirische Kulturwissenschaft (DGEKW), Warburg-Haus Hamburg, 08.–09. September 2023

LEA KOOP-MEYER

Im Mittelpunkt der Tagung stand die medizinanthropologische Erforschung der alltäglichen Erfahrungen und körperlichen Dimensionen von Krisen. Angesichts der aktuellen gsellschaftlichen Dynamiken und der Vielzahl von Krisenerfahrungen, darunter auch die Auswirkungen von SARS-CoV-2, werden Fragen nach den Verkörperungen permanenter Krisenerfahrungen und den Veränderungen sinnlicher Wahrnehmung und Erfahrung aufgeworfen. In diesem Zusammenhang wird das Spannungsverhältnis zwischen Degeneration und Resilienz als Verlust oder Gewinn an Kompetenz thematisiert. Zentral ist die Diskussion kollaborativer und partizipativer Forschungsansätze, die die traditionelle Unterscheidung zwischen Forschenden und Beforschten in Frage stellen. Die Tagung bot somit eine Plattform, um die Herausforderungen und Potenziale medizinanthropologischer Forschung im Kontext von Krisen zu diskutieren, einschließlich neuer Methodologien und digitaler Forschungsmethoden.

PANEL I: Krisen und Körper in Geschichte und Gegenwart

PHILIPP OSTEN (UKE Hamburg) beleuchtete die Rolle historischer Pandemien für das Verständnis und die Bewältigung gegenwärtiger und zukünftiger Krisensituationen. Er betonte, dass Pandemien nicht isoliert betrachtet werden können, sondern in einem kontinuierlichen historischen Kontext stehen. Anhand historischer Medienberichte über Pandemien wie Pest und Cholera illustrierte Osten die Veränderungen in der Medienlandschaft und der öffentlichen Wahrnehmung. Insbesondere zeigt er auf, wie sich im Laufe der Zeit die Kommunikationsmethoden und der Umgang mit Pandemien durch den Medienwandel verändert haben: Von religiösen Appellen bis hin zu modernen Impfkampagnen. Gleichzeitig betont Osten auch die soziale Dimension von Pandemien. Sein Beitrag verdeutlicht die Relevanz einer medizinhistorischen Perspektive auf Pandemien für ein umfassendes Verständnis und einen angemessenen Umgang mit aktuellen und zukünftigen Krisensituationen.

TOBIAS BECKER (Universität Hamburg) vertiefte diese historische Betrachtung anhand der Polio-Epidemien der 1950er und 1960er Jahre und zeigte auf, wie Medien und Medizin als wechselseitige Ressourcen fungieren und sich gegenseitig mobilisieren können. Insbesondere betont er die Bedeutung der Medien für die Medizin und das Verhalten der Menschen, indem Mechanismen der Werbung für medizinische Maßnahmen genutzt werden. Becker verdeutlicht den Wandel der Präventionskultur und zeigt anhand von Bildmaterial, wie sich die Anrufung des präventiven Selbst und die Art der Kommunikation von Abschreckung und kollektiver Bedrohung hin zu Hoffnung und persönlicher Ansprache gewandelt haben. Dieser Wandel findet zudem Parallelen in der aktuellen COVID-19-Pandemie.

Nachdem im ersten Panel vor allem die historische Dimension von Pandemien und deren Relevanz für die Bewältigung aktueller und zukünftiger Krisensituationen behandelte, setzte das zweite Panel den Fokus auf Krisen und Institutionen.

PANEL II: Krisen und Institutionen

Im zweiten Panel der Konferenz fokussierte ANDREA KUCKERT (Marien Hospital Düsseldorf) Krisen- und Liminalitätserfahrungen älterer LGBTQI*-Männer, deren Biografien im Rahmen ihrer Studie beleuchtet wurden. Kuckert richtete ihren Blick verstärkt auf die Zusammenhänge zwischen sexueller Orientierung/Geschlechtsidentität, Barrieren im Gesundheitssystem, Versorgungsbedarfen und Ressourcen der Gruppe älterer LGBTQI*-Männer. Ein Schwerpunkt lag dabei auf der Frage, inwiefern die Coronapandemie die Vorstellungen von gesundem Altern verändert hat. Kuckert konnte durch ihre Studie Einblicke in beeindruckende Biographien gewinnen und herausarbeiten, dass das Gesundheitsempfinden multidimensional ist. Deutlich wurde, wie wichtig Partnerschaften als Halt und Unterstützung sind. Gesund älter zu werden, wurde immer wieder auch mit dem Gefühl des Gebrauchtwerdens beschrieben, das Füreinandereinstehen hatte einen hohen Stellenwert. Zentral war auch die Erkenntnis, dass ‚gutes' Altern bedeutet, mit Hoffnungen, aber auch mit Ängsten umgehen zu können und jeder Mensch die Möglichkeit hat, Alterungsprozesse bewusst und selbstbestimmt zu gestalten.

SOPHIE WITT (Universität Hamburg) stellt nicht nur die Konzeption des Schwerpunktes „Körper, Gesundheit, Gesellschaft: Leben im Anthropozän" im Rahmen des neu eingerichteten Studiengangs Liberal Arts & Sciences an der Universität Hamburg vor, sondern betont auch die Relevanz der interdisziplinären Auseinandersetzung mit aktuellen Gesundheitsfragen. Als verantwortliche Leiterin des Vertiefungsbereichs innerhalb des Studiengangs betont sie, dass Gesundheit in diesem Zusammenhang als eine Frage verstanden und erforscht wird, die über den Bereich der Medizin hinausgeht. Die interdisziplinäre Perspektive ziele darauf ab, zu erforschen, was es für Individuen und Gemeinschaften bedeutet, ‚gesund' zu sein, und welche Körper- und Gesellschaftskonzepte damit verbunden sind. Es werde analysiert, aus welchen Blickwinkeln, mit welchen Erkenntnissen und möglichen Leerstellen das Wissen der verschiedenen Disziplinen erscheint. Die verstärkte Integration der Geistes- und Sozialwissenschaften in die Medizin ermöglicht aus Sicht von Witt nicht nur ein umfassenderes Verständnis von Gesundheit, sondern auch eine vertiefte Erforschung der Wechselwirkungen zwischen Körper, Gesellschaft und Umwelt. Witt sieht die Notwendigkeit, die starren Grenzen zwischen den Disziplinen aufzubrechen und ein hegemoniales Verständnis von Wissensformen zu überwinden. Dazu müssen die jeweiligen Disziplinen in ihrem Selbstverständnis kritisch hinterfragt werden.

Das zweite Panel thematisierte daher den Umgang mit Unsicherheiten und Machthierarchien – einerseits in Bezug auf den Umgang mit älteren LGBTQI*-Männern im Gesundheitswesen, andererseits in Bezug auf die Reflexion disziplinären Handelns und hegemonialer Wissensverhältnisse.

PANEL III: Ethnografische Annäherungen an Krisen und Körper

MAREN HEIBGES (TU Berlin) unterstrich die Begrenzungen traditioneller Entscheidungsmodelle angesichts von „radikaler Unsicherheit" in komplexen medizinischen und gesellschaftlichen Szenarien und plädierte für eine reflektierte Herangehensweise an wissenschaftliche Zweifel. In solchen Fällen können traditionelle Entscheidungsmodelle, die von vollständiger Information und rationalen Akteur*innen ausgehen, unzureichend sein. Heibges betonte die Verbindung zwischen dem Unsicherheitsparadigma und der (Europäischen) Ethnologie und präsentierte prominente Kritikpunkte am Risikoparadigma in der Medizin. Im Zentrum ihres Vortrags stand das Spannungsverhältnis in heutigen Gesellschaften, die durch zunehmende wissenschaftliche Informiertheit und gleichzeitig wachsende wissenschaftliche Skepsis gekennzeichnet sind. Heibges betonte, dass Zweifel omnipräsent sind und reflektiert werden müssten. Dennoch plädierte sie für die Idee einer „bounded uncertainty": Ungewissheit existiert, aber innerhalb bestimmter Grenzen oder Einschränkungen, die helfen können, mit ihr umzugehen und fundierte Entscheidungen zu treffen.

PATRICK BIELER (HU Berlin) beschäftigte sich mit der wechselseitigen Bedingtheit von Umwelt und Mensch und deren Auswirkungen auf die psychische Gesundheit, die er als Ergebnis dieser wechselseitigen Bedingtheit ansah. Während soziales Kapital und soziale Isolation bereits intensiv erforscht worden seien, sei die Bedeutung flüchtiger sozialer Bindungen bisher vernachlässigt worden. Gleichzeitig seien vor allem die direkten sozialen Kontakte aggregiert worden, wodurch die Spezifika urbaner Lebenswelten verloren gegangen seien. Bieler konzentrierte sich daher speziell auf nachbarschaftliche Begegnungen in urbanen Räumen und untersuchte mit einem ethnographischen Ansatz, was Vorstellungen von einem ‚wohltuenden Leben ausmacht. Detaillierte und dialogische Analysen wurden durchgeführt, um die Ambivalenzen in diesem Kontext aufzuzeigen. Dieser methodische Ansatz ermöglichte ein vertieftes Verständnis der Bedeutung flüchtiger sozialer Interaktionen für die psychische Gesundheit. MAREN HEIBGES und PATRICK BIELER präsentierten im Panel eine umfassende Analyse der Herausforderungen und Dynamiken im Bereich der Gesundheitsforschung. Beide Vorträge verdeutlichten die Notwendigkeit eines multiperspektivischen Ansatzes und einer differenzierten Betrachtung sozialer und medizinischer Dynamiken für ein umfassendes Verständnis von Gesundheit.

HELLA VON UNGER (LMU München) analysierte zunächst die verschiedenen Ansätze partizipativer Forschung in der Sozialwissenschaft und präzisierte die Merkmale, die für sie eine partizipative und qualitativ-forschende Gesundheitsforschung ausmachen. Gleichzeitig zeigte sie die zentralen Herausforderungen auf, mit denen sowohl Forschende als auch Beforschte konfrontiert sind. Anhand von zwei Studienbeispielen, die sie selbst partizipativ durchgeführt hat, illustriert von Unger die Herausforderungen, denen sie in ihrer Arbeit begegnet ist. Zum einen betonte sie, dass Communities vielfältige Machtstrukturen aufweisen und keine homogene Einheit darstellen. Zum anderen wies sie auf strukturelle Hindernisse hin, die oft zur unbewussten Reproduktion von Machtstrukturen beitragen. Sie betonte, dass die Bedingungen in der Forschung oft dem entgegenstehen, was für einen dialogischen Prozess in der partizipativen Gesundheitsforschung notwendig ist. Des Weiteren thematisierte von Unger die Schwierigkeit, partizipative Forschung in den wissenschaftlichen Diskurs zu integrieren. Hier machte sie deutlich, dass Diskurse in der partizipativen Forschung unterschiedlich funktionieren und nicht immer rein wissenschaftlichen Logiken folgen. Gleichzeitig betonte von Unger die Stärken der partizipativen Zusammenarbeit, insbesondere die multiperspektivische Betrachtung einer Fragestellung.

Der erste Tag der Konferenz bot spannende Einblicke in die historischen Wurzeln von Krisensituationen und die sich wandelnde Rolle von Medizin und Medialisierungsprozessen. Das zweite Panel des Tages vertiefte das Verständnis von Krisen, indem es sich auf die Unsicherheiten im medizinischen Bereich und die Bedeutung sozialer Interaktionen für die psychische Gesundheit konzentrierte, während HELLA VON UNGER die Herausforderungen und Stärken partizipativer Forschung hervorhob und einen Einblick in ihre eigene partizipative Arbeit gab.

PANEL IV: Räume und Narrative von Körpern in der Krise

Der zweite Tag der Tagung startete mit einem Beitrag von ANITA HAM (Leiden University Medical Centre/The Hague University of Applied Science) und ANDREA KUCKERT (Marien Hospital Düsseldorf). Sie veranschaulichten in ihrem Beitrag exemplarisch die Herausforderungen der Forschung, indem sie auf die schwierige Erreichbarkeit von Menschen mit Migrationshintergrund und niedrigem sozioökonomischem Status in Bezug auf Mammographie und Gebärmutterhalskrebsvorsorge in den Niederlanden eingingen. Das Participatory Action Research (PAR) Projekt zielte daher darauf ab, informierte Entscheidungen über die Teilnahme an bevölkerungsbasierten Früherkennungsprogrammen zu fördern. Es wurde ein partizipativer Ansatz gewählt, der auf einer engen Zusammenarbeit mit Mitgliedern der lokalen Bevölkerung, professionellen Gesundheitsdienstleister*innen und Studierenden basierte. Die Forschung konzentrierte sich insbesondere auf die Hindernisse, die der Erreichbarkeit dieser Zielgruppe entgegenstehen. Besonders hervorgehoben wurde die Notwendigkeit, spezielle Anlaufstellen für Frauen einzurichten, um einen adäquaten Zugang zu gewährleisten. Darüber hinaus wurde die Bedeutung einer wertebasierten Versorgung hervorgehoben, die individuelle Wertvorstellungen berücksichtigt und darauf aufbaut.

Im Mittelpunkt des Vortrags von MANUEL BOLZ (Universität Hamburg), MONA MOTAKEF (TU Dortmund), HOLLY PATCH (TU Dortmund), SABINE WÖHLKE (HAW Hamburg) stand die Lebenssituation von trans* Personen, ihre zunehmende Aufmerksamkeit und rechtliche Sichtbarkeit in Gegenwartsgesellschaften. Insbesondere wurde auf die hart umkämpften Rechte von trans* Personen in Deutschland eingegangen und die Herausforderungen in der transgeschlechtlichen Gesundheitsversorgung diskutiert. Des Weiteren wurden die unterschiedlichen Lebenslagen von trans* Personen im Kontext der explizit und implizit prägenden cis-normativen Rahmenbedingungen beleuchtet. Anhand von den Perspektiven „Verhindern", „Verschieben" und „Werden" wurden verschiedene Aspekte von trans* Erfahrungen aus drei Forschungsprojekten vorgestellt, die eine Linearität von Zeitlichkeit in Frage stellen. Es wurde darauf hingewiesen, dass eine empirisch fundierte Auseinandersetzung mit Zeitlichkeiten in Bezug auf trans* Personen notwendig ist und die lineare Vorstellung von Zeitlichkeit kritisch hinterfragt werden sollte, um Normalisierungspraktiken bewusst zu machen.

PANEL V: Krisen und Körper kuratieren, musealisieren, ausstellen

Was kann Weiblichkeit sein und was bedeutet sie aus medizinischer Sicht? Diesen Fragen ging AMELIE SACHS in ihrer multiperspektivischen Betrachtung der Lebenserfahrungen von Frauen mit dem polyzystischen Ovarsyndrom (PCOS) nach. Dabei lenkte sie den Blick auf die strukturelle Prägung der Gynäkologie durch männliche Einflüsse und die bisher vernachlässigte Berücksichtigung eines ganzheitlichen Behandlungsansatzes. Sachs widmete sich der Darstellung der Krankheit und des weiblichen Körpers, die immer auch mit Machtverhältnissen verbunden ist. Für ihr Fotoprojekt wählte sie einen multiperspektivischen Ansatz, bei dem unterschiedliche Sichtweisen aufeinander trafen: Die Perspektive der Betroffenen wurde als Expertise anerkannt und ihre emotionalen Erfahrungen in Bildern veranschaulicht. Diese Bilder wurden als Ausdruck eines dialogischen Prozesses verstanden und durch Expert:inneninterviews ergänzt, um weitere Perspektiven auf das Thema PCOS zu gewinnen.

Trotz unterschiedlicher Schwerpunkte wurden in den Beiträgen gemeinsame Themen herausgearbeitet. Dazu gehören die strukturellen Herausforderungen im Gesundheitswesen und die Notwendigkeit eines multiperspektivischen Ansatzes für ein umfassendes Verständnis von Gesundheit.

Abschlussdiskussion

Eine facettenreiche Diskussion zentraler Aspekte der Gesundheitsforschung zeigte sich in der Abschlussdiskussion der Tagung. Trotz der Vielfalt der behandelten Themen wurde deutlich, dass es Möglichkeiten gibt, Verbindungen und Verknüpfungen zwischen den verschiedenen Bereichen herzustellen. Besonders hervorgehoben wurde die Bedeutung des Umgangs mit Unsicherheit und Machthierarchien für eine effektive Gesundheitsförderung. Darüber hinaus wurde die Notwendigkeit betont, Geisteswissenschaften und Medizin enger miteinander zu verknüpfen, um zu einem umfassenderen Verständnis von Gesundheit zu gelangen und disziplinäre Grenzen aufzubrechen. Ein weiterer Schwerpunkt der Diskussion lag auf partizipativen Formen der Zusammenarbeit, die als entscheidend für ein ganzheitliches Verständnis von Gesundheit angesehen wurden. Es wurde betont, dass alternative Zugänge zu den Zielgruppen, z.B. über Kunst, Musik oder andere innovative Ideen, neue Perspektiven für die Erforschung und Gestaltung von Gesundheitsfragen eröffnen.

LEA KOOP-MEYER studiert derzeit im Masterstudiengang Health Sciences an der Hochschule für Angewandte Wissenschaften Hamburg (HAW Hamburg). Ihr Bachelorstudium der Sozialen Arbeit absolvierte sie an der Alice Salomon Hochschule Berlin. An der HAW Hamburg arbeitete sie als wissenschaftliche Hilfskraft in der Arbeitsgruppe „Gesundheitswissenschaften und Ethik" unter der Leitung von Prof. Dr. Sabine Wöhlke. In den Projekten PANDORA und ORIENTATE sammelte sie wertvolle Erfahrungen zur Patient*innenbeteiligung in der (quantitativen) Forschung und entwickelte ein starkes Interesse an partizipativer Gesundheitsforschung. Derzeit leitet Lea Koop-Meyer die Frauenwerkstatt in Sulingen, die Frauen bei der Entwicklung beruflicher Perspektiven unterstützt. In ihrer beruflichen Praxis beschäftigt sie sich mit den Themen soziale Ungleichheit, Frauengesundheit und gesundheitsbezogene Lebensqualität.

Hochschule für Angewandte Wissenschaften Hamburg
Fakultät Life Sciences
Department Gesundheitswissenschaften
e-mail: Lea.Koop-Meyer@haw-hamburg.de

REZENSIONEN
BOOK REVIEWS

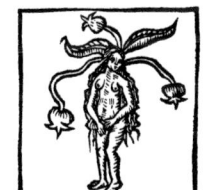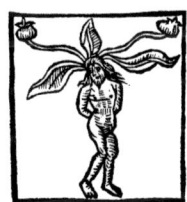

Diana Espírito Santo 2023. Spirited Histories. Technologies, Media, and Trauma in Paranormal Chile.
London & New York: Routledge, 202 pp.

Diana Espírito Santo is Associate Professor of Social Anthropology at the Pontificia Universidad Católica de Chile. She has already delivered several contributions to the anthropological study of spirits and mediumship, for example, on the Cuban Espiritismo and the social life of spirits. Her current work has been published in Routledge's series "The Anthropology of History" (edited by Stephan Palmié and Charles Stewart), and accordingly, she focuses on alternative histories and micro-histories developed in paranormal and para-patrimonial practices. She explores occult topographies rearticulated as alternative forms, understandings, and productions of history as less representational than actual affective and experiential endeavors. With her focus on paranormal investigators throughout three years of ethnographic data collection (participant observation and interviews), she understands history as a continuous social practice.

Nonetheless, her report is also of value to medical anthropologists due to the initial question of how far paranormal practices may help to deal with individual and collective trauma produced throughout Pinochet's violent dictatorship in Chile (1973–1990). According to the author, lingering trauma is connected to spaces or sites where human violations occurred. It keeps boiling beneath functional surfaces once that it has often been ignored in official strategies of remembrance due to the post-dictatorship democracy's emphasis on reconciliation and forgiveness, rather than justice or retribution. Diana Espírito Santo identifies ghosts as ripples in a particular space-time continuum, such as disappearances, affective absences, and the effort to break repression and silencing. She wonders how we can understand individual and collective suffering in this way and extends her focus from the dictatorship to earlier colonial violence and contemporary neoliberal inequalities, including the repression of protests against COVID-19 policies.

According to her, there are manifold traumas to be dealt with in Chile. Whereas she identifies political repression of the highest order, gravest violations of human rights, and brutalization resulting in death and disappearances throughout the dictatorship, contemporary neoliberal economic models result in the massive privatization of fundamental rights, such as housing, education, and health. Referring to what she calls the dictatorship's B side, Diana Espírito Santo detects roaming questions of, e.g., what happened to the souls of those who were brutally assassinated and/or disappeared. Ghosts may be a symptom of what is missing, but also the means to tease it out. In this regard, she compares history to photography that captures random events and fragments, excluding both completeness and transience. It is about exploring the emotions and embodied affective stances of the victims.

The monography is subdivided into seven chapters (Introduction/Ghosts – Machines – Noise – Affect – Aliens – Play – Afterword) in which the author focuses on cosmology, discourse, and practices within social phenomena such as mediumship, paranormal investigation in historical spaces, and ghost tours in places such as former psychiatric hospitals, labor camps, or prisons as sites of torture, human experiments, murder, etc. She presents many vivid case studies and reports from her participant observation, including instances of autoethnography. These are framed by dense theoretical and philosophical discussions (e.g., on space-time, multidirectory dynamics of time, the plurality of history, hauntology, interference, noise/voice/sound, media/technology) that, in their complexity, may overwhelm the recipient at first sight. However, a thorough reading of her account reveals the central argument that periods of Chilean history are laid bare in paranormal investigations and ghost tours. Ghosts pull us into structures of feeling and produce resonance systems, activating and altering memories and setting in motion a collective will to know and commemorate; memory is constructed through affective involvement.

Accordingly, paranormal activities draw on a plastic reading of history, a history whose traumas are marked by unsilenceable traces, evoked as fragments of sound and images through specific apparatuses that, as a further development of

19th century's Spiritualist technologies, mark the digital turn in paranormal investigations. Wherever an increased activity is detected, the dead demand some reparation, operating through electromagnetic currents. The example of ghost tours in Santiago de Chile illustrates how such interferences create thrill and fear, generating affective atmospheres and sensations, moving people into certain physical and mental states, and producing historical experiences in correspondence with existent evidentiary formats of documents and archives.

In the end, the answer to the question of how exactly history and trauma are being recovered remains open. DIANA ESPÍRITO SANTO does not investigate the effectiveness of practices but argues for a perspective of history as unfinished and in-the-making, as sensational and embodied internal work that provides clues helping to understand past, present, and future individual and socio-political trauma fully.

In an excursus, the author also explores two cases of alleged Alien communication. The first are geoglyphs in the Atacama desert that are interpreted as information from and about ancient astronauts who supposedly interfered in the development of human culture, and the second are mediumistically received messages from hybrid human-aliens of the future that warn humankind of its self-induced annihilation. It illustrates the multidirectionality of histories in the past-present-future continuum. However, particularly the latter example can also be interpreted as a meta-commentary on contemporary neoliberal and capitalist structural violence, introducing alternative human development strategies from affliction to insight. Psycho-social trauma and political suffering thus may become a "metaphorical noise on a continual loop," and the author stresses the performative character of media and mediation in its broadest sense – the forming of forms interfering with environments, generating communion and facilitating communication with and about the past and the future. Enactments may trigger social memory and individual perceptions, excavating the past and envisioning the future in an empathetic approach. They provide a life of their own to alleged paranormal phenomena as narratives and (hi)stories. It is about historical possibilities rather than ontological realism.

It is a complex book due to its thorough discussion of variant theoretical and philosophical perspectives and their entanglement with the provided data. DIANA ESPÍRITO SANTO delivers a must-read for an interdisciplinary collegium and lay people interested in Spirit(ual)ism, mediumship, and paranormal phenomena affecting our well-being-in-the-world. Notably, her focus on affective atmospheres, corporeal engagements, and the aesthetical importance of voices/noises and (inner) visualizations makes it an essential contribution to an anthropology of the senses/sensory ethnography that, in the reviewer's opinion, is crucial to contemporary (medical) anthropology.

HELMAR KURZ, Münster

Inga Scharf da Silva 2022. Trauma als Wissensarchiv. Postkoloniale Erinnerungspraxis in der Sakralen Globalisierung am Beispiel der Zeitgenössischen Umbanda im Deutschsprachigen Europa.
Marburg: Büchner, 514 S.

Inga Scharf da Silva hat Ethnologie und Kunstgeschichte an der Freien Universität Berlin sowie an den staatlichen Universitäten von Salvador da Bahia (UFBA), Recife (UFPE) und São Paulo (USP) studiert. Sie hat am Institut für Europäische Ethnologie der Humboldt Universität Berlin promoviert und bisher u.a. zum Synkretismus der brasilianischen *Umbanda* und im Kontext der Disability Studies publiziert. Sie ist außerdem bildende Künstlerin innerhalb des Atelierhaus Sigmaringer1art (Berufsverband Bildender Künstler) in Berlin/Wilmersdorf und hat 2019 das Titelbild (aus ihrem Zyklus „Die Suche" 2009–2010) zur *Curare* 42 (2019) 3+4 Schwerpunktausgabe „Ästhetiken des Heilens: Arbeit mit den Sinnen im Therapeutischen Kontext" beigesteuert. Auch viele Abbildungen der hier rezensierten Monographie entstammen ihrem künstlerischen Zyklus „Orixás" (seit 2012).

Dementsprechend nehmen sinnlich-ästhetische Kommunikations- und Wahrnehmungsformen der brasilianischen Religion *Umbanda* und ihrer Ableger in Deutschland als Wissenswelten, die sich mit dem Intellekt, der Intuition, den Emotionen und dem Körper wahrnehmen lassen, einen zentralen Raum ein. Zugeschriebene Trancezustände werden als „lebendige Archive erfahrener emotionaler Wissensbestände" begriffen und durch eine „Methodik des Mit-Gefühls" erschlossen. Insbesondere interessiert sich die Autorin für subtiles Wissen kolonialhistorischer Lücken als Gefühlsarchive, welche kulturelles Gedächtnis über den Körper transportieren können (vgl. zu einer vergleichbaren Perspektive auf paranormale Praktiken in Chile die Rezension von Diana Espírito Santos „Spirited Histories" von 2022 in dieser Ausgabe).

Sie betrachtet aber insbesondere auch materielle bzw. technisch-künstlerische Medien und deren Kapazität, einen „Geist" bzw. ein Bewusstsein zu transportieren, welches sich ggf. in Objekten und Körpern manifestiert. Die Kommunikation bzw. Vermittlung von spiritueller Erfahrung und Ergriffenheit wird dabei sowohl auf kognitiv-imaginäre, als auch auf körperlich-sinnliche Weise geschult und bedient u.a. auch das Konzept der Archetypen Jungianischer Psychologie und Körpertherapieformen, wie z.B. systemische Aufstellung, mit dem Ziel, inneren Konflikten, nicht Integriertem und biografisch Unaufgearbeitetem einen Raum der Umwandlung von Ohnmacht zu aktiver Handlungsmacht zu bieten.

Als zentrales Argument ihrer auf fünfjähriger ethnografischer Arbeit basierenden Monografie nennt Inga Scharf da Silva die Bearbeitung von Traumata als Archive von Erinnerungen, wobei sie auf die Vielschichtigkeit individueller und kollektiver Traumata hinweist. Für den brasilianischen Kontext zieht sie eine in verschiedenen interdisziplinären wissenschaftlichen Diskursen oft angeführte Verinnerlichung eines kollektiven Traumas bzgl. der Zerstörung indigenen Lebens und Glaubens sowie der Versklavung afrikanischer Menschen durch die Gewaltherrschaft des Kolonialismus heran. Durch die globale Ausbreitung der *Umbanda* werden diese Inhalte u.a. auch in das deutschsprachige Mitteleuropa transportiert, wobei viele AdeptInnen keine BrasilianerInnen sind, bzw. solche die es waren, oftmals wieder austraten, da sie einen „brasilianischen Rückzugsort" erwarteten (siehe zum vergleichbaren Phänomen des Kardecismus in Deutschland Kurz 2024).

Stattdessen erkennt die Autorin auch im Kontext „teutonischer *Umbanda*" den Versuch einer Auseinandersetzung mit kollektivem Trauma durch eine Spiritualität, die interessanterweise an die genuin afrikanisch generierte Tradition der *orixás* (westafrikanische Gottheiten, die innerhalb der *Umbanda* einen afro-brasilianischen Bezug repräsentieren) anknüpfen, statt historische europäisch-spiritistischen Ansätze zu bedienen. Sie nennt zwei Gründe hierfür: Neben anderen Qualitäten vereinen die westafrikanischen Gottheiten Elemente der Natur in sich, die im deutschsprachigen Kontext hervorgehoben werden und somit eine Rückannäherung an die Umwelt als Reaktion auf ihre zunehmende Zerstörung und Ausbeutung andeuten. Viel tiefgreifender erscheint INGA SCHARF DA SILVA jedoch eine sich abzeichnende geistige Transformation innerhalb europäischer Gesellschaften, die bewusst „fremdes" Wissen annimmt und eine globale Zugehörigkeit imaginiert, um Diskursen und Praktiken eines real erfahrenen (Neo-)Kolonialsimus entgegenzutreten. Zwar könnte man hier durchaus den aktuellen verbreiteten aber fragwürdigen postkolonialen Vorwurf „kultureller Aneignung" heranziehen, doch die Autorin argumentiert ganz im Gegenteil für eine antikoloniale Bewegung, die sich als nonkonforme Gemeinschaft gegen normative Repräsentationen wendet.

Sie geht allerdings noch einen Schritt weiter und erarbeitet am Fallbeispiel eines gemeinsamen Besuchs einer KZ-Gedenkstätte, dass es im hiesigen Kontext auch um Traumata der Weltkriege und deutschen Diktaturen mit inhärenten Erfahrungen von Unterdrückung, Folter, Massenmord und Flucht geht, die auf *Umbanda*-Praktiken projiziert bzw. durch sie reflektiert werden. Zwar erscheinen Opfer historischer und zeitgenössischer diskriminatorischer Regime nicht als eigenständige Geist-Entitäten in der medialen Trance, obwohl die brasilianische *Umbanda* durchaus eine Matrix bzgl. marginalisierter Bevölkerungsgruppen dafür liefern würde (z.B. „Zigeuner", Homosexuelle, Prostituierte, Drogensüchtige etc.). Stattdessen werden aber persönliche, alltägliche Belange in Bezug gesetzt zu einer historischen bzw. überzeitlichen, kollektiven, kulturellen und spirituellen Erinnerungspraxis als Schaffensprozess, der zugunsten einer Implementierung von „Liebe, Güte und Kraft" auf Schuldzuweisungen und die Darstellung von Leid verzichtet:

> Alle Aktivitäten behandelten die Thematik von kollektivem Trauma und der innewohnenden Struktur des Speichergedächtnisses, das über den gemeinsamen Dialog in der Form einer aktiven Erinnerung wieder ins Bewusstsein gerufen werden sollte. In diesem Prozess sind nicht nur die gemeinsam geteilten Wahrnehmungen von Bedeutung gewesen, sondern auch die vielfältigen individuellen Familienerzählungen, denen durch Aufstellungen ein seelischer Raum geöffnet worden ist. Der Ansatz war stets, der seelischen, ‚äußere[n] und inneren Erstarrung aus Grauen und Wahnsinn' [...] zu begegnen (454).

Eine solche „politische Spiritualität" verwandle Negatives durch kritische Betrachtung, (Lebens-)Affirmation und affektive Zugänge in eine positive Erinnerung als Solidarität und Lösung seelischer Erstarrung. Das weitere Beispiel eines Stadtrundgangs „Auf den Spuren des Kolonialsismus" (auch hier bietet sich der Vergleich an mit „Ghost Tours" in DIANA ESPÍRITO SANTO's (2022) „Spirited Histories", rezensiert in dieser Ausgabe) indiziert für die Autorin länderübergreifende Ansätze der postkolonialen Aufarbeitung bzw. eines Katalysators zur Hinterfragung kultureller Selbstverständlichkeiten, welche die europäische Kolonialzeit für abgeschlossen halten. Ziel sei eine „Dekolonialisierung des Geistes", wobei der Begriff des „Kolonialen" natürlich sehr weit gefasst ist und fast gleichsetzbar ist mit europäisch-christlicher (bzw. monotheistischer und damit eine einzige Wahrheit beanspruchender) Überheblichkeit, Gewalt, und Ab-/Ausgrenzung in unterschiedlichen aber vergleichbaren Kontexten. Beispielhaft herangezogen werden aktuelle Flüchtlingstragödien auf dem Mittelmeer, der allgegenwärtige Missbrauch von Macht und die zunehmende Verletzung individueller, ethnischer, oder nationaler Integrität, wo eine klare Trennung von Tätern und Opfern nicht mehr möglich ist. Gemäß dieser Argumentation generiert die *Umbanda* im deutschsprachigen mitteleuropäischen Kontext Schutzräume der Archivierung von Vergessenem und wieder neu Erinnertem als Versuch einer Integration individuell und sozial generierter Leerstellen und unterdrückter Gedanken und Gefühle. In Abgrenzung zu einer westlich dominierten Psychotherapie und ihren Verweisen insbesondere auf die altgriechische Mythologie (veranschaulicht am Beispiel der *Medusa*, vgl. die Rezension zu URSULA WIRTZ' [2018] „Stirb und Werde" in *Curare* 42 (2019) 3+4) setzt INGA SCHARF DA SILVA in ihrer Analyse gesundheitsrelevanter Praktiken innerhalb der *Umbanda* einem passiven Ertragen (metaphorisch als Versteinerung und Immobilisierung) Transformationsprozesse im Sinne einer aktiven Auseinandersetzung und spirituellen Umwandlung historischer Kontinuitäten imperialistischer und rassistischer Ideologien und Praktiken gegenüber. Hinzu kommt, so die Autorin, eine parallele (Re-)Integration des Menschen in durch Kapitalismus und Sozialismus „versaute" Naturkontexte als Strategie einer ganzheitlichen „gesunden" Zukunftsgestaltung.

Als Rezensent der Arbeit einer Kollegin, mit der ich u.a. auch in der gemeinsamen Vorstandsarbeit der Regionalgruppe „Afro-Amerika" innerhalb der DGSKA verbunden bin, möchte ich an dieser Stelle aber auch konstruktive Kritik üben, indem ich eigene Perspektiven auf der Basis langjähriger Auseinandersetzungen mit dem Forschungsgegenstand heranziehe. Ich bewerte den Fokus auf Traumabewältigung (oder einen vielleicht auch nur zu weit gefassten Traumabegriff) bzw. die Hypothese einer Repräsentation des Leidens marginalisierter Menschen kritisch, wie m.E. auch die von der Autorin aufgezeigte Vielschichtigkeit und Diversität der Zugänge zur *Umbanda* nahe legt. Obwohl INGA SCHARF DA SILVA mehrmals ausführt, dass sich die *Umbanda* in einem spiritistischen Kontinuum zwischen *Kardecismus* und *Candomblé* bewegt und Kategorisierungen bzgl. Klasse, Rasse und/oder Geschlecht nicht gerecht wird, zeichnet die Autorin zum einen das Bild einer „weiblichen" Spiritualität (was auch immer das sein mag) und hebt aufgrund ihres ethnografischen Beispiels im deutschsprachigen mitteleuropäischen Kontext afrikanische Teilaspekte hervor. Dies entspricht durchaus einer in populären und wissenschaftlichen existierenden Identifikation als *Yoruba*-Religion, widerspricht (bzw. verwirrt den Rezensenten zunächst) andererseits den detaillierten Darstellungen mehrheitlich brasilianisch-indigener Entitäten für den südamerikanischen Kontext in anderen Kapiteln des Buches. Letztendlich spiegelt aber auch dies die Heterogenität der *Umbanda* wider, und auch im Feld war der Rezensent mehrmals verwirrt aufgrund augenscheinlich widersprüchlicher Aussagen von Forschungspartnern, die diese aber selbst keineswegs als solche wahrnahmen.

Im ethnografischen Beispiel unterstreicht sie nachvollziehbar den Einfluss der afro-brasilianischen Religion *Candomblé* ohne diese jedoch auf eine Praxis der Traumabewältigung reduzieren zu wollen. Sie erlaubt damit auch eine breitere Diskussion, inwiefern afro-brasilianische Religionen generell als eine kritische Auseinandersetzung zu verstehen sind mit dem was ist und was sein könnte/sollte, also einer Widerstandsform gegen Strukturen, die lediglich symbolisch, performativ, bzw. als Metakommentar und Metapher Bezug auf koloniale Wirklichkeiten (und ggf. deren Fortführung) nehmen (vgl. KURZ 2013).

Über die wichtigen wissenschafts-theoretischen Interpretationen hinaus bleibt aber eine der vielen Stärken dieser Arbeit die detaillierte und facettenreiche Darstellung der *Umbanda* als transkulturelles Phänomen verschiedener afrikanischer, indigener und europäischer Aspekte, die in ihrer „sakralen Globalisierung", innerhalb ihrer Netzwerke translokalen Widerstand als Graswurzelbewegung „von unten" generiert und insbesondere aktuelle Migrationskontexte thematisiert. Hier zeigt sich eine metaphorische und praktische Integrationsfähigkeit, die sich gegen soziale (und spirituelle) Ausgrenzungen des „Fremden" zur Wehr setzt – nicht in Form eines politischen Aktivismus, sondern in der Hinwendung zu spirituellen Lösungsansätzen. Entsprechend stellen sich Räume der *Umbanda* (sowohl in Brasilien, als auch im deutschsprachigen Europa) als Refugium der Entschleunigung dar, wo individuelle Krankheiten, Leiden oder Schicksalsschläge als Auslöser für Hinwendung, Sinngebung, Ganzheitlichkeit, Gemeinschaft und Integrationsfähigkeit fungieren können. Es erscheint daher auch nicht überraschend, dass viele Mitglieder Angehörige lokaler Gesundheitsansätze sind, beispielsweise als VertreterInnen „psychologischen coachings" und von Naturtherapien.

INGA SCHARF DA SILVA liefert eine umfangreiche Darstellung zeitgenössischer *Umbanda*-Forschung inklusive detaillierter Beschreibungen kosmologischer, praktischer und sozialer Kontexte, die sie als Multi-Sited Ethnography mit autoethnografischen und -biografischen Aspekten (inkl. persönlicher Bezüge der SchwerHörigkeit/Behinderung) anreichert. Ihr Ansatz eines kollaborativen Forschens, die Einbindung persönlicher Vignetten sowie die Einflechtung von literarisch-künstlerischen Formaten liefert ein umfangreiches und gleichzeitig fragmentiertes emisches und etisches Wissensarchiv, das dem Forschungsgegenstand in seiner Diversität gerecht wird. Wie die Autorin selbst eingangs klarstellt, beschreibet sie einen Grenzweg zwischen Religion, Wissenschaft und Kunst, und ihre multiplen Zugänge entsprechen der Vielschichtigkeit des Felds: wissenschaftlich, intellektuell, persönlich, emotional, und körperlich sowie interdisziplinär zwischen klassischer und europäischer Ethnologie, Religionswissenschaft und Theologie, Psychologie und Philosophie. Es ist ein Meilenstein deutschsprachiger Brasilienforschung mit so vielen unterschiedlichen aber verwobenen Aspekten wie Geschichte, Religion, Medizin, Migration, und Translokalität. Wie auch schon eine frühere Arbeit (SCHARF DA SILVA 2004) wird es über den wissenschaftlichen Stellenwert hinaus wohl auch ein Standardwerk für nichtwissenschaftliche Interessenten an der Religion der *Umbanda* werden, wobei der persönlich-emische Ansatz der Autorin als solcher identifizierbar bleibt und von Generalisierungen absieht.

HELMAR KURZ, Münster

Referenzen

ESPÍRITO SANTO, DIANA 2022. *Spirited Histories. Technologies, Media, and Trauma in Paranormal Chile*. London: Routledge.

KURZ, HELMAR 2013. *Performanz und Modernität im Brasilianischen Candomblé. Eine Interpretation*. Hamburg: Kovač.

--- 2024. Spiritism in Germany. A Resource of Integration for Brazilian Migrants? *JLAR*. DOI: https://doi.org/10.1007/s41603-024-00233-0 (Open Access).

SCHARF DA SILVA, INGA 2004. *Umbanda: Eine Religion zwischen Candomblé und Kardecismus. Über Synkretismus im städtischen Alltag Brasiliens*. Münster: LIT.

WIRTZ, URSULA 2018. *Stirb und Werde. Die Wandlungskraft Traumatischer Erfahrungen*. Ostfildern: Patmos.

ZUSAMMENFASSUNGEN
ABSTRACTS
RÉSUMÉS

Zusammenfassungen der Beiträge der *Curare* 46 (2023) 2
Ambivalenzen von Heilungskooperationen in biomedizinischen Settings

HERAUSGEGEBEN VON CORNELIUS SCHUBERT & EHLER VOSS

ANNA HÄNNI: Die stationäre Psychiatrie als Ort der Ambiguitäten. Therapeutische Begegnungen aus sensorischer und verkörperter Perspektive   S. 11–26, verfasst auf Englisch

Im sozialanthropologischen Kanon gibt es nur wenige Forschungen, welche die sensorischen und zwischenmenschlichen Aspekte von stationären psychiatrischen Kliniken beleuchten. Ausgehend von Vignetten aus meiner ethnographischen Feldforschung in zwei psychiatrischen Kliniken in der Schweiz werden zwei Forschungsinteressen dargelegt und miteinander in Dialog gebracht. Einerseits analysiere ich die therapeutischen Interaktionen und Praktiken in der Klinik aus der Perspektive der sensory ethnography und verkörperter Wahrnehmung. Andererseits zeigt sich anhand der Daten, dass es innerhalb der Klinik verschiedenste „Kulturen des Therapeutischen" gibt, die parallel nebeneinander existieren – teils mit divergierenden Zielsetzungen und Grundannahmen über Psychopathologie und Heilung. Daraus geht eine Vielzahl zwischenmenschlicher Beziehungsmöglichkeiten hervor, von welchen viele durch Ambivalenz gekennzeichnet sind. Was als „therapeutisch" erfahren wird und was, im Gegenzug, als eine Bedrohung der menschlichen Integrität und Gesundheit erscheint, kann nahe beieinander liegen und individuell variieren. Ich diskutiere, wie eng Erfahrungen der Ambivalenz – sei es unter Patient:innen oder Mitarbeitenden – mit Räumlichkeit, verkörperter Erfahrung und Zeitlichkeit verknüpft sind. Anhand der sensory ethnography und Harmut Rosas Konzept der Resonanz wird deutlich, dass im stationären psychiatrischen Setting Zwischenmenschlichkeit untrennbar mit dem Nichtmenschlichen verwoben ist.

Schlagwörter   Sensorische Ethnographie – Psychatrie – Medizinethnologie – Phänomenologie – Therapie

NICOLE ERNSTMANN, SOPHIE ELISABETH GROSS, UTE KARBACH, LENA ANSMANN, ANDRÉ KARGER, HOLGER PFAFF, MARKUS WIRTZ, WALTER BAUMANN & MELANIE NEUMANN: Patienten-Arzt-Beziehung in der Krebsbehandlung. Relevanz und Ambivalenzen aus der Sicht von Onkologen   S. 27–41, verfasst auf Englisch

Eine Hauptfunktion der Kommunikation zwischen Patient*innen und Ärzt*innen besteht darin, eine vertrauensvolle Beziehung und eine therapeutische Allianz aufzubauen. Der Aufbau vertrauensvoller Beziehungen ist jedoch mit Ambivalenzen behaftet. Es gibt Rollenerwartungen, wie die Erwartung der affektiven Neutralität, die im Gegensatz zu dieser Funktion stehen. Darüber hinaus wird die Umsetzung im Versorgungsalltag durch Zeitmangel oder fehlende Unterstützung erschwert. Zusätzlich kann der Aufbau einer vertrauensvollen Beziehung eine persönliche Herausforderung darstellen. Diese qualitative Studie, basierend auf semi-strukturierten Interviews mit Onkolog*innen, wurde durchgeführt, um deren Wahrnehmungen und Erfahrungen hinsichtlich der Relevanz vertrauensvoller Beziehungen zu ihren Patient*innen sowie mögliche Ambivalenzen zu explorieren. Die Ergebnisse zeigen, dass eine vertrauensvolle Arzt-Patient-Beziehung für Onkolog*innen eine wichtige Voraussetzung für eine erfolgreiche Krebsbehandlung darstellt. Dies betrifft die Bereiche offene Kommunikation, Anpassung der Behandlung an die Patientenbedürfnisse, Adhärenz, Kontrolle von Nebenwirkungen, Aktivierung der Patientenressourcen, Vertrauen in die Behandlung, Reduktion von Ängsten, Berücksichtigung der Bedürfnisse von Angehörigen sowie die Krankheitsbewältigung. Die Unterstützung von Patient*innen mit fortgeschrittenen Erkankungsstadien wird sowohl als bereichernd wie auch als belastend erlebt. Von Patient*innen abgelehnt zu werden, wenn die Therapie nicht anschlägt, wurde von einigen Onkolog*innen als schmerzhaft empfunden. Es besteht somit ein Bedarf an Unterstützung für Onkolog*innen, um vertrauensvolle Arzt-Patient-Beziehungen aufzubauen und aufrechtzuerhalten. Diese Unterstützung muss die Kontextfaktoren, die Kommunikationsfähigkeiten und die Haltung berücksichtigen, die erforderlich sind, um der persönlichen Herausforderung des Aufbaus vertrauensvoller Arzt-Patienten-Beziehungen zu begegnen. Sie sollte auch eine geschützte Umgebung bieten, um über die eigenen Ängste und Herausforderungen im Aufbau von Beziehungen zu Patient*innen zu reflektieren.

Keywords Vertrauen – Beziehung – therapeutische Allianz, Onkologie – Ambivalenzen

NICK J. FOX: Digitale Heilung? Digitaler Kapitalismus? Neoliberalismus, digitale Gesundheitstechnologien und „Bürgergesundheit" S. 45–55, verfasst auf Englisch

Das Aufkommen digitaler Gesundheits- und Krankheitstechnologien und die Digitalisierung der kapitalistischen Wirtschaftsproduktion spiegeln die zunehmende Cyborgisierung der organischen Materie in aktuellen wirtschaftlichen und sozialen Beziehungen wider. In meinem Aufsatz nähere ich mich „digitaler Gesundheit" mit einem materialistischen und posthumanistischen Ansatz, um die mikropolitischen Auswirkungen von digitalen Technologien und Apps im Kontext zeitgenössischer sozialer Beziehungen und der Entstehung des digitalen Kapitalismus zu erforschen. Dies ermöglicht neue Einblicke in die Auswirkungen des Digitalen auf die Produktion des Sozialen und macht den Beitrag menschlicher und nicht-menschlicher Materie sowohl zur digitalen Gesundheit als auch zur umfassenderen Ökonomie und Politik der neoliberalen Gesundheitsversorgung verständlich. In meinem Aufsatz analysiere ich vier digitale Gesundheitstechnologien, um zu untersuchen, welche Kapazitäten sie in Körpern erzeugen und welche mikropolitischen Auswirkungen die Technologie in Bezug auf Macht, Widerstand und soziale Ordnung hat. Anschließend gehe ich der Frage nach, wie diese Mikropolitik durch die Umgestaltung des Kontextes oder anderer Kräfte verändert werden könnte, und lege dar, dass dies Wege für den Einsatz digitaler Technologien zur Förderung radikaler und transgressiver Möglichkeiten eröffnet, indem die Wechselwirkungen zwischen Technologien und anderen materiellen Gegebenheiten neu gestaltet werden. Abschließend erörtere ich den „digitalen Aktivismus". Ich untersuche, wie Technologien und Apps entwickelt werden können, um Daten zu demokratisieren: um kollektive Reaktionen auf Gesundheitsprobleme zu ermöglichen, um die Gesundheitspolitik in Frage zu stellen und um sich gegen Gesundheitskonzerne, Umweltverschmutzer und Anbieter von Fast Food und Fertiggerichten zu organisieren. Dieses kollektive buttom-up-Modell der „Bürgergesundheit" (RIMAL et al. 1997) wirkt sowohl der Vermarktung der Gesundheit als auch dem Paternalismus der Gesundheitsversorgung entgegen.

Schlagwörter Kapitalismus – Bürgergesundheit – Digitale Gesundheit – Mikropolitik – Neuer Materialismus

MÁRCIO VILAR: Über den Tellerrand fühlen: Ambivalenzen unerwarteter Besserung bei erkrankten medizinischen Fachleuten durch verlagerte Kooperationen in Brasilien pp. 55–73, verfasst auf Englisch

Wie fühlen sich Menschen mit diagnostizierten Autoimmunerkrankungen und was tun und denken sie, wenn sie unerwartet auf ein unangemeldetes Medikament stoßen, das ihnen helfen könnte, zu heilen, anstatt die Symptome von Autoimmunreaktionen mit konventionellen Immunsuppressiva palliativ zu kontrollieren? Und wie sieht es aus, wenn sie medizinische Fachleute sind, die selbst zu Patienten wurden? Wie beeinflusst eine solche Begegnung ihr Leben, ihre Wahrnehmungen und ihr Tun in Bezug auf ihre jeweilige medizinrechtliche Umgebung? In diesem Artikel analysiere ich Briefe, die ein brasilianischer Arzt und acht seiner Patienten/innen, die ebenfalls medizinische Fachleute sind, hauptsächlich zwischen 1997 und 2000 austauschten. Darin geht es um ihre Erfahrungen mit der Anwendung eines unangemeldeten Medikaments, dem „anti-brucella Vakzin" (VAB), zur Behandlung verschiedener Immunpathologien wie rheumatoider Arthritis. Angenommen, dass VAB-Nutzer/innen in der Lage sind, ihre Krankheits- und Genesungserfahrungen systematisch zu evaluieren und zu kommunizieren, möchte ich die Spannungen bezüglich der Neupositionierung und Haltung betroffener Gesundheitsfachkräfte im Kontext von bahnbrechender biotechnologischen Innovation in Brasilien verstehen und diskutieren. Scheinbar ermöglichen Ihre eigenen Erfahrungen mit VAB ihnen, ihre medizinische Kenntnis und Fähigkeiten im Hinblick auf ihre eigene und die Gesundheit anderer Betroffenen in Antizipation der Mediation, die das konventionelle medizinische Wissen und die entsprechenden Technologien und Verfahren i.d.R. leisten, umzulegen. Außerdem schienen VAB-nutzende Ärzte/innen durch Selbstanalyse und Dialog mit anderen, das Verfassen und Austauschen von Evaluationsberichten über ihre eigene und die Gesundheit anderer sowie ihre therapeutischen Erfahrungen mit VAB medizinische Evidenz implizit zu koproduzieren, die von potenziellen Nutzern/innen berücksichtigt werden kann.

Keywords Immuntherapien – versetzende Kooperationen – therapeutische Narrative – Evidenzproduktion – Brasilien

GIORGIO BROCCO: Verwobene Epistemologien: Eine fragmentarische Untersuchung der post- und dekolonialen Perspektiven in der medizinischen Anthropologie   S. 77–97, verfasst auf Englisch

In den letzten vier Jahrzehnten haben post- und dekoloniale Ideen an Bedeutung gewonnen, indem einflussreiche Werke renommierter Gelehrter und Intellektueller in den Geistes- und Sozialwissenschaften verbreitet wurden. Wegweisende Stimmen wie Franz Fanon, Valentin-Yves Mudimbe und Edward Said sowie Wissenschaftler*innen wie Gayatri Spivak und Verfechterinnen des schwarzen Feminismus wie Sylvia Wynter und Françoise Vergès haben zur Gestaltung dieses Bereichs beigetragen. Die medizinische Anthropologie, die kritische medizinische Anthropologie und andere verwandte Disziplinen innerhalb des breiten Feldes der „Medical/Health Humanities" haben sich aktiv mit diesen kritischen theoretischen Impulsen auseinandergesetzt und epistemologische und methodologische Ansätze verfeinert, die mit post- und dekolonialen Analysen übereinstimmen. Dieser Artikel untersucht die Schnittstellen post- und dekolonialer Perspektiven mit aktuellen anthropologischen Fragestellungen und lenkt die Aufmerksamkeit auf die vielfältigen Forschungswege, die aus solchen Verflechtungen hervorgegangen sind. Insbesondere befasst sich der Artikel mit drei zentralen Forschungsbereichen: (1) der Untersuchung des Einflusses von Ideen über post- und dekoloniale Subjektivitäten in Verbindung mit sich verändernden Vorstellungen von Gesundheit, Krankheit und Behinderung; (2) der kritischen Analyse humanitärer und globaler Gesundheitsinterventionen; und (3) der Erforschung indigener Systeme der Pflege und Heilpraktiken aus dem globalen Süden. Während der fragmentierte, partielle, situierte und selektive Charakter der Auswahl wissenschaftlicher Quellen für diese Diskussion anerkannt wird, zielt der Artikel darauf ab, die dynamischen Wechselwirkungen zwischen post- und dekolonialen Theorien und den vielfältigen und komplexen Landschaften der medizinischen Anthropologie zu beleuchten.

Schlagwörter Dekoloniale Theorie – Medizinanthropologie – Behindertenanthropologie – Subjektivität – Indigenität

ANAHI SY: Erfahrungen des Gesundheitspersonals während der COVID-19-Pandemie in Argentinien. Ein syndemischer Ansatz für Krankenhäuser   S. 101–113, verfasst auf Englisch

Die SARS-CoV-2-Pandemie hat gezeigt, dass es notwendig ist, in syndemischen Begriffen zu denken, da alle Gesundheitsprobleme mit ökologischen, sozialen, wirtschaftlichen und politischen Faktoren zusammenhängen, die Epidemie beeinflussen. In dieser Arbeit schlagen wir das Konzept der „Syndemie" vor, um die Ereignisse in den öffentlichen Krankenhäusern Argentiniens aus einer sozio-epidemiologischen Perspektive zu analysieren. Methodisch wurden halbstrukturierte Interviews mit Arbeitnehmer*innen in zwei Phasen durchgeführt: zu Beginn der Pandemie in Argentinien, über WhatsApp und über virtuelle Meeting-Plattformen. Anhand der Inhaltsanalyse der Erzählungen lässt sich feststellen, dass das Gesundheitspersonal in vielen Situationen die Architekten von Problemlösungsstrategien sind, die während der Pandemie zum Ausdruck kamen: Bewältigung von Engpässen (z. B. bei den Vorräten) und Ausführung von Pflegediensten – selbst unter Gefährdung der eigenen Gesundheit. Auch deliberative Räume des „Dialogs" unter den Arbeitnehmer*innen (Sitzungen, Krisenausschüsse, Gewerkschaftsaktivitäten) – als Umgebungen der Unterstützung, Pflege und/oder Selbstpflege während der Pandemie – werden sichtbar. In diesen Räumen müssen einige Herausforderungen, mit denen der Gesundheitssektor konfrontiert ist, syndemisch betrachtet werden. Wir schließen mit einer Analyse des Potenzials der Anwendung des Konzepts der Syndemie auf Probleme der öffentlichen Gesundheit und der Politik in Krankenhauseinrichtungen aus einer sozio-epidemiologischen Perspektive, wobei wir den Transformationsprozess des Personals zur Bewältigung von Notfallsituationen in den Mittelpunkt rücken. Diese Dimensionen sind von entscheidender Bedeutung für die Entwicklung von Gesundheitspolitiken im Einklang mit anderen Prozessen des sozio-epidemiologischen Wandels, die sowohl in Krankenhäusern als auch in der die öffentlichen Gesundheitsdienste in Anspruch nehmende Bevölkerung stattfinden.

Schlagwörter Krankenhaus – Syndemie – COVID-19-Pandemie – Beschäftigte im Gesundheitswesen – Sozioepidemiologie

Article Abstracts of *Curare* 46 (2023) 2

Ambivalences of Healing Cooperations in Biomedical Settings

EDITED BY CORNELIUS SCHUBERT & EHLER VOSS

ANNA HÄNNI: In-Patient Psychiatric Care as a Space of Ambiguity. Therapeutic Encounters From a Sensory and Embodied Perspective   pp. 11–26, written in English

In social anthropology, there exists only little research about the sensory and intersubjective aspects of in-patient psychiatric care. Proceeding from vignettes from ethnographic fieldwork in two psychiatric clinics in Switzerland, this article outlines two empirical research interests and puts them into dialogue. On one side, therapeutic interactions and practices within the clinical setting are analyzed through the lenses of sensory ethnography and embodiment. On the other side, a multiplicity of "therapeutic cultures" and spaces co-exist within clinical premises. In some cases, they encompass diverging or even conflicting aims and basic assumptions about psychopathology and healing. As a result, various possibilities of human sociality and interaction open up to psychiatric sufferers, many of them characterized by ambivalence. What is being perceived as "therapeutic" and what, to the contrary, as a threat to human integrity and health can lie close together and can vary individually. I discuss how closely experiences of ambivalence – be it among psychiatric sufferers or staff members – are related to spatiality, embodied perception and to temporality. Referring to sensory ethnography and Hartmut Rosa's writing on resonance, I argue that, in in-patient psychiatric settings, the human social is inextricably intertwined with the nonhuman.

Keywords sensory ethnography – psychiatry – medical anthropology – phenomenology – therapy

NICOLE ERNSTMANN, SOPHIE ELISABETH GROSS, UTE KARBACH, LENA ANSMANN, ANDRÉ KARGER, HOLGER PFAFF, MARKUS WIRTZ, WALTER BAUMANN & MELANIE NEUMANN: Patient-Physician-Relationship in Cancer Care. Relevance and Ambivalences as Perceived by Oncologists   pp. 27–41, written in English

A major function of patient-physician-communication is building a trustful relationship and a therapeutic alliance between patient and physician. However, building trustful relationships to patients is subject to ambivalences. There are role expectations including affective neutrality, that stand in contrast to this function. Moreover, translation into every day routine is constricted by lack of time or lack of tools, and building a trustful relationship with the patient is a personal challenge. This qualitative study based on semi-structured interviews with oncologists was conducted to explore oncologists' perceptions and experiences of the relevance of trusting relationships to their patients and to examine sources of ambivalences. The results show that a trusting patient-physician-relationship is for oncologists an important prerequisite for successful cancer treatment in terms of open communication, adjustment of treatment to patients' needs, compliance, control of adverse events, activation of patient's resources, patients' treatment confidence, reduction of patients' anxiety, meeting family and caregiver needs and patients' coping efforts. Supporting critically ill patients can be both enriching and stressful. Being rejected by patients in case the therapy does not work was experienced as painful by some oncologists. There is a need for support for oncologists to establish trustful patient-physician-relationships during their patients' cancer journey. The support will have to address contextual factors, communication skills and the attitude needed to face the personal challenge of building trustful patient-physician-relationships. It should provide a protective environment to reflect on one's own fears and challenges in building relationships with patients.

Keywords trust – relationship – therapeutic alliance – oncology – ambivalences

NICK J. FOX: Digital Healing? Digital Capitalism? Neoliberalism, Digital Health Technologies, and Citizen Health   pp. 43–53, written in English

The emergence of digital health and illness technologies and the digitisation of capitalist economic production reflect the increasing cyborgisation of organic matter within current economic and social relations. In this paper I employ a materialist and posthuman approach to 'digital health', investigating micropolitically what digital technologies and apps actually do, within the contexts of contemporary social relations and the emergence of digital capitalism. This enables new insights into the impacts of the digital upon social production, making sense of the contribution of both human and non-human matter both to digital health and to the wider economics and politics of neoliberal health care. The paper evaluates four digital health technologies to consider what capacities they produce in bodies and the micropolitical impact of the technology in terms of power, resistance and social order. I then consider how these micropolitics might be changed by altering the contexts or other forces, and argue that this opens up ways for digital technologies to be used to promote radical and transgressive possibilities, by re-engineering the interactions between technologies and other materialities. I conclude by discussing 'digital activism'. I examine how technologies and apps may be engineered to democratise data: to enable collective responses to health issues, to challenge health policy and to organise against health corporations, environmental polluters, and purveyors of fast and processed foods. This collective, bottom-up model of 'citizen health' (RIMAL et al. 1997) counters both the marketisation of health and the paternalism of health care.

Keywords capitalism – citizen health – digital health – micropolitics – new materialism

MÁRCIO VILAR: Feeling out of the Box. Ambivalences of Unexpected Amelioration among Sickened Health Professionals through Displacing Cooperations in Brazil   pp. 55–73, written in English

How do people with diagnosed autoimmune diseases feel, and what they do and think when they unexpectedly encounter an unregistered drug that may help them to heal, instead of palliatively controlling symptoms of autoimmune reactions through conventional immunosuppressants? What then if they are health professionals who became patients? How does such an encounter affect their lives, their perceptions and attitudes towards their respective medico-legal environments? In this article, I analyse letters exchanged between a physician in Brazil and eight of his patients, who are also health professionals, mainly between 1997 and 2000, concerning their experiencing of using an unregistered medicine, the "anti-brucellic vaccine" (VAB), to treat different immunopathologies such as rheumatoid arthritis. Considering VAB users as capable of systematically evaluating and communicating their experiences of illness and recovery, I seek to understand and discuss the tensions surrounding the repositionings and attitudes of affected health professionals within the co-production of medical evidence in the context of disruptive biotechnological innovation in Brazil. Apparently, their own experience with VAB seemed to have enabled them to reground their medical knowledge and skills in relation to their own and someone else's health in anticipation of the mediation regularly played out by conventional medical knowledge, technologies and procedures. Furthermore, when VAB-using physicians self-analyse and dialogue with others, writing and exchanging evaluative reports about their own and others' health and therapeutic experiences of using VAB, they seemed to implicitly co-produce medical evidence that can be taken into consideration by potential users.

Keywords immunotherapies – displacing cooperation – therapeutic narratives – evidence making – Brazil

ARTICLE ABSTRACTS

GIORGIO BROCCO: Connected Epistemologies. A Fragmented Review of Post- and Decolonial Perspectives in Medical Anthropology pp. 77–97, written in English

Over the last four decades, post- and decolonial ideas have gained prominence through the dissemination of influential works by renowned scholars and intellectuals in the humanities and social sciences. Pioneering voices such as Franz Fanon, Valentin-Yves Mudimbe, and Edward Said, along with scholars like Gayatri Spivak and advocates of Black feminism such as Sylvia Wynter and Françoise Vergès, have contributed to shaping this realm. Medical anthropology, critical medical anthropology and other related disciplines within the broad field of "medical/health humanities" have actively engaged with these critical theoretical impulses, refining epistemological and methodological approaches that align with post- and decolonial analyses. This article explores the intersections of post- and decolonial perspectives with current anthropological agenda, drawing attention to the manifold research avenues that have emerged from such entanglements. Specifically, the paper delves into three key research areas: (1) the examination of the influence of ideas about post- and decolonial subjectivities in connection to changing notions of health, disease, and disability; (2) the critical analysis of humanitarian and global health interventions; and (3) the exploration of indigenous systems of care and healing practices from the Global South. While acknowledging the fragmented, partial, situated and selective nature of the selection of scholarly sources for this discussion, the article aims to shed light on the dynamic interplays between post- and decolonial theories and the multifold and complex medical anthropology landscapes.

Keywords decolonial theory – medical anthropology – disability anthropology – subjectivity – indigeneity

ANAHI SY: Healthcare Workers' Experiences during the COVID-19 Pandemic in Argentina. A Syndemic Approach to Hospitals pp. 99–111, written in English

The SARS-CoV-2 pandemic put into evidence the need to think in syndemic terms, as all health issues co-exists with environmental, social, economic and political factors that exacerbate any epidemic. In this work we propose the concept of "syndemic" to analyze what happened in public hospitals of Argentina, from a socio-epidemiological perspective. In methodological terms, semi-structured interviews with workers were carried out in two stages: at the start of the pandemic in Argentina, via WhatsApp and through virtual meeting platforms. The content analysis of the narratives makes it possible to identify how health workers, in many situations, are the architects of problem-solving strategies that emerge during the pandemic: managing shortages (of supplies, for example) and providing care – even at risk to their own health. We also identified deliberative spaces of "dialogue-work" among workers (meetings, crisis committees, union activities), recognized as environments of support, care and/or self-care during the pandemic. In these spaces some challenges facing the health sector must be seen syndemically. We conclude by analyzing the potential of applying the concept of syndemic to public health problems and policies in hospital institutions from a socio-epidemiological perspective, highlighting the transformative process of workers to attend to emergency situations. These dimensions are crucial in developing health policies in synch with other processes of socio-epidemiological change, which occur both within hospitals and within the population that uses public health services.

Keywords hospital - syndemic – COVID-19 pandemic – healthcare workers – socio-epidemiology

Résumés des articles de *Curare* 46 (2023) 2

Ambivalences des coopérations de guérison en milieu biomédical

SOUS LA DIRECTION DE CORNELIUS SCHUBERT & EHLER VOSS

ANNA HÄNNI: Les soins psychiatriques stationnaires en tant qu'espace d'ambiguïté. Les rencontres thérapeutiques d'un point de vue sensoriel et incarné   p. 11–26, rédigé en anglais

En anthropologie sociale, il n'existe qu'un nombre limité de recherches sur les aspects sensoriels et intersubjectif des soins psychiatriques en milieu hospitalier. A partir de vignettes issues d'un travail de terrain ethnographique dans deux cliniques psychiatriques en Suisse, cet article présente deux intérêts empiriques de la recherche et les met en dialogue. D'une part, les interactions et les pratiques thérapeutiques dans le cadre clinique sont analysées à travers le prisme de l'ethnographie sensorielle et de l'incarnation. D'autre part, il apparaît clairement qu'une multiplicité de «cultures thérapeutiques» et d'espaces coexistent dans les locaux cliniques. Dans certains cas, ils englobent des objectifs divergents, voire contradictoires, et des hypothèses de base sur la psychopathologie et la guérison. En conséquence, les patients ont accès à un vaste éventail de relations et d'interactions humaines, dont beaucoup sont caractérisées par l'ambivalence. Ce qui est perçu comme «thérapeutique» et ce qui, au contraire, est perçu comme une menace pour l'intégrité et la santé humaines peuvent être proches l'un de l'autre et varier individuellement. Je discute de la façon dont les expériences d'ambivalence - que ce soit parmi les patients ou les membres du personnel - sont étroitement liées à la spatialité, à la perception incarnée et à la temporalité. En me référant à l'ethnographie sensorielle et aux écrits de Hartmut Rosa sur la résonance, je soutiens que dans les établissements psychiatriques hospitaliers, le social humain est inextricablement mêlé au non-humain.

Mots-clés   ethnographie sensorielle – psychiatrie – anthropologie médicale – phénoménologie – thérapie

NICOLE ERNSTMANN, SOPHIE ELISABETH GROSS, UTE KARBACH, LENA ANSMANN, ANDRÉ KARGER, HOLGER PFAFF, MARKUS WIRTZ, WALTER BAUMANN & MELANIE NEUMANN: La relation patient-médecin dans les soins oncologiques. Pertinence et ambivalences telles qu'elles sont perçues par les oncologues   p. 27–41, rédigé en anglais

Une fonction majeure de la communication patient-médecin est de construire une relation de confiance et une alliance thérapeutique entre le patient et le médecin. Cependant, établir des relations de confiance avec les patients est soumis à des ambivalences. Il existe des attentes de rôle, telles que l'attente de neutralité affective, qui sont en contraste avec cette fonction. De plus, la traduction en routine quotidienne est limitée par le manque de temps ou d'outils, et établir une relation de confiance avec le patient est un défi personnel. Cette étude qualitative, basée sur des entretiens semi-structurés avec des oncologues, a été menée pour explorer les perceptions et les expériences des oncologues sur la pertinence des relations de confiance avec leurs patients et pour examiner les sources d'ambivalences. Les résultats montrent qu'une relation de confiance patient-médecin est pour les oncologues une condition préalable importante au succès du traitement du cancer en termes de communication ouverte, d'adaptation du traitement aux besoins des patients, de compliance, de contrôle des effets indésirables, d'activation des ressources du patient, de confiance des patients dans le traitement, de réduction de l'anxiété des patients, de réponse aux besoins des familles et des soignants et des efforts de coping des patients. Soutenir les patients gravement malades peut être à la fois enrichissant et stressant. Être rejeté par les patients lorsque la thérapie ne fonctionne pas a été vécu comme douloureux par certains oncologues. Il est nécessaire de soutenir les oncologues pour établir et maintenir des relations de confiance avec leurs patients. Le soutien devra aborder les facteurs contextuels, les compétences en communication et l'attitude nécessaire pour faire face au défi personnel de construire des relations de confiance patient-médecin. Il devrait fournir un environnement protecteur pour réfléchir à ses propres peurs et défis dans la construction des relations avec les patients.

Mots-clés confiance - relation – alliance thérapeutique –oncologie – ambivalence

NICK J. FOX: Guérison numérique ? Capitalisme numérique? Néolibéralisme, technologies numériques de la santé et «santé citoyenne»   p. 43–53, rédigé en anglais

L'émergence des technologies numériques de santé et de maladie et la numérisation de la production économique capitaliste reflètent la cyborgisation croissante de la matière organique dans les relations économiques et sociales actuelles. Dans cet article, j'adopte une approche matérialiste et posthumaine de la « santé numérique » et j'étudie de manière micropolitiquement ce que les technologies numériques et les applications font réellement dans le contexte des relations sociales contemporaines et de l'émergence du capitalisme numérique. Cela permet d'apporter un nouvel éclairage sur les impacts du numérique sur la production sociale, en donnant un sens à la contribution de la matière humaine et non humaine à la santé numérique et à l'économie et la politique plus larges des soins de santé néolibéraux. Cet article évalue quatre technologies de santé numérique afin d'examiner les capacités qu'elles produisent dans les corps et l'impact micropolitique de la technologie en termes de pouvoir, de résistance et d'ordre social. J'examine ensuite comment ces micropolitique pourraient être modifiées en changeant les contextes ou d'autres forces, et je soutiens que cela ouvre la voie à l'utilisation des technologies numériques pour promouvoir des possibilités radicales et transgressives, en réorganisant les interactions entre les technologies et d'autres matérialités. Je conclus en discutant de l'« activisme numérique ». J'examine comment les technologies et les applications peuvent être conçues pour démocratiser les données : pour permettre des réponses collectives aux questions de santé, pour remettre en question les politiques de santé et pour s'organiser contre les entreprises de santé, les pollueurs environnementaux et les fournisseurs d'aliments rapides et transformés. Ce modèle collectif et ascendant de « santé citoyenne » (RIMAL et al., 1997) s'oppose à la fois à la marchandisation de la santé et au paternalisme des soins de santé.

Mots-clés capitalisme – santé citoyenne – santé numérique – micropolitique – nouveau matérialisme

MÁRCIO VILAR: Se sentir hors de la boîte : Ambivalences d'une amélioration inattendue chez des professionnels de santé malades suite à des coopérations délocalisées au Brésil   p. 55–73, rédigé en anglais

Que ressentent les personnes atteintes de maladies auto-immunes diagnostiquées, que font-elles et que pensent-elles lorsqu'elles découvrent de manière inattendue un médicament non homologué susceptible de les aider à guérir, au lieu de contrôler des symptômes de réactions auto-immunes par des immunosuppresseurs conventionnels du traitement palliatif ? Qu'en est-il alors s'il s'agit de professionnels de santé devenus patients ? Comment une telle rencontre affecte-t-elle leur vie, leurs perceptions et leurs attitudes envers leurs environnements médico-légaux respectifs ? Dans cet article, j'analyse des lettres échangées entre un médecin brésilien et huit de ses patients, également professionnels de santé, principalement entre 1997 et 2000, concernant leur expérience de l'utilisation d'un médicament non homologué, le « vaccin anti-brucellique » (VAB), pour traiter différentes immunopathologies telles que la polyarthrite rhumatoïde. Considérant les utilisateurs de VAB comme capables d'évaluer et de communiquer systématiquement leurs expériences de maladie et de rétablissement, je cherche à comprendre et à discuter des tensions entourant les repositionnements et les attitudes des professionnels de santé concernés dans le cadre de la coproduction de preuves médicales dans le contexte d'innovations biotechnologiques disruptives au Brésil. Apparemment, leur propre expérience avec VAB semble leur avoir permis de réorienter leurs connaissances, leur expérience et leurs compétences médicales en lien avec leur propre santé et celle d'autrui, en anticipant la médiation régulièrement exercée par les connaissances, les technologies et les procédures médicales conventionnelles. De plus, lorsque les médecins utilisateurs de VAB s'auto-analysent et dialoguent avec d'autres, rédigeant et échangeant des rapports d'évaluation sur leur propre santé et celles d'autrui, ainsi que sur leurs expériences thérapeutiques liées à l'utilisation de VAB, ils semblent coproduire implicitement des preuves médicales pouvant être prises en compte par les utilisateurs potentiels.

Mots-clés Immunothérapies – coopérations que déplace – thérapeutique narratives – production de évidences – Brésil

Giorgio Brocco: Épistémologies enchevêtrées. Un examen fragmentaire des perspectives post et décoloniales en anthropologie médicale   p. 77–97, rédigé en anglais

Au cours des quatre dernières décennies, les idées postcoloniales et décoloniales ont gagné en importance grâce à la diffusion des travaux influents de chercheurs et d'intellectuels renommés dans les sciences humaines et sociales. Des voix pionnières telles que Franz Fanon, Valentin-Yves Mudimbe et Edward Said, ainsi que des chercheurs comme Gayatri Spivak et des défenseurs du féminisme noir tels que Sylvia Wynter et Françoise Vergès, ont contribué à façonner ce domaine. L'anthropologie médicale, l'anthropologie médicale critique et d'autres disciplines connexes dans le vaste domaine des « sciences humaines médicales/sanitaires » se sont activement engagées avec ces impulsions théoriques critiques, affinant des approches épistémologiques et méthodologiques qui s'alignent sur les analyses postcoloniales et décoloniales. Cet article explore les intersections des perspectives postcoloniales et décoloniales avec les programmes anthropologiques actuels, attirant l'attention sur les multiples voies de recherche qui ont émergé de ces enchevêtrements. Plus précisément, l'article se penche sur trois domaines de recherche clés : (1) l'examen de l'influence des idées sur les subjectivités postcoloniales et décoloniales, en lien avec les notions changeantes de santé, de maladie et de handicap ; (2) l'analyse critique des interventions humanitaires et de santé mondiale ; et (3) l'exploration des systèmes de soins et des pratiques de guérison indigènes du Sud global. Tout en reconnaissant le caractère fragmenté, partiel, situé et sélectif de la sélection des sources scientifiques pour cette discussion, l'article vise à éclairer les interactions dynamiques entre les théories postcoloniales et décoloniales et les paysages variés et complexes de l'anthropologie médicale.

Mots-clés théorie décoloniale – anthropologie médicale – anthropologie du handicap – subjectivité – indigénéité

Anahi Sy: Expériences des professionnels de santé pendant la pandémie de COVID-19 en Argentine: une approche syndémique dans les hôpitaux   p. 99–111, rédigé en anglais

La pandémie de SARS-CoV-2 a mis en évidence la nécessité de penser en termes de syndémie, car tous les problèmes de santé coexistent avec des facteurs environnementaux, sociaux, économiques et politiques qui exacerbent toute épidémie. Dans ce travail, nous proposons le concept de « syndémie » pour analyser ce qui s'est passé dans les hôpitaux publics d'Argentine, d'un point de vue socio-épidémiologique. Sur le plan méthodologique, des entretiens semi-structurés avec des travailleurs ont été réalisés en deux étapes : au début de la pandémie en Argentine, via WhatsApp et via des plateformes de réunion virtuelles. L'analyse du contenu des récits permet d'identifier comment les travailleurs de la santé, dans de nombreuses situations, sont les architectes des stratégies de résolution des problèmes qui émergent pendant la pandémie : gestion des pénuries (de fournitures, par exemple) et prestation de soins, même au péril de leur propre santé. Nous avons également identifié des espaces de « dialogue-travail » entre les travailleurs (réunions, comités de crise, activités syndicales), reconnus comme des environnements de soutien, de soins et/ou d'autosoins pendant la pandémie. Dans ces espaces, certains défis auxquels est confronté le secteur de la santé doivent être considérés de manière syndémique. Nous concluons en analysant le potentiel d'application du concept de syndémie aux problèmes et aux politiques de santé publique dans les établissements hospitaliers d'un point de vue socio-épidémiologique, en soulignant le processus de transformation des travailleurs pour faire face aux situations d'urgence. Ces dimensions sont cruciales pour élaborer des politiques de santé en phase avec d'autres processus de changement socio-épidémiologique, qui se produisent tant au sein des hôpitaux que parmi la population qui utilise les services de santé publique.

Mots-clés hôpital – syndémie – pandémie de COVID-19 – professionnels de santé – socio-épidémiologie

Ziele & Bereiche

Die Zeitschrift *Curare* bietet seit 1978 ein internationales und interdisziplinäres Forum für die wissenschaftliche Auseinandersetzung mit medizinanthropologischen Themen, die sämtliche Aspekte von Gesundheit, Krankheit, Medizin und Heilung in Vergangenheit und Gegenwart in allen Teilen der Welt umschließt.

Alle wissenschaftlichen Forschungsartikel werden nach einer ersten Durchsicht durch das Redaktionsteam einer externen Begutachtung im Doppelblindverfahren unterzogen. Alle anderen Beiträge werden von der Redaktion intern begutachtet. Neben Forschungsartikeln werden auch Tagungsberichte und Buchbesprechungen veröffentlicht. Die Rubrik Forum bietet darüber hinaus Raum für essayistische Beiträge, Interviews und ethnographische Vignetten.

Curare publiziert Beiträge auf Englisch und als einzige Zeitschrift für Medizinanthropologie auch auf Deutsch. Sie unterstützt die Publikation von Schwerpunktheften durch Gastherausgeberschaften.

Bei Interesse an der Veröffentlichung eines Beitrages oder der Übernahme einer Gastherausgeberschaft freuen wir uns über eine Email an: curare@agem.de.

Nähere Informationen zu den Bedingungen von Artikeleinreichungen und Gastherausgeberschaften finden Sie unter www.curarejournal.org.

Aimes & Scope

Since 1978, *Curare* has provided an international and interdisciplinary forum for the scientific discussion of topics in medical anthropology, understood as encompassing all aspects of health, disease, medicine and healing, past and present, in different parts of the world.

After a first internal review by the editorial team, all research articles are subject to a rigorous, double-blind external review procedure. All other submitted manuscripts are internally reviewed by the editorial team. In addition to research articles, the journal publishes conference reports and book reviews. Furthermore, the journal's forum section offers space for essayistic contributions, interviews and ethnographic vignettes.

Curare is unique among medical anthropology journals in that it publishes articles in English and German. *Curare* also supports the publication of guest-edited special issues.

If you are interested in submitting an article or a special issue proposal, please send an email to curare@agem.de.

For further information on manuscript submission and guest editorships, please see www.curarejournal.org.